Vital Man

OTHER BOOKS BY STEPHEN HARROD BUHNER

Sacred Plant Medicine:
Explorations in the Practice of Indigenous Herbalism

One Spirit Many Peoples

Sacred and Herbal Healing Beers:
The Secrets of Ancient Fermentation

Herbal Antibiotics:
Natural Alternatives for Drug-Resistant Bacteria

Herbs for Hepatitis C and the Liver

The Lost Language of Plants:
The Ecological Importance of Plant Medicines to Life on Earth

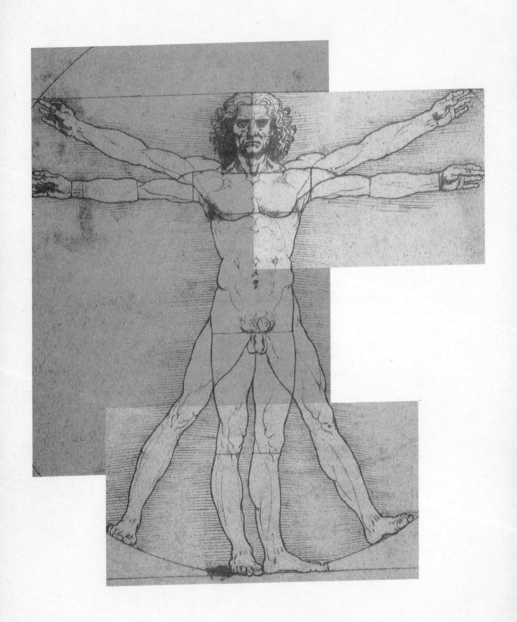

Vital Man

Natural Health Care for Men at Midlife

S T E P H E N   H A R R O D   B U H N E R

Avery
a member of Penguin Putnam Inc.
New York

Most Avery books are available at special quantity discounts for bulk purchase for sales promotions, premiums, fund-raising, and educational needs. Special books or book excerpts also can be created to fit specific needs. For details, write Putnam Special Markets, 375 Hudson Street, New York, NY 10014.

a member of
Penguin Putnam Inc.
375 Hudson Street
New York, NY 10014
www.penguinputnam.com

Library of Congress Cataloging-in-Publication Data

Buhner, Stephen Harrod.
    Vital man : natural health care for men at midlife / Stephen Harrod Buhner.
       p.   cm.
    Includes bibliographical references and index.
    ISBN 1-58333-136-0
       1. Middle aged men—Health and hygiene.   2. Alternative medicine.
    3. Health.   I. Title.
RA777.8.B84   2003   2002074603
613'.04234—dc21

Printed in the United States of America
10 9 8 7 6 5 4 3 2 1

Book design by Lee Fukui
Technical editor: David Hoffmann

For every man

who has looked in the mirror

and one day found

his father's face.

Thanks especially to James Hillman for helping me find the heart of this book, and to Michael Murray for the excellence of his research. Thanks are also due to: Robert Bly, Edward Abbey, Andrew Weil, James Duke, John Duff, Ethan Ellenberg, John Dunning, Dave Gersen, my uncle David Carl Buhner, my father John Harrod Buhner, my grandfather Carl Buhner, my great-grandfather C. G. Harrod, and Laura Shepherd, the only pretty face among these aged turks. (Well, . . . except for Michael Murray.)

CONTENTS

Part III
Diet, Exercise, and Other Unmentionables

Part IV
Final Words, Suggested Readings, and Resources

Part I
About This Book

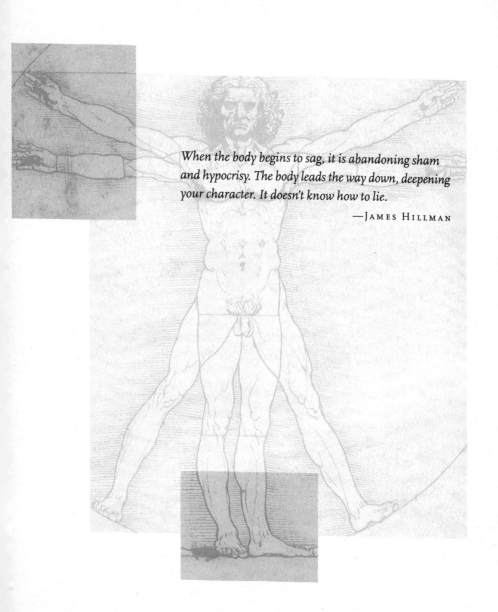

When the body begins to sag, it is abandoning sham and hypocrisy. The body leads the way down, deepening your character. It doesn't know how to lie.

—JAMES HILLMAN

PREFACE

About This Book and the Maturing of Men

Youth is glorious, but it isn't a career.
—Unknown old person

Although this book is about men's health, it is also about men and being a man. I cannot write about men's health without also writing about being a man; the two are inextricably intertwined. Even if I simply wrote about the challenges and aids to a man's health, my core beliefs and perspectives about what it means to be a man, to suffer disease, to age, would still be (as with all writers) embedded in my choice of words—those I used and those I did not. My beliefs would be woven throughout my sentence structure, the topics I choose, and the way I phrase my statements: in short, whatever a person believes is made plain in both what they do and do not say. In the end, you would feel the impact of those unspoken thoughts; they would stir in your feelings and thoughts as you read this book. I might as well, then, just talk about it all plainly.

During my research for this book, I read a great many texts dealing with various aspects of men's health. With few exceptions, they all viewed men's health from one of two perspectives. Either they asserted that: (1) Aging and its effects are a disease and everything must be done to reverse it. We, as men, must always be as we were at age twenty-five. So we must exercise, not smoke, not drink, eat a really great diet, have regular checkups with our physician, and take vitamin supplements. Or they thought that: (2) Our aging and decline are inevitable. We all possess a one-way ticket to a nursing home, incontinence, and semicoherently babbling to a nurse whom, to the dismay of our families, we call "Mama." The only thing we can do is put off this inevitable process as long as possible. So we must exercise, not smoke, not drink, eat a really great diet, have regular checkups with our physician, and take vitamin supplements.

Neither perspective evidenced much sense of humor.

A third perspective, belonging to an older way of viewing the world, was presented by just a few writers. In James Duke's *The Green Pharmacy* (Rodale Press, 1997) this third perspective is presented indirectly, inherent in Duke's words, phrasing, and embedded perspectives. In James Hillman's *The Force of Character and the Lasting Life* (Random House, 1999), it is quite direct. Both of them view the aging of the self as a natural process that allows qualities, capabilities, and aspects of ourselves to emerge in specific ways at their proper times in life. In other words, there is something we are becoming that cannot occur without this aging process; there are talents and behaviors that are not available to us in our younger stages of life. In short, aging is an important maturation of the human soul—it is neither a disease nor an inevitable descent into incontinence and Alzheimer's. It is perhaps not a coincidence that both of these writers are in their seventies. They were born in a time when that third perspective was culturally integrated as a more accepted view of the human condition. I saw it myself in the faces of my great-grandparents, most especially my great-grandfather's.

My great-grandfather was a physician in rural Indiana who, for most of his career, used botanic medicines. He often treated people in their homes, and before the purchase of his first automobile in 1918, he really was a horse-and-buggy physician. There was an expression I often noticed in his face; not so much something that would come over him in response to a joke, a comment, or some transient difficulty, but rather it was something that seemed built in. It *emerged* from his face, an integral part of who he was, a reflection that came out of the deep interaction of his life with the human predicament. It was only in middle age that I understood the basic element of that expression, the experience that gave it birth. In some fashion, he had come to an acceptance of the truth that pain is an integral part of each human life. It can no more be removed than our skins, our personalities, or our constant respiration. This perspective, of course, flies in the face of all that we now wish and are often taught to believe.

During an interview, *20/20* correspondent Chris Wallace once remarked off camera to me that it is impossible to put a rubber bumper around life. This occurred in spite of the fact that his show often attempts to do so. Still his insight is noteworthy. A significant portion of the underlying beliefs of the New Age movement, of modern medicine, of the content of current talk shows, and of many lawsuits is, in one form or another, believing that it is possible to avoid all pain in life (or righteous anger in response to pain that does occur). While suffering may in some instances be an indulgence, it is not an optional element of life. Truly, it is not so important that pain or suffering happens to us but what we do with it after. Modern medicine, unlike the medicine practiced in my great-grandfather's time, is less about the alleviation of suffering than it is about the destruction of disease through the arsenal of medicine so that everyone can live a disease-, and suffering-free, life. To alleviate suffering means only to make it better, more manageable—to ease it, not to end it. The concept of "alleviation" takes into account that there are many stages in our lives, some of which include pain.

A number of New Age colleagues also have insisted that there is a difference between pain and suffering. Pain, they have said, is a hot rock dropped in the palm. Suffering is not immediately dropping the hot rock to the ground. The fact that there are times in our lives when fate drops a hot rock into our palm and does not allow us to drop it has seemingly escaped them (as examples: long-term chronic illness; the long, slow death of a loved one; long-term inability to find a job through no fault of one's own; divorce and years-long child support payments; or even being falsely or unfairly imprisoned). My fifteen years as a psychotherapist and decade as a clinical herbalist were, more often than I knew at the time, motivated by those same beliefs. It was only as I moved into middle age, only when I took the time to look back over the second part of my life—my young adulthood—that I could begin to understand this. I suspect that all of us start feeling the impact of this knowledge as we begin to enter the choppy headwaters of our forties or fifties. Really, no matter what scientists and physicians do (and in spite of Star Trek fantasies), there will always be a leading cause of death.

So, most of the writings I explored for this book embodied a deep fear of aging, or rather what the authors thought was going to occur during aging. Out of this fear, they were working to turn back the clock, to make things as they were, to find the elusive secret of eternal youth. I think that perhaps a more useful approach is to instead mourn the young man who has passed away. And, once that mourning is done, to allow ourselves to become who and what we are meant to be at this more mature time in our lives; to find the wisdom, functions, and knowledge that nature intends us to find in order to become ourselves. This entails a process of both grieving and exploration. In the United States, this is commonly called the midlife crisis. I have seen many men go through this process. Most of them are forced to fit it in between work and family responsibilities. They often feel tremendous pressure from their society, families, work environments, and culture to remain the young men they were. This natural process of the maturation of the human soul then becomes difficult—there is little support for it, yet it inevitably affects all of us. I am not the only man to have unused exercise equipment in the garage, to have considered hair transplants, to have the occasional fantasy about other women, or to suddenly have considered the acquisition of a sports car.

It has been said, I think it was Dorothy Parker, that the only way a man can escape his past is in the reflection from a younger woman's eyes. I never knew what this meant until I mildly flirted with a young woman, much as I had done since adolescence, and the reflection that her eyes returned to me said: "You are old enough to be my father." Suddenly I wanted to find a young woman whose eyes reflected something else, a reflection that would allow me to escape my accumulating years. It was in that moment that my middle age began and I started to clearly see the passing of my younger self. My whole body knew in that moment that things were different and that they would never be the same again.

I have subsequently found that most men and women have this experience, one way or another, sometime in their life. At the moment it occurs, we are being asked a question about ourselves and about our place in the world. Most of us try to run from the question rather than grapple with the difficulty of finding an answer. Many years ago, I read a comment by the Holocaust survivor and great analyst Victor Frankl that went something like:

There comes a time in every man's life when he walks out in the night, looks up at the stars, and asks, "God, what is the purpose of my life?" He almost always does so without understanding that he is not the questioner but the questioned.

The answer to this question is of profound importance to all of us. At the great passages of our lives—adolescence, middle age, old age, death—it takes on special importance and must be answered anew. At each transition stage, we have the opportunity to refine the answer, to deepen it, or even to answer it for the first time.

Later adolescence and young adulthood—the time from eighteen to forty—is *a* time of power and strength, not *the* time of power and strength. Different qualities of mind, life, power, and interest come into play at middle age, qualities that we need in order to become who we are, qualities our families and cultures need to be whole and healthy. If we refuse to make that transition, refuse to let go of that younger self, we become, as Nan DeGrove, one of my mentors, commented, only a caricature of a human being.

The patterns we learn through our bodies in young life—holding firmly as we lift something, the drive to succeed, to reproduce—are encoded in our bodies and minds and become patterns for other, less physical actions in later life. In that later time when our strength lessens, we may no longer grip as firmly with our hands but now have the capacity to grip tightly with our minds and souls. We may no longer inseminate women but instead may reproduce our lives in other forms—through art, or writing, or new work. We begin seeding new generations, passing on what it means to be male to younger men, allowing our life force to flow into the world and generate different kinds of life. We no longer are so insistent on being the top dog, having learned that although it is true that if you are not the lead dog, the view never changes; if you are always the lead dog, others' view of *you* never changes.

So then . . . if this transition of our bodies is so natural, why write a book on health care for men? Basically, because there are a number of factors at work in the world that I believe are interfering with our healthy transition as men through the stages of our lives and I want to address them. I believe the four factors most impacting men's passages through the stages of their lives are: (1) The cultural attitudes present in the United States do not support men developing as men in any other form except that of the young adult aged eighteen to forty; (2) the wide variety of plant foods normally used by human beings over the course of their many millennia-long development as a species are either no longer present or abnormally rare in our diets, causing significant problems with our health; (3) the presence of estrogenic pollutants and mimics throughout our ecosystems is causing severe problems in our aging and health as men; and (4) while technological medicine is exceptionally good at treating trauma and for certain surgical techniques, I believe it is ill-suited for nondisease conditions such as women's menstruation, menopause (male or female), chronic diseases such as arthritis, or creating wellness. In fact, technological medicine can often do more harm than good by defining as a disease something that is not (menopause), by the extreme overuse of pharmaceuticals (the fourth leading cause of death in the United States), or by engaging in unnecessary surgeries (e.g., prostate surgery) instead of less invasive, more human-supporting therapies (herbs).

I believe very strongly in plant medicines. *Harper's* magazine estimates that 1,900 Americans die from properly prescribed pharmaceuticals each week. Confirming *Harper's* figures, a study in the *Journal of the American Medical Association* also estimates that 2.2 million Americans (42,300 per week) are either permanently disabled by or hospitalized with serious complications from pharmaceuticals each year. In contrast, NBC Prevention News (in information supplied by the American Botanical Council) estimates that of the 60 million Americans who use herbal medicines, each year only *two* die from properly prescribed botanicals. (*One* person is estimated to die from properly prescribed vitamins.)

These are the basic perspectives out of which this book is written and these attitudes and beliefs (however well based they may or may not be in fact) shape everything I write and say in this book.

The sections and chapters that follow offer a rich diversity of approaches for enhancing male health. I hope you find them useful.

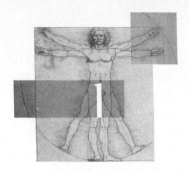

The Importance of
Natural Hormone Support for Men

*All of us have two lives: the life we learn with and the
life we live with after.*

—GLENN CLOSE IN *The Natural*

*The big shock in becoming middle-aged is that you
discover you keep on growing older, even after you are
old enough.*   —DON RADDLE

One of the more amusing stories I have heard about scientific research details the yearlong, $100,000 program to determine why children fall off their tricycles. After the well-designed study was completed and the well-credentialed researchers had compiled and analyzed their data, they found that children fall off their tricycles because they lose their balance.

This story often comes back to me when I read various pronouncements from the medical profession and never more so than when I read that there is no such thing as male menopause. Essentially, they say, because no study has found it, it does not exist. The observations of millions of men that they just don't feel themselves, that something is wrong, are passed off as being psychological—our minds are playing tricks on us. This same kind of denial has occurred with the symptoms that accompany many women's reproductive conditions as well—menstruation, pregnancy, and menopause. In response, women have pioneered research and exploration into the changes that occur for them during these periods of their lives and none more so than their passage into menopause. Men are long overdue for their own exploration into this territory, for the changes that we experience are just as profound, just as life altering, just as pervasive as those experienced by women. While it is true that men at advanced ages can still participate in creating children and older women cannot, there are significant alterations in men's hormonal chemistries, just as there are in women's.

Sudden shifts in our body chemistries occur for all of us during the major passages in life: birth, adolescence, middle age, old age, and death. These shifts have tremendous physical and emotional impacts. During adolescence (as at all other passages), the body's shape changes significantly, the skin alters, hair grows in places it had not grown before, the voice deepens—in short, a person's entire appearance changes. How the world sees him also changes.

During adolescence, all of us had to get used to a new "image," a new "face." The person we saw when we looked in mirrors, those on our walls and those in people's eyes, was changing. Part of us was leaving, a new someone coming to take his place. At the same time, a similar process was occurring in our minds and spirits. New options for life were opening up, the world of sex lay before us, vast horizons of reproductive options and attractive bodies in endless variation. We were learning new interaction styles—where we wanted to go and what we wanted to do, who we wanted to be as adults. A certain force of personality, an older self began to take us over and come into being.

These developmental elements of adolescence have a certain life span—a period of growth, development, maturity, and then senescence, or ending. A transition process, in many ways similar to adolescence, occurs again when we enter the middle of life. We look in the mirror and notice that someone new is taking the place of that young man we were. We look in attractive women's eyes and the reflection we see is strange, distorted, middle-aged. Their eyes tell us we are old enough to be their fathers. A certain shock runs through our systems, and we begin to grapple with our own aging processes and the ending of an earlier, important period of male life. As with adolescence, there are emotional and spiritual components as well. We begin to examine our lives, to see what we have done and have not done, to sum up, to take stock. Our function as a man begins to change. In middle age, a man's function is not so much concerned with the reproduction of children but something else—something that our society is not so clear about and so it is harder to identify, making it harder to resolve the shifting ground of midlife. Still, we notice our body *is* older. The impact of twenty or thirty years of riotous, reproductive living, raising children, learning our trades, surviving our mistakes have all taken their toll. Parts of our bodies are not working as well as they once did. Our bodies, as they were in adolescence, are ready for something else, some other function—again a function that our society is not so clear about, so, too, we struggle with that during this midlife change.

The United States is a young country. In many ways our culture is still an adolescent and, as such, is concerned with adolescent things: sex and reproduction, protection of territory, the making of money, asserting our independence, the freedom to do and say what we want, to be top dog. All these things are integral to the movement into adolescence and young adulthood. But in middle age something else begins to happen. Because our culture is so unclear about what that is, each of us struggles perhaps more than we should with who and what we are becoming and the new tasks that lie before us.

Historically, many cultures have understood this transition much better than we do now. Middle age was recognized for its importance as were the tasks that lay before the newly awakening middle-aged man. The Jungian analyst James Hillman is one of the few writers struggling to understand the territory of middle and old age and its importance. In his book *The Force of Character and the Lasting Life,* he calls the movement from youth into middle age the transition from *lasting to leaving.* He makes a deeply insightful point when he remarks:

> The transition from lasting to leaving is first of all psychological, and to me it means this: It is not we who are leaving, but a set of attitudes and interpretations regarding the body and the mind that have outlasted their usefulness—and their youthfulness. We are being forced to leave them behind. They can no longer sustain us, not because we are old, but because *they* are old.[1]

Middle and old age are not simply the wearing out of the body but the movement into new territories of self, into new tasks as human beings. As Hillman goes on to say, "Aging is no accident. It is necessary to the human condition, intended by the soul." Emotionally, we are in fact coming to terms with our youth, thinking it over, integrating its lessons. The dreams of who we would be when we were grown, made during our adolescence, are pulled out of the cupboard, dusted off, and examined. We compare them to what we have actually done. And, of course, for many reasons, we grieve.

In time we begin to look over who we are now and what we want to do from now on. It is common for many men to be less interested in the accumulation of power, in reproduction, or the making of money and more interested in the respect of peers, intimacy, and developing a new wealth of experience of the world. Often, men become more interested in learning, travel, and helping younger generations through their own struggles with young adulthood. We see our children into adulthood and our parents out. We look at who we are and discover important things that we must still accomplish and often we leave one career and begin another, one more concerned, quite often, with deeper aesthetic values—writing, or art, or teaching.

After this transition, men remain vital and strong, possessed of new insights, tasks, skills, and strengths. Yet we *are* different; a new form of maleness has emerged. And although our culture's lack of understanding of this transition interferes with its natural development, there is another factor, perhaps even more pervasive, that interferes with the successful transition into a healthy, vital middle age—the pervasiveness of chemistries throughout the ecosystem that mimic the actions of female hormones or estrogens. The powerful and historically unique presence of these chemistries in our ecosystems and on our bodies cannot be overstated.

During our shift into middle age (just as it did when we shifted into adolescence) our body chemistry begins to change. Testosterone and other androgen (male hormone) levels start to shift in important ways. Our bodies broaden out; our ears grow bigger; hair, once again, begins to appear in unusual places (and disappear in others). These are normal changes; they, and many others, are elements of our shift into another kind of maleness. But something is interfering with this natural shift of our bodies. Researchers now know that environmental estrogenic pollutants and substances are entering our bodies in tremendous quantities. When they do so, they shift the balance between our testosterone (and other androgens) toward the estrogen side of the equation. Like women, we do have estrogens in our bodies (just as they have testosterone), we just don't have the same quantities and we have a great deal more testosterone than they do. What is most important is the ratio of androgens to estrogens. Anything that upsets that balance changes who and what we become. We are not our chemistry, but we certainly are affected by our chemistry. The power of our androgenic chemistry to shape who we are begins while we are still in the womb.

SEXUAL HORMONES AND
THE SHAPING OF OUR LIVES

Essentially, there are four kinds of hormones in our bodies and they are typed depending on what kind of molecule they are built from. Sexual hormones such as testosterone are built around a specific type of molecule, a sterol, from which the word *steroid* comes. The name of the particular sterol that is used for sexual hormones is familiar—chole*sterol*. It is in fact cholesterol from which all steroid hormones are made.

Epinephrine (aka adrenaline) is another kind of hormone. It serves as a source of energy during the fright-flight-or-fight response. It is built around an amino acid called tyrosine (as is the thyroid hormone thyroxine) in the adrenal gland. Another type of hormone, insulin, which is highly important in the body's ability to utilize glucose (or sugar) effectively, is built in the pancreas using complex proteins. And still others, like angiotensin, are built around short-chain amino acids called peptides.

Hormones regulate much of the functioning of our bodies. Through complex biofeedback loops our bodies determine exactly what their needs are at any one moment in time and either make or release hormones to shift their functioning in the direction they need to go. As an example of this kind of generalized biofeedback, there is no central thermostat in our bodies that keeps them a certain temperature. In spite of the famous 98.6 redlined on so many Fahrenheit thermometers, the temperature of our bodies shifts constantly. It is always in flux. The various systems of our bodies compare notes, as it were, and together, in some manner not understood by scientists, come to a conclusion about how temperature needs to shift and then shifts it. We are more a collection of cooperating parts, each with its own innate intelligence, than a mechanical system, the brain its intelligent overseer.

Women's sexual hormones are collectively known as estrogens, the most important ones being estradiol, estrone, and estriol. Estradiol is the most pervasive and the strongest in its effects, much like testosterone is considered to be in male bodies. Progesterone, not usually considered an estrogen, is instead a progestin, another female steroid hormone that most people have heard of.

Mens' sexual hormones are collectively known as androgens, the primary ones being testosterone, androstenedione (Andro), androstene-diol, dihydrotestosterone (DHT), dehydro-epiandrosterone (DHEA), and a slightly more complex form of (body-stabilized) DHEA called DHEA sulfate (DHEAS).

The original precursor to all these hormones is cholesterol, which is converted into the gender-neutral steroid hormone pregnenolone and then into 17a-hydroxypregnenolone. Essentially, pregnenolone is the primary steroid hormone that is converted, or metabolized, into all the other steroid hormones in both women and men; for this reason it is sometimes referred to as a prohormone. Other people sometimes refer to it as the "mother" steroid (which I guess would make cholesterol the "grandmother").

The whole sequence of testosterone production begins when specialized nerve cells in the hypothalamus release a hormone, gonadotropin-releasing hormone (GnRH), sometimes also called luteinizing release hormone. GnRH travels through direct blood vessel connections to the anterior pituitary gland, where it stimulates the release of luteinizing hormone (LH). LH flows into the bloodstream, travels to the testes, and attaches to receptors on the testes' Leydig cells. This causes the P-450cc enzyme (cholesterol-side-chain-cleavage enzyme) to initiate a series of five enzymatic processes that convert cholesterol into testosterone. This testosterone is then used in the Leydig cells in the generation and maturation of sperm and is also released into the bloodstream, increasing overall testosterone levels. All women have some androgens; all men have some estrogens. They are all important in the healthy functioning of our bodies.

Women's estrogens are made primarily in their ovaries, adrenal glands (which sit on top of the kidneys), and brain. (Increasingly, research is revealing that both androgens and estrogens also act as potent neuro-hormones, strongly affecting central nervous system activity.) Men's androgens are made in their testes, adrenal glands, brain, and peripheral tissues and cells. The majority of a man's testosterone is made in the testes, most of the rest is made in the adrenal glands and peripheral tissues. Other androgens (such as DHEA and DHEAS) are made in the brain from precursors or prohormones like pregnenolone. The two sexual hormones that seem to be the most important, at least on the surface, are estradiol in women and testosterone in men.

Everyone knows that testosterone makes a man a man. Its presence in our bodies literally does make us men. Testosterone levels peak three times in our lives. During the second trimester of fetal development blood testosterone rises to about 4.0 nanograms per milliliter. (A nanogram is a billionth of a gram and a milliliter is .034 of an ounce.) This is a tremendously tiny amount yet this initial rise in testosterone causes the fetus to develop as male. After the second trimester testosterone levels drop nearly to zero. Then, just after birth, they rise again, peaking around six months of age at about 2.5 nanograms per milliliter. By one year of age, testosterone has again dropped to near zero. (Part of the purpose of this surge in testosterone after birth is to initiate the formation of the prostate gland. Still, the prostate remains tiny, weighing only one to two grams.) The final rise in testosterone begins between ages ten and eleven and rises slowly to a peak of about 5.0 nanograms per milliliter around the age of eighteen, then it holds relatively steady until sometime around the age of forty-five, when it very slowly declines throughout the rest of life. During this last increase in testosterone in adolescence, the penis, scrotum, and prostate gland all enlarge, the voice deepens, facial hair appears, sperm production begins, muscles rapidly develop, the bones enlarge and lengthen, and the body expands rapidly to a much larger size.

Because the overall level of testosterone remains roughly the same after age forty-five, because men can still father children, and because there is not the sudden shift in body function that women experience during the cessation of menstruation, many physicians and researchers have insisted that there is no such thing as a male menopause (sometimes called andropause). Newer researchers, not accepting this perspective, have, however, found two interesting things. The first is that while the overall levels of total testosterone remain relatively constant, *free* testosterone levels do change considerably. The second is that the androgen/estrogen *ratio* shifts considerably as well.

Of the testosterone in the male body, 70 to 80 percent of it is bound to a protein—*sex hormone binding globulin* (SHBG). Another 20 percent or so is bound to a different protein—*albumin.* Bound testosterone is used up, not available, doing something else. Only free testosterone, 1 to 3 percent of the body's total testosterone levels, is completely biologically available and active at the receptor sites in testosterone target cells. As we age, the amounts of these testosterone types alter considerably. SHBG-bound testosterone increases nearly 80 percent by age ninety. By age one hundred, free testosterone will usually disappear entirely. In Massachusetts, the Male Aging Study found that in healthy men the amount of free testosterone declines an average of 1.2 percent per year between the ages of thirty-nine and seventy. During this same period, albumin-bound testosterone declines around 1 percent per year while SHBG-bound testosterone (and body levels of SHBG) increases 1.2 percent per year. During the same time period, the quantity of testosterone that is converted to other substances increases as well.

Testosterone itself is not an end product. It too gets converted into other hormones that the body needs. An enzyme called *aromatase* converts testosterone to the estrogenic hormone *estradiol,* and another enzyme, *5 alpha reductase,* converts testosterone to dihydrotestosterone (DHT). DHT is the most potent androgen (the actual hormone that does most of what testosterone has long been thought to do), while estradiol is the most potent estrogen. Neither can be converted into other hormones.

In small amounts, estradiol is crucial for supporting the health and growth of the neural filaments in the brain (they connect brain cells to each other). Mental clarity, memory function, and the creation and maintenance of the essential brain neurotransmitter acetylcholine are all dependent on estradiol. Estradiol and other estrogens in the male body also play important roles in healthy sexual function, blood and arterial flow, and skin health. As we age as men, our bodies start to have more estrogens than they did earlier in life and fewer androgens. The ratio between the two hormonal substances changes.

The increasing loss of free testosterone beginning in middle age creates significant alterations in our bodies and our experiences of ourselves. Remember, we are male simply from exposure to tiny nanogram quantities of testosterone while we were in the womb. At the same time that free testosterone levels are dropping, we are experiencing *more* estrogenic hormones, which, at the same tiny nanogram levels, make women who they are. It is no wonder that so many men's experience of themselves and their lives changes so much when they begin entering their forties and fifties.

It is this shift in free testosterone levels *and* the changing androgen/estrogen ratio together that signals our movement into middle age. Hormonal shifting as we move into new stages of life is something that our bodies naturally do. These hormonal shifts occur at different ages for every man and no one can predict why, how, or when they will naturally occur. It is an expression of our unique selves: genetic history, body chemistry, environment, beliefs, stresses, foods, hopes, dreams, aspirations, losses, grievings, loves, and destiny. It is a natural occurrence, not an inevitable *decline*, not a disease. Simply a shift into a new way of being, a new expression of maleness.

Unfortunately, this is where environmental pollutants become a problem. There is significant evidence that scores of substances, usually synthetic chemistries that are either estrogens or that mimic estrogens, are entering men's bodies and significantly altering the androgen/estrogen ratio far beyond the normal range that men have historically experienced. Some of these environmental pollutants act as *anti*-androgens. They bind with free testosterone or even interfere with its creation, thus altering the proper testosterone levels in our bodies. These environmental pollutants are also affecting younger men, often through estrogenic impacts in the womb prior to their birth. Some of the impacts are extremely sobering. As a result of these external (or exogenous) estrogens, Peter Montague, of *Rachael's Environment and Health News Weekly*, observes that

> Each year more men in the industrialized world are getting cancer of the testicles [and prostate], birth defects affecting the penis, lowered sperm count, lowered sperm quality, and undescended testicles.[2]

The *degree* of this shift in male androgen levels is, historically, a relatively new occurrence. It began in a very mild way in Europe in 1516 with the passage of the German Beer Purity Act (see Hops in the next chapter), spread very slowly for three hundred years, and then began escalating with the discovery and production of synthetic chemistries in industry.

Researchers have linked the significant alteration in androgen levels and ratios that men are now experiencing to the hundreds of synthetically

produced estrogenic chemicals, estrogen mimics, and androgen antagonists that are present in the environment. The past sixty years have seen
an evolutionarily unprecedented proliferation of these kinds of synthetic
chemistries. One-third of American men, about thirty million of us, are estimated to be experiencing some form of erectile dysfunction or impotence.
But the males of every species, not just ourselves, are paying the price of
these estrogenic pollutants.

The Effects of Estrogen Mimics and Anti-androgens on Male Health

*It is not a debate about whether [endocrine disruption] is happening or
not. It is happening. We just have to decide to what degree we want to
let it continue to happen.* —Louis Guillette

During the past fifty years, scientists have recorded a frightening shift in
men's reproductive health. Sperm counts have shown a significant decline
worldwide, testicular cancer has grown at approximately 2 to 4 percent
per year in men under fifty years of age, there has been a general increase
in cryptorchidism (undescended testes) in young males, and cases of
hypospadia (deformities of the penis) are on the rise.[3] The increases in testicular cancer have been found to parallel almost exactly the historical
production of synthetic chemicals—both industrial, agrochemical, and pharmaceutical. From 1880 to 1920, there was virtually no change in testes cancer risk; thereafter it has steadily risen in direct proportion to worldwide
production of synthetic chemistries.[4]

These same kinds of reproductive problems are now found in the
males of scores of species throughout the world: panthers, birds, fish, alli-
gators, frogs, bats, and turtles. Louis Guillette, a reproductive endocrinologist and professor of zoology at the University of Florida, is an expert on the
study of endocrine-disrupting chemicals in the environment. He has spent
decades studying the effects of environmental endocrine disruptors (chemicals that interfere with sexual hormonal activity). His research on male alli-
gators, he notes, has consistently shown that androgen levels, androgen
ratios, and free testosterone levels are all significantly altered by environmental pollutants and have been for some time. "In males," he writes, "this
abnormality in testosterone persists, so there is a dramatic change in circu-

lating levels of testosterone. DHT is altered as well, and some males have elevated levels of estrogens. So there are feminized males."[5] He comments that the levels of chemicals needed to produce such changes are incredibly tiny: "We did not [test] one part per trillion for the contaminant, as we assumed that was too low. Well, we were wrong. It ends up that everything from a hundred parts per trillion to ten parts per million is ecologically relevant . . . at these levels there is sex reversal. . . . [And our research] shows that the highest dose does not always give the greatest response. That has been a very disturbing issue for many people trying to do risk assessment in toxicology.[6]

Pharmaceutical-quality steroids are in fact extremely pervasive in world ecosystems. They are entering soil, air, and water in the millions of tons from farming and the heavy use of estrogenic pharmaceuticals by women worldwide. Birth control pills and menopausal hormone replacement therapies are especially pervasive sources of estrogenic pollution. The synthetic estrogen Premarin, for example, is the most widely prescribed pharmaceutical in the United States. Pharmaceuticals such as these are excreted out of the human body and enter the environment where they continue to be active as steroidal chemicals. Researchers commonly find synthetic estradiol, the most potent estrogen, and estrone, another type of estrogen, in sewage plant wastewater streams. The usual concentration of estradiol found in wastewater is 14 parts per trillion and of estrone 400 parts per trillion. The male fish downstream all exhibit sexual reproductive problems, many of them becoming female. Researchers testing the potency of these estrogens have found that intersex changes begin at the incredibly tiny levels of 0.1 parts per trillion of estradiol and 10 parts per trillion of estrone.[7]

Other chemicals, such as DDT, organochlorines, and PCBs (and their metabolites), are strongly active as estrogen mimics and are prevalent throughout the world's soils, water, and air. Millions of tons of these estrogen mimics are used as pesticides on farms throughout the world. They are especially prevalent in huge agribusiness operations.

DDT, while no longer used in the United States, is still common in other parts of the world. In fact, in 1995 more DDT was used than at any previous time in history.[8] Chemicals like DDT circulate in the atmosphere and oceans; DDT is a globally pervasive chemical. Recent studies have regularly found DDT in North American wildlife blood samples at average concentrations of 1 nanogram per milliliter. This is about 1,000 times higher than the normal levels of free estradiol (which DDT mimics) that should be found in wildlife.[9] A breakdown byproduct of DDT, p,p'-DDE (pronounced "p, p-prime D D E"), has been found to be a powerful anti-androgen, strongly interfering with male androgen balances and levels in any species that encounters it.[10] And the common pesticide vinclozolin, used, for instance, on cucumbers, grapes, lettuce, onions, bell peppers, raspberries, strawberries, tomatoes, and Belgian endive, is also a powerful anti-androgen. Sold under the trade names Ronilan, Ornalin, Curalan, and Voralan and mixed as a part of Hitrun, Kinker, Ronilan M, Ronilan T Combi, Silbos, and Fungo-50, it is widely available for agricultural and gardening use. One of its breakdown byproducts (a metabolite) has been found to be 100 times more anti-androgenic than vinclozolin itself.[11] Some of the environmental pollutants are so strong, the fungicide propiconazole for example, that numerous researchers have begun exploring them as potential male contraceptives.[12] Pyrimidine carbinol fungicides are so potent that they can actually inhibit all hormone production. They completely block the synthesis of sterols, including cholesterol, from which all steroid hormones are made.[13]

Phthalates, widely used in medicine to make plastics flexible, also significantly affect androgen-dependent tissues.[14] Health Care Without Harm, an organization helping to minimize the negative impacts from hospitals and medical technology on human health, has found that while some phthalates act as estrogen mimics, others are powerful anti-androgens. One phthalate, DEHP, and its metabolite, MEHP, both show testicular toxicity, especially to the testes' Sertoli cells. The Sertoli cells nurse immature sperm to maturity and this kind of chemical toxicity results in decreased sperm production. Simply using medical devices (such as plasma bags or tubing) that contain DEHP can result in significant drops in sperm health as the phthalates readily leach out of the plastic and into the human body.[15] PVC plastic and dioxins produce similar kinds of impacts on male health.[16]

Greenpeace has raised concern about just a few of the synthetic chemicals that are known to be hormone disruptors: eleven common pesticides and their metabolites, PCBs (still environmentally present even though no longer produced), dioxins and furans (by-products of chlorine production and the chlorinated plastic PVC), bisphenol A (an ingredient used to coat the inside of tin cans and reusable milk bottles and in dental fillings), phthalates (used to make plastic flexible—used in such things as check-book covers, medical tubing, baby teething rings), and butylated hydroxy-anisole (BHA) (a food additive).

Increasingly, these substances are being found to have direct impacts on male reproductive health. As the authors of *Our Stolen Future* comment, "Several studies report that infertile men have higher levels of PCBs and other synthetic chemicals in their blood or semen, and one analysis found a correlation between the swimming ability of a man's sperm and the con-centration of [PCBs] found in his semen."[17]

Scientific organizations and environmental agencies in countries throughout the world have come to the inescapable conclusion that male health in every species on Earth is being negatively affected by these syn-thetic chemicals.

As only one example, the Danish Environmental Protection Agency in Copenhagen, Denmark, April 18, 1995, released a report entitled "Male Re-productive Health and Environmental Chemicals with Estrogenic Effects." The 175-page report identifies numerous consumer products that contain known hormone-disrupting chemicals: "pesticides, detergents, cosmetics, paints, and packaging materials including plastic containers and food wraps."[18] Ten classes of chemicals containing hundreds of different types of products are listed as agents of concern.

Peter Montague reflects that the report makes clear, that "in contrast [to natural hormones], many industrial chemicals that enter the body are not readily broken down so they circulate in the blood for long periods—in some cases many years—mimicking natural hormones."[19] What is worse, these hormonally active substances can combine with each other in ways that are not understood, are not predictable, and have never been studied.

As men, the impacts of these kinds of chemistries on our lives and our movements through the stages of our lives cannot be overstated. It is tremendously important to recognize that many of the difficulties that men are experiencing in middle age or even as young adults are from the perva-sive intake of nanogram quantities of these chemicals. Prostate problems, erectile dysfunction, sterility, sperm motility problems, loss of energy, li-bido, and even atherosclerosis (fat-clogged arteries), heart disease, and many more common physical problems can be tied to the disruption of the androgen/estrogen balance and the dropping levels of free testosterone in our bodies. In fact, nearly all the primary medical problems now affecting men can be directly tied to alterations in their androgen levels. This has had severe impacts on our length of life. In 1920, men in the United States had the same life expectancy as women. As increasing amounts of estrogen-like chemistries have entered the environment and our bodies, our life expectancy has faltered, until we now lag by some six years behind women.

The pervasive problem of these chemistries is being compounded by the historically significant shift in the foods we eat. Over the million years of our evolutionary history, human beings lived as a part of their forest and savanna homes. Normally human beings ate several hundred to several thousand plants each year as a regular part of their diet. Our human bodies have been used to that kind of food intake for at least a million years—they expect it and need it. The majority of those types of wild plants are filled with hundreds to thousands of potent natural chemistries that we need to remain healthy. Normally, in the industrialized nations, we now eat from five to twelve vegetables per year. Most of them have been modified for taste, which has reduced or eliminated many of the most potent chemistries.

The combination of these converging historical events is ensuring that men do not enter middle age in vital health as we historically have done. This is why it becomes important for many of us to actively work in some fashion to restore our natural levels and ratios of androgens.

Part II
Natural Health Care for Men

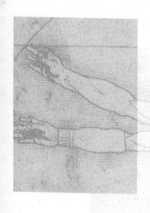

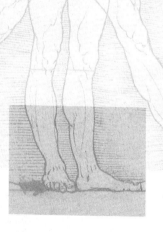

[As the body ages] it seems to have a lot to say to the soul. It begins to act up, break down, and speak out. Like a plant we tend, or an animal, the part lets us know what it likes and how it can best be favored: with which teas, which temperatures, which poultices, and which positions. —JAMES HILLMAN

As they fell from heaven, the plants said, "whichever living soul we pervade, that man will suffer no harm." —THE RIG-VEDA

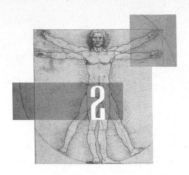

Natural Hormone Replacement Therapy for Men: Phytoandrogens, Androgenic Foods, and Supplements

How old would you be if you didn't know how old you was? —Satchel Paige

Old age is like everything else. To make a success of it you've got to start young. —Felix Marten

The litany of problems that women experience when their hormonal balance shifts is well known. Not so well known are those that men experience. Though they are not commonly compared, surprisingly, they are nearly the same as shown in the table on page 26.[1]

As increasing numbers of physicians and researchers have been realizing, these changes in men are directly related to altered hormonal levels, just as with women. Researchers are also finding that many, if not most, of the physical problems facing men in middle and old age can be reversed by increasing their free testosterone levels and their androgen-to-estrogen ratio.[2] While many of the researchers have focused on testosterone injections or patches to accomplish this, there are a number of plants that are high in androgenic hormones (including testosterone), many natural androgenic supplements and vitamins, and many androgen-stimulating foods. (See "Natural Androgen Replacement" below.) Testosterone replacement can

EFFECTS OF HORMONAL SHIFTS
IN WOMEN AND MEN AS THEY AGE

Women	Men
Reduced libido	Reduced libido
Disturbed sleep	Disturbed sleep
Depression	Depression
Fatigue	Fatigue
Irritability	Irritability
Heart disease	Heart disease
Atherosclerosis	Atherosclerosis
Osteoporosis	Osteoporosis
Thinning skin	Thinning skin
Slow wound healing	Slow wound healing
Joint pain/inflammation	Joint pain/inflammation
Poor memory/concentration	Poor memory/concentration
Reduced estrogen	Reduced testosterone
Breast/uterine cancer	Prostate/testicular cancer
Vaginal thinning/dryness	Inflamed prostate
Irregular menstruation	Ejaculatory problems
Painful intercourse	Muscle weakness
Hot flashes	Hot flashes

sometimes cause testicular atrophy; there is no evidence as yet that this occurs with natural alternatives. Incorporating these as a regular part of the diet for three to fourteen months can enhance free testosterone levels and positively alter the androgen/estrogen ratio. Differences can often be felt in as little as two weeks. (Specific problems, such as erectile dysfunction, infertility, and prostatitis, will be dealt with in the next chapter.)

Natural Androgen Replacement

For Three to Fourteen Months

Pine pollen, ½ to 5 grams, one to two times daily or ¼ teaspoon tincture three times a day

David's lily flower, ¼ teaspoon tincture twice a day
Panax/tienchi ginseng tincture, ⅓ teaspoon once a day
Nettle root, 300 to 1,200 milligrams a day
Tribulus, 250 to 500 milligrams three times a day
Pregnenolone, 50 to 100 milligrams a day
Androstenedione, 50 to 100 milligrams, one to three times a day
4-Andiol, 100 milligrams, one to two times a day
DHEA, 25 to 50 milligrams a day
Zinc, 20 to 40 milligrams a day
Juice of 3 fresh celery stalks daily
Oatmeal, corn, and pine nuts in diet frequently

Caution: This protocol may cause irritability, especially if coffee is consumed at the same time. Not for adolescent males.

PHYTOANDROGENS

The concept of using phytoandrogens, or plant sources of androgens, is relatively new. Phyto*estrogens,* or estrogens from plant sources, have been more extensively studied by scientists and are better known to the public. Phytoandrogens can be used to increase the body's levels of free testosterone and shift the androgen/estrogen balance more toward the androgen side of the equation by directly supplying androgens such as testosterone, stimulating the body's production of various androgens, or interfering with the breakdown (or conversion) of androgens into estrogens.

PINE POLLEN

Pine pollen is a yellow, flourlike substance produced in the millions of tons each year by the pine forests of the Earth. (*Pollen* is Latin for "flour.") Unlike the majority of flowering plants, pine trees are wind-pollinated. That is, they don't have a pollinator to help them reproduce but rely on the wind carrying the pollen to the pine cone (the female part of the plant). Every spring, the trees release the pollen from their male catkins, each of which can produce six million grains of pollen.

Under magnification, individual pine pollen particles look a lot like Mickey Mouse—a big head with two huge, cupped ears. The wind catches

ANDROGENS IN BLACK PINE POLLEN (PER 10 GRAMS)

Androsterone, .2 mcg

Androstenedione, .75 mcg

Testosterone, .7 mcg

Dehydroepiandrosterone (DHT), .1 mcg

While these amounts might seem small, recall that it takes as little as 4 nanograms (.004 mcg) to change our sex to male while in the womb. At .7 mcg pine pollen is, in comparison, high in testosterone. The normal dose in China is 5–10 grams per day of pollen, stirred into warm milk.

in the cupped ears and the head acts as a sort of keel hanging underneath for balance. The pollen flows through the air until it finds its way inside the overlapping scale of a cone. (The needles around the cones and the cones themselves literally alter wind-flow patterns to more accurately funnel the pollen into place so that fertilization can take place.) Under each little overlapping scale of a cone, a pine seed or pine nut will grow.

Pine pollen contains large quantities of exceptionally potent sterols. One such, brassinoloide, is a powerful growth stimulant to plants. As little as one nanogram applied to a bean sprout can cause tremendous plant growth. Plants that grow around pine forests have come to depend on this potent nutrient source. In fact, brassinosteroids regulate many plants' gene expression. The pollen that falls to the ground and water is generally taken up very quickly by all the living organisms in the area, including insects and animals. The brassinosteroids in pollen are also very similar in structure to many animal steroid hormones and produce similar steroidal activity. In addition to these kinds of sterols, pine pollen also contains significant human male hormones such as testosterone and androstenedione and relatively large quantities of amino acids and other essential nutrients.

Chinese pine pollen (*Pinus massoniana*) has been used in traditional Chinese medicine (TCM) for at least a thousand years as a health restorative, longevity tonic, and antiaging nutrient. Chinese physicians prescribe it for moistening the lungs, relieving rheumatic pain, relieving fatigue, increasing endurance, strengthening the immune system, improving the skin, strengthening the heart, increasing agility, and decreasing weight.

Korean pine pollen (*Pinus koraiensis*) is used in Korea much the same way, usually as a tea or an ingredient in food.

Interestingly, many of the actions attributed to pine pollen in both Korea and China are functions of testosterone and other androgens. While it has an extensive history in China, the use of pine pollen in Western medicine is still in its infancy. What researchers have found, however, bears out the Chinese use of pine as an antiaging medicine for men. Pine pollen is extremely high in androgens and the amino acids that support healthy endocrine function.

Black pine pollen (*Pinus nigra*) is high in androsterone, androstenedione, testosterone, and dehydroepiandrosterone (DHT).

Scots pine (*Pinus sylvestris*) pollen has been found to contain androstenedione, testosterone, and epitestosterone in comparable quantities.

Montana pine (*Pinus montana*) pollen contains the following amino acids: arginine (6.4 grams/100 grams), leucine (6.5 grams/100 grams), lysine (5.1 grams/100 grams), methionine (1.5 grams/100 grams), phenylalanine (2.1 grams/100 grams), tryptophan (0.8 grams/100 grams), tyrosine (2.1 grams/100 grams), plus trace amounts of alanine, amino-butyric acid, aspartic acid, cystine, glutamic acid, glycine, hydroxyproline, isoleucine, proline, serine, threonine, and valine.

All these amino acids contribute to human health and well-being. Phenylalanine, for instance, is linked with neurotransmitters in the brain and strongly affects mood. Both phenylalanine and tyrosine are L-dopa precursors. L-dopa is metabolized into dopamine in both the heart and brain. Dopamine is a neurotransmitter without which communication among the nerves within the brain would be impossible. L-dopa has also been found to increase sexual interest and activity and to facilitate erections in men. It is used for treating anorgasmia (a woman's inability to have an orgasm). Tyrosine is also the precursor for the important thyroid hormone thyroxine and the adrenal gland hormones epinephrine (aka adrenaline) and norepinephrine. Arginine is a precursor of nitric oxide (an erection stimulant and vasodilator) and possesses wound-healing and immune-enhancing properties. Arginine boosts human growth hormone (HGH) release, improves fertility, and is a specific spermigenic, or sperm-producing, amino acid when taken in quantities of 4 grams per day.

Pinus montana also contains the following B vitamins: riboflavin (5.6 milligrams/gram), nicotinic acid (79.8 milligrams/gram), pantothenic acid

> ### BENEFITS OF OTHER PARTS OF THE PINE TREE
>
> **Pine Seeds:**
> Moderately androgenic, strongly nutritive.
>
> **Actions of Pine Bark:**
> Mildly androgenic, potent antioxidant, free-radical scavenger, and lipid peroxidation inhibitor, anti-inflammatory, collagen and elastin stabilizer.

(7.8 milligrams/gram), pyridoxine (3.1 milligrams/gram), biotin (.62 milligrams/gram), inositol (9 milligrams/gram), and folic acid (.42 milligrams/gram).

These B vitamins are essential to male health. Pantothenic acid (aka vitamin B_5), for example, is essential in maintaining the health of the adrenal glands and their production of male hormones.[3]

Dosage
Take up to 5 grams of pine pollen two times daily.

Chinese pine pollen may be purchased as tablets (500 milligrams each) or in powder form. Usually, it is harvested in and then imported from China. (It is also often included as an ingredient in many of the power bars used by weight lifters.) One to three 500-milligram tablets one to three times per day or up to 5 grams of the powder in warm milk two times daily is traditionally used. Dosage for other pine pollens is the same.

Korean pine pollen is sold in Korea in boxes, similar to those that contain baking powder in the United States. It is used copiously in cooking and as a tonic, often taken as a tea.

P. sylvestris and *P. nigra* are more difficult to find. See the Resources section for sources.

Cautions
Some people are sensitive to pine products—seeds, pollen, bark, resin, and so on. Negative reactions can run from mild allergies to anaphylactic shock. **If you have a history of allergies to pollen or severe reactions to bee stings,**

do not use without consulting your health-care practitioner. Adolescents should not take pine pollen.

DAVID'S LILY

The lily is a huge family of plants, containing 294 genera and some 4,500 species of herbs. Garlic and onion, *Allium* species, are members of the lily family, and like most lilies possess edible bulbs—what we call onions and garlic cloves. Like onions and garlic, the bulbs of most lilies are pungent and are rarely eaten fresh. They are almost always cooked, usually baked or boiled. As with onions and garlic, this softens the pungent nature of the plants and, for many types of edible lilies, makes them a delicious food. Native Americans, Greeks and Romans, Europeans, and the Chinese have all regularly eaten lilies. Even Henry David Thoreau in his journal of July 1857 commented that he "dug some, and found a mass of bulbs pretty deep in the earth, two inches in diameter, looking and even tasting somewhat like raw green corn on the ear."

David's lily (*Lilium davidii*) is native to and is used primarily in China, where it is grown in huge quantities as a medicinal and gourmet food. The plant grows three to five feet tall with a showy spray of up to twelve or so bright orange, black-spotted flowers, and flower fanciers have spread it throughout the world. Usually the root is baked or boiled, sometimes stuffed with a blend of pork, onions, and garlic.

Modern analysis has found significant levels of testosterone in this species of lily's petals, anthers, pollen, and pistils, making it one of a handful of plants currently known to possess testosterone as a constituent. The flower and pollen have also been found to contain beta-sitosterol, stigmasterol, and emodin (a fairly potent anti-inflammatory, antiviral, and antibacterial that has a broad range of actions against various types of cancer). Beta-sitosterol and stigmasterol have many of the same actions, but beta-sitosterol is also a gonadotrophic compound, meaning it stimulates the testes and ovaries, increasing and normalizing steroid production. For men, it is both androgenic and antiestrogenic.

The bulb of David's lily has been used in (usually western) China to clear the lungs, and for coughs and sore throats, lung and breast cancer, low-grade fever, insomnia, restlessness, irritability, and calming the spirit. The flower has been used as a relaxant for the nerves and a general strengthening tonic. The herb is considered slightly stronger than a tonic medicinal and is generally used over long periods of time to help maintain health. Some people consider the plant to be interchangeable with the more widely used Chinese lily *Lilium brownii*. Generally, the flowers are collected when they are mature and the pollen is well developed. The bulbs are usually harvested in autumn or winter.

There has been, as yet, very little clinical research on the plant. It is interesting, however, that both garlic and onion, the two most famous members of the lily family, are exceptionally potent in maintaining the health of the cardiovascular system and the male reproductive system. Garlic, like David's lily, has been found to possess androgenic-stimulating constituents. (See "Garlic" on page 51.)

For millennia, lily flowers (scores of species) have been used to soothe pain, as anti-epileptics, for relaxing nerves, as diuretics, as a treatment for dropsy (i.e., the accumulation of water in the lower extremities from a poorly functioning heart), and for strengthening the heart and lungs. The most commonly used lily in herbal medicine is now Brown's lily, *Lilium brownii*.[4]

Dosage

Tincture: Take ¼ teaspoon two times daily. The flowers, prepared or fresh, are very hard to find; see the Resources section for sources.

Cautions

Do not confuse David's lily with tiger lily; the pollen of tiger lily is toxic. Some people have been known to experience extreme sensitivity and/or side effects to lily pollen. Adolescent males should not take David's lily.

RED ASIAN GINSENG

This type of ginseng is a native of Asia and most of it grows on the mountain slopes of China's northeastern ranges and in adjacent regions of Korea and Russia. Due to heavy medicinal use in China over thousands of years the wild plant is exceptionally rare and most Asian ginseng is now farm raised. The older the roots, the stronger and more potent their chemistries; generally, ginseng roots are not harvested until after at least the fifth year.

Research has shown that the ginsenoside (an important active constituent) content of the roots becomes high at that time (at which time the root also doubles in weight).

Chinese physicians have been using ginseng for at least two thousand years; the earliest mentions in medical texts are found in the first century. The Chinese process Asian ginseng in at least fifteen different ways, the two most common resulting varieties being "white" and "red." White ginseng is the whole, carefully dried root. Red ginseng is processed by steaming the roots for three hours, drying them over a low fire, and compressing them into bricks. Red ginseng is hard, brittle, almost glasslike, with a red, translucent look to it. Grinding it prior to tincturing sounds like grinding broken glass. While possessing similar medicinal activities, there are slight differences between these two forms of Asian ginseng. Red, for example, shows more antioxidant activity. There are also significant differences between American ginseng (*Panax quinquefolius*) and Asian ginseng (*Panax ginseng*). The Chinese consider American ginseng more *yin* (female, cool, soft, yielding) and Asian ginseng more *yang* (male, hot, hard, aggressive). Scientific research has verified this in a number of ways, the most elementary being that American ginseng contains the female hormone estradiol, an estrogen, and Asian ginseng does not. For androgen replacement purposes, Asian ginseng should be used, *not* American ginseng.

Nearly three thousand scientific studies have been conducted on Asian ginseng over the past fifty years. The kind of research that has been done has often differed depending on the country of origin. Steven Foster notes in *Herbal Emissaries* that "Chinese researchers, as is the case with medicinal plants in general, have focused on *how* ginseng works, whereas Western researchers focus on *if* it works. . . . In Asia, the efficacy of an herb is already established in a cultural context. In the West we presuppose that traditional or folk uses have no rational scientific basis."

Still, a great deal of important research has been done. As Foster goes on to note, Asian ginseng has been found to possess "radioprotective, antitumor, antiviral, and metabolic effects; antioxidant activities, nervous system and reproductive performance [effects]; effects on cholesterol and lipid metabolism; and endocrinological activity." It is an adaptogen (increasing general strength and resistance to stress), an antifatigue, stimulates the adrenal cortex, supports skin regeneration, and has hypoglycemic activity.

What is most important are the studies supporting its use for balancing androgen shifts and for helping with many of the common problems men experience in middle age, especially reproductive problems.

European clinical studies have shown consistent shortening of reaction time to visual and auditory stimuli, heightened alertness, increased
concentration, increased mental clarity, better grasp of abstract concepts,
heightened visual and motor coordination, and stronger respiration after
the use of Asian ginseng. Research also shows clear activity for male reproductive systems.

In one human trial with a saponin fraction (several constituents) of
Asian ginseng, after the use of 4 grams per day for three months with sixty-
six men, researchers found that they showed an increase of plasma testosterone, DHT, follicle stimulating hormone (FSH, which stimulates the
maturation and health of sperm), luteinizing hormone (LH, which stimulates the synthesis and secretion of testosterone into the bloodstream),
number of sperm, and sperm motility. Russian researchers found in a number of clinical studies that ginseng is effective for impotence in both diabetic and nondiabetic populations.

In vivo studies (meaning "in living animals," usually rats and mice)
have consistently shown increases in levels of testosterone after powdered
ginseng root was included in their diet, mixed with food. Both *in vivo* and
in vitro (in the lab—usually in petri dishes) studies show that ginseng
and the ginsenosides present in Asian ginseng stimulate the release of luteinizing hormone as strongly as the luteinizing release hormone (called
gonadotropin-releasing hormone, GnRH) produced by the body.[5]

Dosage

Asian ginseng can be taken as tablets, 1 to 9 grams per day, or as a tincture.
Normal (American) dosage range for the tincture is: Kirin (dark red)—5 to
20 drops per day; white—20 to 40 drops per day. Asians often consume it in
much higher quantities.

Cautions

Ginseng can be quite stimulating and should be used in small doses initially and increased once you are used to it. It can sometimes cause hypertension, especially with large, sustained doses, and is contraindicated in

those with high blood pressure. Under a health practitioner's supervision, it can be used with care if you have moderate hypertension. Sustained overuse can cause insomnia, heart palpitations, muscle tension, and headache. It may cause difficulty in sleeping if taken before bedtime. Because it affects androgen and testosterone levels, it should not be used by adolescent males.

TIENCHI GINSENG

I prefer to combine Asian ginseng with another type of ginseng called Tienchi ginseng (*Panax pseudoginseng*), of which there are several varieties. The subspecies *notoginseng* has been found in a number of studies to possess definite androgenic effects.[6] I generally use a combination of Tienchi and Asian ginseng, half and half, ⅓ teaspoon per day in water. Usual ginseng cautions apply. Tienchi is a prepared root—small, black, and marble-sized—with the same glasslike properties as Kirin red.

SIBERIAN GINSENG

Siberian ginseng (*Eleutherococcus*), a persistent, aggressive shrub from three to fifteen feet in height, grows throughout parts of China, Russia, Korea, and even a bit in the northern islands of Japan. Due to its popularity as a medicinal, it is undergoing heavy planting in the United States and will no doubt escape captivity soon, becoming, like a number of important medicinals, a naturalized aggressive weed with qualities unknown to those it irritates.

Though used in China for several thousand years, Siberian ginseng, or eleuthero as some people prefer to call it, was brought to prominence by intensive Russian research in the latter half of the twentieth century. A number of clinical trials have shown significant immune-enhancing activity, including significant increases in immune cells, specifically T lymphocytes (helper white blood cells). Tests of the herb have repeatedly shown that it increases the ability of human beings to withstand adverse conditions, increases mental alertness, and improves performance. People taking the herb consistently report fewer illnesses than those who do not take the herb. Part of its power is its ability to act as a stimulant on the adrenal glands, normalizing adrenal activity. Basically, this reduces stress, increases male androgen levels, and normalizes physiological functioning throughout the body.

These overall effects make Siberian ginseng a good herb for men with low libido, loss of energy, or problems with androgen levels in middle age. Siberian ginseng also contains two known androgenic substances: eleutheroside-B-1 and eleutheroside-E.[7] Preliminary work on the effects of Siberian ginseng on male reproductive health has shown that it increases the weight of prostate and seminal vesicles (SV) in castrated rats (118 percent and 70 percent respectively) and that it also prevents the atrophy of the prostate gland and SV if given to rats before castration. Essentially, Siberian ginseng can apparently keep levels of male androgens high enough so that even when the primary source of testosterone is lost through castration, the rest of the sexual organs remain normal. Presumably this occurs in part through its ability to stimulate testosterone production in the adrenal glands.

Dosage

Most of the Russian studies were conducted using a 1:1 tincture. (A 1:1 tincture means that the manufacturer uses one part herb to one part of an alcohol/water mixture—in this case a mixture that contains about 30 percent alcohol. The majority of tinctures are made 1:5, that is, one part herb to five parts of an alcohol/water mix.) The dosage ranged from 2 to 20 milliliters per day (the smaller dose is about ½ teaspoon of tincture). This means people were taking from one-sixteenth to two-thirds of an ounce (and in some instances up to one and a half ounces) of tincture per day. At an average cost of seven to twelve dollars per ounce of tincture, this can be prohibitively expensive at the upper dosage ranges.

The Russians generally took 2 to 16 milliliters, one to three times a day for sixty days, with a two- to three-week rest period in between. Ill patients received less, .5 to 6 milliliters one to three times a day for three days, then a two- to three-week rest period in between. Russian researchers, at these kinds of dosages, saw responses within a few days, or even hours, of administration. Some of the American companies that utilize the Russian approach for tincturing also like to standardize their formulas for specific eleutheroside content as well.

I have generally used, and prefer, a weaker tincture, as do many American herbalists and herbal companies, 1:5, 60 percent alcohol, full dropper

(⅓ teaspoon) of the tincture one to three times a day for up to a year. In my experience, this dosage and pattern of use is less stimulating to the system and the long-term effects are better. The body gradually uses the herb to build itself up over time, the herb acting more as a long-term tonic and rejuvenative than an active stimulant. With this type of tincture it is not necessary to stop every one to two months, and I have not seen any of the side effects that can occur with the stronger Russian formula. The Chinese, much less given to tincturing anyway, use 4.5 to 27 grams, often as a decoction or powder.

Cautions

Siberian ginseng is nontoxic and the Russians have reported the use of exceptionally large doses for up to twenty years with no adverse reactions. It is especially indicated for people with pale, unhealthy skin, lassitude, and depression. The herb may temporarily increase blood pressure in some people, but this tends to drop to normal within a few weeks. Caution should be exercised for people with very high blood pressure, especially if combined with other hypertensives like licorice. With extreme overuse, tension and insomnia can sometimes occur.

NETTLE ROOT

One of nettle root's (*Urtica dioica*) best attributes is that it interferes with the binding of androgens to sex-hormone-binding globulin (SHBG), thus keeping the body's levels of usable, or free, androgens higher. It also prevents the conversion of testosterone to estradiol, again keeping the body's levels of androgens higher.

Nettle root has been found to be a general SHBG-binding inhibitor of multiple androgens in both human and *in vitro* studies. Interestingly, nettle root contains *secoisolariciresinol,* a substance that, to date, has been found to be the third most powerful SHBG-binding substance known. Nettle root has also been found to possess strong anti-aromatase action in the human placenta and in animal and *in vitro* studies. In other words, it deactivates the enzyme (*aromatase*) that converts testosterone to estradiol, keeping testosterone levels higher. Rather than containing androgens itself, nettle acts to protect the androgens already in the body from being deactivated or metabolized.

The herb is also important in that it supplies a number of minerals and vitamins necessary for male reproductive health and acts as a tonic for the health of the male reproductive system, especially the prostate. Nettle root is specifically indicated if you suffer *both* BPH and low testosterone levels. (See BPH in Chapter 3.)[8]

Dosage

Take 300 to 1,200 milligrams of nettle root per day.

Cautions

Mild side effects have occasionally been reported with the root, usually mild gastrointestinal upset. With the plant, only mild side effects are noted: skin afflictions such as rashes and mild swelling. *The Physicians' Desk Reference for Herbal Medicines* lists a contraindication for the plant in cases of fluid retention from reduced cardiac or renal action. No contraindications are noted for the root.

TRIBULUS

Numerous studies have found that tribulus (*Tribulus terrestris*) increases serum levels of testosterone, stimulates the hypothalamus to release more LH or luteinizing hormone (which stimulates the testes' Leydig cells to make more testosterone), increases the production and release of follicle-stimulating hormone or FSH (which increases the production of sperm), and significantly increases the body's DHEA and DHEAS levels. Eighty percent of men who take the herb consistently show increases in or enhancement of libido, erection, ejaculation, sperm health, and orgasm. Perhaps the most intriguing studies have shown that tribulus increases the density of the testes' Sertoli cells, which make testosterone, and that one active constituent of tribulus, protodioscin, enhances the conversion of testosterone into DHT by stimulating 5 alpha reductase activity. This has been found to stimulate the production of red blood cells, muscle tissue, and sperm. All these factors indicate that tribulus may be a useful herb for increasing testosterone levels and rebalancing the androgen/estrogen ratio. Tribulus is specifically recommended if you suffer *both* low sperm count/low motility (or erectile dysfunction) and low serum testosterone levels. (See Chapter 3.)[9]

Dosage

The usual dosage of tribulus is 250 to 500 milligrams two to three times a day of a standardized extract in pill or tablet form.

Androgenic Supplements

Pharmaceutical manufacturers were some of the original creators of supplemental androgens, now commonly known as anabolic steroids. Initially, there was tremendous excitement among physicians and athletes (weight lifters and muscle builders primarily) and pharmaceutical steroids were widely prescribed. Unfortunately, many of the people who used the synthetic steroids (testosterone propionate, testosterone cypionate, testosterone enanthate, testosterone undecanoate, and so on) became quite ill some years later, some dying from liver disease or cancer. The negative impacts from these artificial steroids came from how they are produced.

As with many synthetic pharmaceuticals, the natural molecule, testosterone, had been altered just enough (to make it longer-lasting, more assimilable, or more potent) so a patent could be obtained. What they basically did was tack on an extra molecule to the testosterone molecule. The body then takes what it knows from its long evolutionary history—i.e., the testosterone molecule—separates it from any alien chemicals, uses the testosterone, and is left with the problem of getting rid of the remaining constituents. These leftover molecules are often processed in the liver and are the source of the toxicity associated with anabolic steroids. As Jonathan Wright, M.D., the coauthor of *Maximize Your Vitality and Potency (for Men Over 40)* (Smart Publications, 1999), comments: "Call them what you will, hormone-like drugs are most definitely not hormones, and they *never* work exactly like natural hormones."

Because of the toxicity of artificial hormones, many people are now exploring the use of natural hormones. Natural androgenic substances do not possess the toxicity of synthetic anabolic steroidal drugs. They are *identical* to the hormones produced in the human body. The following five supplements have all been found to increase testosterone levels in the blood and help restore a healthy androgen/estrogen ratio. Some men prefer to use testosterone as injections, patches, implants, creams, or a sublingual pill rather than testosterone precursors or natural androgens, like the ones that follow. If you would like more information on that approach, the two best books are Jonathan Wright's (written with Lane Lenard) and Eugene Shippen's and William Fryer's *The Testosterone Syndrome* (Evans, 1998).

In seeking out natural androgenic supplements, you should make sure you are getting pure pharmaceutical-grade supplements and nothing else. Many of these supplements are made from the Mexican wild yam (*Dioscorea spp.*) and some confusion has arisen as a result. Some people recommend the use of wild yam itself as a steroidal precursor; however, the human body cannot alter the compounds in wild yam into testosterone or any testosterone precursors. Wild yam is completely ineffective as a natural hormone for men or women unless its compounds have been extracted and chemically altered or processed in a laboratory.

PREGNENOLONE

Pregnenolone is the first metabolite of cholesterol, or the first thing cholesterol is made into. Thus, it is the primary steroid hormone (in both women and men) from which all the others are made. For this reason, it is sometimes called a prohormone, or the "mother" steroid. In spite of its being recognized as an important steroidal metabolite of cholesterol, there hasn't been much research on pregnenolone in raising androgen levels. While it is commonly used by many people to increase androgen levels, it is not known whether in fact it does so. The primary effect of pregnenolone that is widely agreed upon is that it appears to enhance mental functioning—it acts as a mood elevator and a mild sharpener to the memory and senses. One placebo-controlled trial has shown that pregnenolone (50 milligrams per day) will reduce general fatigue levels by half and that the reduction will continue for at least two weeks. In airline pilots, 50 milligrams of pregnenolone has been found to significantly enhance performance. It has also shown beneficial effects for arthritis and Alzheimer's disease.[10]

Dosage
Generally, 5 to 50 milligrams of pregnenolone per day is recommended. Anecdotal evidence has reported that doses as high as 500 milligrams per day may in some instances help with extreme memory loss and mental fatigue from chronic fatigue syndrome. This dosage, however, is not usually recommended because of pregnenolone's side effects (see below).

Cautions

Hyperalertness, irritability, mood changes, headaches, and insomnia some-times occur, especially at high doses. *This can be markedly exacerbated by cof-fee intake.* Reduce dosage or discontinue use if they occur.

ANDROSTENEDIONE

Androstenedione, often called andro, is one of two androgens in the body that is converted directly into testosterone, making it a metabolic precursor of testosterone. The body converts DHEA to andro and then turns it (usu-ally) into testosterone and (sometimes) into estrone, an estrogen. Andro and testosterone convert back and forth between each other using the zinc-dependent enzyme *17-beta-hydroxysteroid dehydrogenase.* (Interestingly, echinacea [*Echinacea purpurea*] has been found to *increase* levels of 17-hydroxysteroids in the body and has shown activity in the kidneys and adrenals as a 17-hydroxysteroid stimulant.) Androstenedione is also some-times made through an entirely different process in the body, which uti-lizes the enzyme *17,20-lyase.* Anything that reduces the levels of those enzymes (or the zinc the first pathway needs) results in lower levels of testosterone. Licorice, as noted later in this chapter, inhibits the 17,20-lyase enzyme and reduces both serum testosterone and andro levels.

Andro, compared to testosterone, is a *weak* androgen. Its importance for men is that it has been shown to increase testosterone levels. German researchers have found that a 50-milligram dose of andro can raise testos-terone levels in testosterone-normal men from 140 percent to 183 percent above normal and an East German study showed increased testosterone levels up to 250 percent. However, the peak only lasts a few minutes and testosterone levels slowly drop to baseline in a few hours. A more recent study by a California urologist found that after taking andro, men experi-enced a rapid rise in testosterone levels (from 22 to 56 percent) within ninety minutes. A placebo-controlled trial (1997) showed that, compared to placebo, only those taking andro experienced increases of testosterone, about a 24 percent increase on average.

Men who take andro commonly report feelings of increased well-being and more energy and strength. Because andro causes a predictable peak in testosterone, some men take it ninety minutes prior to sex in order to stimulate sexual arousal and response or prior to exercise in order to get maximum effect from a workout.

Testosterone tends to peak in the body in midmorning, in midafternoon, and between three and five A.M. During aging, the height of these peaks lowers, sometimes considerably, especially in those who are testosterone-compromised. Some people recommend that andro be taken upon rising, again at noon, and again before bed, to simulate the body's normal patterns.[11]

Dosage
Normally 50 to 100 milligrams is taken one to three times a day. Some people prefer to allow the pill to dissolve under the tongue so that it enters the bloodstream directly instead of going through the liver and digestive system. Some research has indicated this is more effective.

Cautions
Since 1996, an estimated 50 million doses of andro have been taken with no reported side effects. Andro, like all androgens, should not be used by adolescent males.

ANDROSTENEDIOL

Androstenediol (andiol, androdiol, 4-andiol) has generated interest because, unlike androstenedione, it cannot be converted into estrone, *only* into testosterone. Andiol is converted to testosterone through the action of an enzyme, *3-beta-hydroxysteroid dehydrogenase*. Although not much research has been conducted on andiol, the little that has occurred has shown it to be a more significant testosterone booster than andro. Researchers at Eastern Michigan University found in one study that 100 milligrams of andiol increased testosterone levels by 50 percent. And East German research has shown that andiol converts to testosterone three times more efficiently than andro. The most easily accessible strong androgen that can be purchased is 4-andiol.

There are actually two types of andiol: *4-androstenediol* and *5-androstenediol*. Normally 4-andiol is used, as it is the only form that is generally considered to be a testosterone booster. It is a much stronger androgen by itself than andro and converts much more readily to testosterone than andro. On the other hand, 5-andiol is not considered by many researchers to be a useful androgenic supplement. Most studies show that less than 1 percent of 5-andiol is converted to testosterone; most of it converts back into DHEA, from which it originates. What little research has been done has shown 5-andiol to be a very weak androgen. It is mostly useful for increasing DHEA levels.[12]

Dosage

Dosage ranges for 4-andiol are from 25 to 500 milligrams, generally 100 to 300 milligrams. Most people take one 100-milligram capsule one time per day. Though it is a bit harder to find than andro, 4-andiol can be easily located on the Internet, usually through muscle-building sites. See the Resources section for sources.

Cautions

No long-term or toxicity studies have been conducted on androstenediol use. As yet, no adverse reports have been found from use within these dosage ranges, as it is a natural androgen found readily in the body. Adolescent males should not use 4-andiol.

DIHYDROTESTOSTERONE (DHT)

There is a growing controversy about DHT, its presence in the male body, what it does as men age, and whether it should be used as a supplement.

DHT is made from testosterone through the action of two enzymes—Type I and Type II *5 alpha reductase*. DHT is, in fact, much more powerful than testosterone. It binds ten times more powerfully to the body's androgen receptors, it cannot be metabolized into estrogens (as can testosterone), and it inhibits the action of aromatase (the enzyme that converts testosterone to estradiol). DHT, in fact, seems to be a strong regulator of the androgen/estrogen balance in the body. The controversy over DHT arises because a number of people believe that DHT is responsible for the current epidemic of prostate problems in men in the United States. As a result, many people strongly advise that men not use DHT supplementation and heavily support the use of pharmaceuticals that interfere with the action of 5 alpha reductase to decrease DHT levels in the body. There is growing evidence, however, that these perspectives about DHT are incorrect.

Some physicians, like the French endocrinologist Bruno de Lignieres, have suggested that the best treatment for an inflamed prostate may, in fact, be DHT. His research has indicated that prostate problems may be occurring not from the presence of DHT but from the imbalance in the androgen/estrogen ratio. A growing body of research indicates that high estradiol levels are indeed a more likely initiator of prostate inflammation than DHT. Because DHT is not convertible to estradiol through the action of aromatase, it could in fact help relieve prostate inflammation if this is correct. (For more on prostate inflammation, see Prostatitis and Benign Prostatic Hyperplasia [BPH] in Chapter 3.) A number of studies with DHT have verified this.[13] Research has shown *no* correlation with DHT use and prostate enlargement in older men. Estradiol, not DHT, has been found to act with sex-hormone-binding globulin (SHBG) to cause an eightfold increase in intracellular cAMP (cyclic adenosine monophosphate, a stimulator of cellular activity) in human BPH tissue, which causes increased growth of the prostate. DHT, which blocks the binding of estradiol to SHBG, completely negates the effect of estradiol. In fact, the use of DHT in clinical trials was found to lower both estradiol and SHBG levels.

Clinical trials have also shown that during supplemental administration of DHT, men did not experience prostate enlargement and blood serum PSA (prostate specific antigen—an indicator for prostate disease) did not increase, while urine stream strength did increase (showing that the enlarged prostate was shrinking). In other words, there *was* relief in the obstructive symptoms experienced by the BPH patients, not an increase as there would be if DHT were the cause of prostate enlargement.

In human trial and clinical use, DHT has been found to increase androgen levels and feelings of well-being, counter many of the effects of low testosterone, and support better erections and libido. DHT topical gel (70 milligrams) was found safe and effective when used in a three-month, double-blind, placebo-controlled, randomized clinical trial with thirty-three men over age sixty; all had low testosterone levels. The men experienced improved blood cholesterol levels, decreases in fat mass, and increases in muscle strength. The report notes "standard markers of prostate or cardiovascular diseases were not adversely affected by the DHT treatment."

DHT is exceptionally important in the health of the body and there are growing reports that the widespread use of 5 alpha reductase inhibitors is having mild negative effects on muscle mass and even stronger negative impacts on normal male androgenization. DHT is in many ways the most important hormone in the development of male characteristics, not testosterone. Men who are born lacking the 5 alpha reductase enzyme develop little or no pubic hair, have an underdeveloped prostate and penis, and experience disrupted libido and sexual capacity. Weight lifters who take testosterone with 5 alpha reductase blockers have experienced reduced muscle enhancement in their muscle-building programs instead of more. DHT, it turns out, is crucial for the central nervous system and brain. DHT is vital in the organization and functioning of neural cells in the brain and has a greater neural impact than testosterone. Both testosterone and DHT increase androgen receptor proliferation in neural cells but testosterone begins to fade after three hours, and DHT maintains the increase up to twenty-one hours later. The brain converts the testosterone to estrogens when it needs estradiol to maintain healthy brain function but it also converts testosterone to DHT in the brain through the use of 5 alpha reductase. The use of 5 alpha reductase blockers may, in fact, produce negative impacts on brain function because they are generic in their action, not specific to the prostate. DHT is also made in a number of peripheral target cells in order to carry out essential functions of the body. By blocking the action of 5 alpha reductase, pharmaceutical blockers prevent the brain and all other peripheral tissues from converting testosterone to DHT when they need it.

These new findings about DHT in the brain suggest that, like the prostate, it is the balance of androgens to estrogen that creates the healthiest brain function. Research has also begun to suggest that DHT and testosterone affect the body (and prostate) through very different mechanisms. Testosterone alone may be insufficient in keeping the body healthy; DHT is proving essential. In the rush to blame DHT as the culprit for an enlarged prostate, its general impacts on male health are being overlooked.

Unfortunately, DHT appears to be available only in France. There is a DHT prohormone (other than testosterone), 5 alpha androstanidiol (aka 5AA), which is apparently converted directly into DHT. Unfortunately, only about .15 percent makes it through the liver after ingestion. Sold in the U.S. in 50-milligram capsules, it has been estimated that one gram needs to be ingested (definitely not recommended) to overcome its travel through the liver. It has also been hypothesized that allowing the capsule to dissolve under the tongue (thus allowing direct entry into the bloodstream) could be more efficacious. DHT can also be taken directly in patch or cream form.

One of the major benefits of 5AA is that it is strongly inhibitory of aromatase conversion of testosterone into estradiol. It also frees up a small amount of bound testosterone, thus increasing free testosterone levels in the blood. Also, 5AA is not convertible into estrogens. There are few studies on 5AA, so its route of metabolism in DHT is unknown.

Dosage

While apparently safe, there are no studies on long-term use or potential side effects. The usual recommended dosage is 150 to 300 milligrams daily in three separate doses.

Cautions

Because of the controversy surrounding the use of DHT, you should educate yourself and decide whether you want to use it or not based on all available information. Bearing the controversy in mind, DHT is felt by many people to be contraindicated for men with prostatitis, BPH, and prostate cancer. It is definitely *not* for adolescent males, as it will interfere with normal hormonal development.

DEHYDROEPIANDROSTERONE (DHEA)

DHEA has been studied intensely in the past ten to twenty years; at least ten DHEA-only books have been published, along with scores more that discuss DHEA along with other supplements. While DHEA itself is only a mild androgen, it is the precursor for androstenedione and androstenediol, the precursors of testosterone, making it essential for testosterone production. In addition, it has shown significant positive effects on human health in almost every organ system in the body.[14]

DHEA is the most abundant steroid in the human bloodstream; most of it (about 70 percent) is made from DHEA sulfate (DHEAS). The body essentially stores DHEA in a more stable form as DHEA sulfate and converts it to DHEA (and then other androgens) whenever it is needed. Like testosterone, both DHEA and DHEAS levels decline over time, but much more quickly. Levels of DHEA reach a peak around a man's twenty-fifth year, then decline by about 2 percent per year; by age eighty, there is only 10 to 15 percent of age twenty levels. Normal levels of DHEA in the blood are 250 to

650 micrograms per deciliter (about one-tenth of a quart) of blood; DHEAS levels are 500 to 1,000 times higher. (DHEAS and DHEA can be considered interchangeable when talking about the health effects of DHEA.) People with levels of DHEA below 100 micrograms per deciliter consistently show higher levels of cancer, heart disease, diabetes, and arthritis.

Most DHEA is synthesized in the adrenal glands; about 10 percent is made in the testes, while the rest is made in the brain, heart, and liver. Because of its synthesis in the brain, DHEA is also considered to be a neurosteroid, having potent effects on the central nervous system and brain function.

Contrary to earlier medical perspectives, it is now known that the brain can synthesize sex steroids. To some extent, this occurs in response to erotic imagery. Scents also can lead to increases. This has been demonstrated in rats, where the smell of a female in estrus leads to significant increases of DHEA in the hypothalamus. (Men exposed to tiny quantities of the sweat of a woman who is sexually aroused also experience increases in testosterone.) However, the brain creates potent androgens for many reasons other than sex. They play crucial roles in memory and neural activity in the brain and central nervous system. DHEA is a crucial precursor to the creation of both androgens and estrogens in the brain.

DHEA is also metabolized in peripheral tissues to more active androgens, and these levels never appear in the bloodstream. Basically, peripheral tissues in the human body make more active androgens from DHEA whenever they need them. Peripheral tissues in the body normally contain all the enzymes necessary to convert DHEA to androstenedione and then to testosterone. This allows potent androgenic chemicals to be used at the site where they are most needed and perhaps explains how DHEA is able to affect so many different parts of the body. In essence, the androgens synthesized from DHEA exert their effects within the same cells where synthesis takes place and these synthesized androgens are rarely released into general blood circulation (thus never showing up in blood tests). The parts of the body that are engaging in androgen synthesis are essentially using an extremely sophisticated biofeedback loop to determine exactly what levels of androgens are necessary and then making exactly what they need from the DHEA that normally circulates in the body. At least 30 to 50 percent of the total androgens in men are synthesized in peripheral tissues in just this way. The enzymes that are used for this androgen synthesis (or metabolic conversion) and the basic androgenic precursors, especially DHEA, are, thus, absolutely necessary for overall health.

Because DHEA can be converted to the estrogens estrone and estradiol, some people feel that DHEA is a potential problem when used in androgen replacement therapy. No research has found this to occur; estrogen levels in men consistently remain unaffected by DHEA intake. For example, one study of sixty- to seventy-year-old men who received intramuscular DHEA injections showed increased levels of DHEA and androstenedione in their blood. No change was found in their levels of estrone and estradiol. Even with extremely high oral dosing in young, healthy men (1,600 milligrams a day), estrone, estradiol, and SHBG levels remain level.

DHEA supplementation will generally increase levels of DHEA in the blood as well as increase serum androstenedione and testosterone. In one study, 25 milligrams a day of oral DHEA for one year led to higher serum DHEAS levels and higher levels of testosterone in a young man suffering from hypogonadism (severely low-functioning testes). Overall, DHEA supplementation increases androgen levels in peripheral tissues, increases serum androstenedione, and improves functioning in most organ systems of the body. The majority of chronic diseases associated with male aging can be significantly helped with DHEA supplementation.

DHEA use has been shown to be associated with higher levels of energy and well-being, lower obesity/waist-to-hip ratio, enhanced libido and erectile ability, reduced depression, enhanced cognition, reduced death from coronary heart disease, and improved insulin sensitivity and glucose tolerance. More can be found on DHEA in later chapters dealing with those conditions.

Dosage

The average dosage of DHEA supplementation is 50 milligrams per day. For men over fifty, this dosage will usually raise blood levels of DHEA to the same levels they experienced in the early twenties within two weeks. Some people have taken dosages as high as 1,600 milligrams per day for extended periods, but this dosage is not recommended. Side effects even at this high a dosage level are extremely rare.

When buying DHEA, make sure you are purchasing a pharmaceutical-grade supplement, which is at least 98 percent pure. There is also food grade (95 percent pure) and animal grade (70 percent pure). DHEA is widely available.

Cautions

Some clinicians think DHEA can exacerbate the mania stage of manic depression, others believe it is contraindicated for men whose PSA (prostate-specific antigen—an indicator for prostate disease level) is high. The only literature-noted side effect is masculinization (facial hair, etc.) in some women and the case of one woman who developed jaundice and liver problems after one week of use. It is not known if the latter side effect was related to the use of DHEA. Women seem most at risk of side effects.

ZINC

Zinc has significant effects on male sexuality, including on sperm motility and production, erection, and even testosterone levels (see Chapter 3). Because the transformation of andro to testosterone depends on a zinc-dependent enzyme, zinc intake significantly affects testosterone levels in the body. One study found that 60 milligrams of zinc daily for fifty days increased serum testosterone levels. Because DHT is metabolized from testosterone, a subsequent rise in DHT levels was also seen. Testosterone and DHT levels increased *only* in those men whose testosterone levels were low. Normal men experienced no increase.[15]

Dosage

A dose of 20 to 40 milligrams of zinc per day is recommended for men over forty.

Cautions

Over time, zinc intake can cause copper depletion in the body. To counteract this, most zinc supplements come with copper added. At very high doses, zinc can cause nausea and upset stomach, skin rashes, depression, folate deficiency, and lower tolerance to alcohol. It is generally recommended to not exceed 40 milligrams of zinc per day.

Androgenic Foods

A significant number of foods have been found to possess androgenic actions and to help with restoring androgen levels or the androgen/estrogen balance in men. These are some of the strongest. Try to use only organic foods in order to minimize the amount of possible estrogenic pollutants in your food.

CELERY AND PARSNIP

Researchers have found moderate levels of a male steroid in both celery and parsnip. The chemical (5 *alpha*-androst-16-en-3 *alpha*-ol) and its related 3-ketone combine together to form the chemicals that stimulate sexual arousal in a number of female animal species; they are a sign of elevated sexual hormones in the male and its readiness to mate. The two compounds are closely related in structure to both androstenedione and testosterone. (It was the researcher's wives who discovered this, by the way. Upon visiting their husbands' laboratory, they commented that the chemicals smelled just like celery.)[16]

Parsnips and celery each contain about .008 microgram of these substances per gram of fresh weight. Although parsnips can be regularly added to the diet, perhaps the best way to ingest these compounds is by drinking 2 to 3 freshly juiced celery stalks each day. (These chemical constituents are perhaps the reason that celery has historically been thought to be good for male sexuality and reproductive health.) Fresh juices are more concentrated and go quickly into the bloodstream, bypassing much of the digestive process. For a great combination try 5 carrots, 1 small beet, and 2 to 3 stalks of celery. (Or if you need kidney/adrenal support, try celery/corn juice daily. See Chapter 6.)

CORN

Corn has profound effects on the male hormonal system, especially the adrenal glands. In addition, corn juice stimulates the production and release of luteinizing hormone (LH),[17] which promotes the production of testosterone and its release into the bloodstream. (See also Chapter 6.)

OATS

Green oats (*Avena sativa*) (basically the fresh green oatmeal plant in seed) have been found to increase testosterone levels in men in at least one study; various other studies support this androgenic activity as well. *In vivo* research has found that oats, dried and added to animal diets, increase the release of luteinizing hormone (LH), which stimulates the creation and release of testosterone into the bloodstream.

Oats were official as a sexual tonic and stimulant in older German pharmacopoeias and are listed as a common doctor-prescribed unofficial herb for this use in the current German Commission E Monographs on herbal medicine.

Oats also contain a number of alkaloids (trigonelline and avenine) that have central nervous system relaxant activity and that help relax the people who eat them regularly. This relaxant activity makes oats one of the best long-term foods for stressed nerves, tension, chronic nervousness, debility, and exhaustion. This kind of stress reduction in many instances helps male sexual function.

Oats are also high in vitamin E, an essential vitamin for sexual health, as it helps prevent atherosclerosis and prostate disease. Oatmeal also contains about 7 percent fiber and is very high in polyunsaturated fatty acids. Both these factors contribute greatly to lowering cholesterol levels in the blood and rectifying or preventing atherosclerosis (fat clogging the arteries and veins), one of the major factors affecting erectile function.

Oats are best used long term; the effects build up over time and increase in effectiveness the longer oats are eaten. In general, effects begin to be noticed after three months and increase throughout the first year. Eat one bowl of noninstant oatmeal per day.[18]

GARLIC

Garlic (*Allium sativum*), a member of the lily family, has a long history as a sexual tonic for men. After ginseng, it is perhaps one of the most intensely studied medicinal plants on Earth. Garlic has consistently been shown to increase testosterone levels, stimulate sperm production, increase sexual desire, reduce atherosclerosis, and alleviate cardiac arrythmia, diabetes, hypertension, and immunodepression. There have been a substantial number of clinical trials, including double-blind, placebo-controlled, crossover studies. Garlic and its close relative, onion, which has many of the same properties, should be liberally added to the diet. Garlic supplements can also be used. Follow the directions on the bottle.[19]

PINE NUTS

For thousands of years, and among such different cultures as the Romans, Greeks, Arabs, and Asians, pine nuts have been considered an aphrodisiac. The Greek physician Galen suggested that a mixture of honey, almonds, and pine nuts, eaten on three consecutive evenings, would produce an increase in male vitality. And Ovid, the Roman poet, provides a list of aphrodisiacs in his *Ars Amatoria* (*The Art of Love*), which includes "the nuts that the sharp-leaved pine brings forth." There is good reason for this long-standing recognition that pine nuts can increase male vitality.

Like pine pollen, pine nuts contain testosterone, and they are also highly nutritious. Although the nutrients in pine nuts vary between species, a good indication of their nutritional power can be seen from a look at the nut of the American piñon pine. One ounce of piñon nuts contains 161 calories, 3.3 grams of protein, 5.5 grams of carbohydrates, 2.7 grams of saturated fat, 6.5 grams of monounsaturated fat, 7.28 grams of polyunsaturated fat, 2.3 milligrams of calcium, 10 milligrams of phosphorus, 20 milligrams of sodium, 178 milligrams of potassium, .88 milligrams of iron, 8.2 international units (IU) vitamin A, .35 milligrams of thiamine, .05 milligrams of riboflavin, and 1 milligram of niacin. As an example of how they can vary, Spanish pine nuts (pignolias) contain nearly 7 grams of protein, 144 milligrams of phosphorus, but only 1 milligram of sodium, the other constituents being about identical. All pine nuts are high in omega-3 oils and amino acids, such as arginine.[20]

The green cones are picked by hand from autumn to spring and piled to dry. As they dry, the cones open and allow the hull-covered seed nuts to be extracted by either mechanical or hand thrashing. They are then further dried and the nuts hulled by milling. The primary species used (in order) are *Pinus pinea*, *Pinus koraiensis*, and *Pinus edulis* (the piñon pine), while at least ten others are used for food around the world. Unfortunately, it is often impossible to find out which species you are buying as few nut suppliers list the tree species on their packages. Sometimes, to make it even more difficult, the different nuts are intermingled for sale. (Some Internet companies do say which species they sell.) Pine nuts can go rancid, so they should be used moderately quickly; unrefrigerated—three months; refrigerated—six months. Pine nuts are readily available in supermarkets and can be purchased on the Internet from nut companies.

Cautions
Pine nuts also contain the female hormones estrone and estradiol.[21] Anecdotal evidence indicates that their presence is not usually a problem affecting male androgen levels.

Erotic Stimulation

Though it is somewhat frowned upon in our society, there are good reasons for men with androgenic imbalances to allow themselves to regularly view erotic images. A study at the Max Planck Institute in Germany in 1974 revealed that three-fourths of the men who were shown a mildly erotic film experienced significant increases of testosterone in their blood levels. These high testosterone levels were found in another study to, not surprisingly, increase resistance and immunity to many diseases.[22]

Foods and Substances to Avoid

Just as there are substances that increase androgen levels and androgenic activity in men, there are also substances that can significantly lower or suppress them. If you are having trouble with your levels of testosterone or your androgen/estrogen ratio, you should especially avoid consuming any quantity of licorice, black cohosh, and hops.

LICORICE

Licorice (*Glycyrrhiza glabra*) is an exceptionally good herb for a great many things; however, it should be used sparingly, if at all, and only for conditions for which nothing else will do as well. Licorice has highly negative effects on men's androgen levels and hormonal functioning. In numerous human studies, for example, it has been found to inhibit 11-beta-hydroxysteroid dehydrogenase (11BOHSD). This is used to convert cortisol to cortisone and back again as each compound is needed. Cortisol is highly active in the body and a specific ratio is naturally maintained between cortisol and cortisone in order to minimize the negative effects of cortisol. (Natural cortisone is structurally different than pharmaceutical cortisone preparations. The body actually converts both types of cortisone to cortisol to make them active.) By inhibiting 11BOHSD licorice upsets the cortisol/cortisone ratio. Any imbalance in this ratio will usually have strongly negative side effects.

High cortisol levels have been linked to impaired immune health, reduced ability to utilize glucose in the blood, increased bone loss, osteoporosis, increased fat accumulation around the hips and waist, impaired memory and learning, destruction of brain cells, and impaired skin growth and regeneration. Cortisol levels sometimes rise in the bodies of intensively training weight lifters and will cause muscle tissue breakdown because cortisol actually converts the protein structure in the muscles into glucose as a source of energy. High cortisol levels also cause a lowering of testosterone levels in the body; basically, cortisol appears to suppress testosterone. Part of the reason for this is that pregnenolone is converted to cortisol through enzymatic activity. If it is not converted to cortisol, pregnenolone is instead turned into testosterone and other DHEA-based androgens. The shifting of the body to cortisol production tends to lower DHEA production and, as a result, testosterone levels.

Also, licorice actually restricts the conversion of 17-hydroxyprogesterone into the androgen androstenedione (which itself becomes testosterone and DHT) by inhibiting the 17,20-lyase enzyme. As a result, human studies have found that the use of licorice decreases both serum testosterone and androstenedione levels while raising the levels of progesterone. This directly results in decreased libido and various forms of sexual dysfunction. To compound this dynamic, licorice also contains at least seven estrogenic compounds.[23] Two of them are direct estrogens: clycestrone and estriol. Clycestrone is similar to estrone but only 1/533 as potent; estriol is one of the three primary estrogenic steroids produced in the body. Usually, high levels of estriol are present only in women during pregnancy.

To sum up, licorice intake increases cortisol levels in the body, lowers the production of testosterone, and directly increases levels of estrogens in the body. Licorice also possesses a number of other, sometimes serious, side effects from continued use or the use of high levels of the extracts.

Because of these cumulative impacts, men who are concerned about the androgen/estrogen ratio in their bodies should not use licorice except short term for specific conditions such as stomach ulcers (for more see Chapter 5). Although most people do not know it, licorice is used with some frequency in dark beers to increase head, as a coloring agent, and to sweeten the end product (see "Hops").

BLACK COHOSH

Black cohosh (*Cimicifuga racemosa*) is highly estrogenic and often used for normalizing female hormonal levels during menopause and to alleviate menopausal symptoms such as hot flashes. It has shown an antagonist activity toward the production and release of luteinizing hormone (LH), which is essential in testosterone production.[24] It is sometimes used by men for muscle pain as it is an exceptionally good antispasmodic. It should be avoided by men with androgenic imbalances unless no other herb will do.

HOPS

Hops (*Humulus lupulus*) is best known for its use in beer. The majority of physicians and men overlook its potent chemistries and do not realize that beer itself can significantly alter male androgen levels. German beer makers noticed long ago that the young women who picked hops in the fields commonly experienced early menstrual periods. Eventually, researchers discovered the reason—hops is perhaps one of the most powerfully estrogenic plants on Earth. Just 100 grams of hops (about 3.5 ounces) contains anywhere from 30,000 to 300,000 international units of estrogens depending on the type of hops. Most of it is the very potent estrogen estradiol. Estradiol, as it is taken into the male body, actually causes a direct lowering of testosterone levels in the testes and an increase in SHBG levels, which then binds up even more free testosterone in the bloodstream. The estradiol in hops has also been found to directly interfere with the ability of the testes' Leydig cells to produce testosterone.[25] The presence of this highly estrogenic substance in beer is not an accident.

Prior to the German Beer Purity Act of 1516, "beer" almost never contained hops. In fact, over one hundred different plants were used in brewing for at least ten thousand years prior to the introduction of hops in the middle ages. For the last thousand years of that period the most dominant form of "beer" was called gruit, which contained a mixture of yarrow, bog myrtle, and marsh rosemary. These herbs, especially in beer, are sexually and mentally stimulating. (It is rare to become sleepy when drinking unhopped beers.) The Catholic Church had a monopoly on the production of gruit; competing merchants and the Protestants worked together to break that monopoly and force the removal of all sexually stimulating herbs from beer. They replaced them with an herb that puts the drinker to sleep and dulls sexual drive in the male. The legislative arguments of the day all hinged on the issue of the stimulating effects of other herbs that were used in beer: a pilsner, for example, was originally a henbane beer (pilsen means "henbane"), which is an incredibly strong, psychoactive beer, used earlier in history by German berzerkers before battle. The German Beer Purity Act was, in effect, the first drug control law ever enacted by the human species.[26]

Beer, so highly touted as sexy in television commercials, in actuality can powerfully inhibit sexual strength in men. There is a well-known condition in England—brewer's droop—that occurs from middle-aged brewers' extensive handling of hop plants: the plant chemistries readily transmit through men's skin just as they do in women. Very few physicians have looked at any correlation between beer drinking and androgen levels or erectile dysfunction problems in their patients. (How many men on Viagra are heavy beer drinkers?) However, the physician Eugene Shippen in *The Testosterone Syndrome* (Evans, 1998) comments that one of his patients, undergoing pharmaceutical testosterone replacement therapy, showed no response to the testosterone until he reduced his beer intake to one to two beers a night from six to seven. Hops is extremely potent and its consumption should be limited if not completely excluded during all androgen replacement therapy. These effects can be exacerbated if the beers you buy also contain licorice (see above), a fact that will not be noted on the beer label.

It is possible to buy beer that does not interfere with androgen levels though it can be somewhat hard to find. Some microbreweries and brew pubs are now making traditional gruits (check the brew pubs in your town). However, the best source is Bruce Williams, a Scottish brewer who is bringing back the traditional ales of Europe and Scotland (i.e., pre-hopped European beers). He has five in production and they can often be found in larger American cities at any store that carries a wide selection of unusual beers. The heather ale is excellent but perhaps more useful would be the traditional pine ale, made from the Scotch or Scots pine, *Pinus sylvestris,* whose pollen contains testosterone.

It is also best to buy beers that are *bottle* conditioned. Bottle-conditioned beers are carbonated in the bottle and as such contain live yeasts. These yeasts (most commonly *Saccharomyces cerevisiae*) are highly nutritive. They are extremely high in protein, glucose tolerance factor (GTF), and B vitamins—especially niacin and B_1. Brewer's yeast contains the highest levels of GTF of any food; GTF, because it helps regulate blood sugar levels, can help many of the problems associated with diabetes. Brewer's yeasts have been found to reduce serum cholesterol and triglyceride levels and newer research has indicated that *S. cerevisiae* yeasts may have direct enhancement impacts on androgen activity in the body.

And since I am on the subject . . .

ALCOHOL

The United States is undergoing one of its periodic bouts of puritanitis (a spasming or inflammation of the Puritan Reflex). In spite of this, alcohol has been with the human species a long time; it is a *naturally* occurring substance, found throughout nature, and many living organisms are known to imbibe: the birds *and* the bees. Life in fact could not exist without the fermentation that both bacteria and yeasts provide. Nearly all indigenous cultures on Earth ferment and have done so for between ten and thirty thousand years. Beer anthropologists (yes, they exist) have found significant evidence that the Egyptians settled where they did and developed agriculture and cities because they discovered that the naturally growing grain in that region could be fermented. In other words, civilization began when we started *drinking,* not when we starting thinking.

Alcohol is exceptionally good for the body *in moderation.* It stimulates most organ functions, especially the liver and brain, to more optimum levels of health. However, in large quantities, alcohol's well-known negative effects come into play. Overuse leads to highly adverse effects on, not surprisingly, the liver and brain. Basically, a case of overstimulation. Still, it is important to note that alcohol consumption significantly increases the metabolic conversion of androgenic precursors to more potent androgens (basically DHEA to androstenediol). Moderate alcohol consumption has also been found to increase the production of androgens by the adrenal glands and to promote healthy androgen levels in the body. However, ingesting large quantities of alcohol can exhaust the body's androgen levels and even interfere with their production. In rats, high alcohol intake over short time spans causes the leaching of all DHEA from the brain, while in alcoholics, sustained high levels of alcohol have been found to reduce levels of testosterone and other androgens. Consistent high levels of alcohol cause the accumulation of tetrahydroisoquinoline alkaloids (TIQs), which inhibit the testes' Leydig cells' production of testosterone. TIQs have been found to be as potent in that respect as estradiol. They also interfere with the liver's ability to remove estrogen from the body by interfering with the liver's cytochrome P-450 system (the part of the liver concerned with estrogen removal).[27]

Naturally occurring fermentations have been shown to be much healthier for the human body—that is, wines and bottle-conditioned beers, especially beers that do not contain hops. Most studies have shown that one to two drinks of alcohol per day are associated with higher levels of health. More than that and the level of health may begin to decline. Grapes also possess anti-aromatase activity (helping in preventing the conversion of testosterone to estradiol) and antioxidative action (keeping cellular vitality high). Red wines also contain polyphenols, which are exceptionally good at regulating the impacts of fat on the health of the body. Alcohol is normally limited to around 12 percent in nature—levels higher than that kill the yeast. It is primarily when alcohol is concentrated beyond that level (as with distilled drinks), when the yeasts are removed (they counteract many of the side effects of alcohol ingestion—such as the loss of B vitamins), or when it is consumed to excess (as we do with sugar or fat) that side effects begin to be seen.

GRAPEFRUIT

I am pleased to finally find a good reason for my long dislike of grapefruit. Through a number of avenues (especially impacts on the cytochrome P-450 system that breaks down estrogens in the liver), grapefruit interferes with the removal of estrogens from the body, increasing overall estrogen levels. It should be avoided by men following an androgen enhancement protocol . . . well, probably by all men.

OTHER THINGS TO AVOID

There are a number of substances that interfere with the removal of estrogen from the male body. (In essence, they increase estrogen levels by inhibiting the P-450 phase I enzyme in the liver that breaks down estrogen.) If you are struggling with an impaired androgen/estrogen ratio it is important to understand that these substances can have a strong impact on estrogen levels.

- Anti-inflammatories: ibuprofen, ketoprofen, diclofenac, acetaminophen, aspirin, propoxyphene

- Antibiotics: sulfa drugs, tetracyclines, penicillins, cefazolins, erythromycins, floxins, isoniazid

- Antifungal drugs: miconazole, itraconazole, fluconazole, ketoconazole

- Statins (cholesterol-lowering drugs): lovastatin, simvistatin

- Antidepressants: fluoxetine, fluvoxamine, paroxetine, sertraline

- Antipsychotics: Thorazine, haloperidol

- Heart/blood pressure medications: propranolol, quinidine, amiodarone (this also inhibits testosterone production), Coumadin, methyldopa

- Calcium channel blockers: antacids, omeprazole, cimetidine

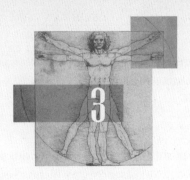

Sexuality

How trapped we are, how inadequate are our times for making sense of our sensuality! Lust in late years has a hard time finding justification. It demands an imaginative perspective. Otherwise, we believe the only impotence is literal, physical, and expect Medicare to provide Viagra. But the enfeebled and lustless imagination may be far more indicative of decline of powers.

—JAMES HILLMAN

Most Americans are shocked when they learn that many people in their eighties and even nineties still enjoy sex regularly. As a friend from France once commented to me, "It has always been hard for your Puritanical American children to imagine their elders' wrinkled bodies slapping together in frenzied sexual ecstasy." And indeed it is. When we are young, the thought of our ancient elders having sex is humorous or disgusting, depending on our upbringing. It becomes a problem, of course, when we ourselves have aged and suddenly possess our own wrinkled bodies. While we may not feel much differently inside, our changed bodies conflict with the internalized assumptions we daily absorb from thousands of television commercials and embedded cultural attitudes. At twenty, a sexually active man is flirtatious, at sixty a dirty old man. And so, as we age, our sexuality hides itself away. The million prescriptions for Viagra that were filled the first year showed just how important, and secret, the deeper dimensions of male sexuality have become in the United States.

The odd perspectives of Americans concerning sex, generated from their history of conservative Protestantism, are continually reinforced in each new generation through the absence of openness about the nature of our sexuality. These attitudes themselves were originally engendered, in part, in response to Christian discomfort with promiscuous Roman sexuality. Fear of syphilis only gave these attitudes a boost during the Middle Ages. The emergence of AIDS has confirmed them once again. Still, these attitudes have little to do with who and how human beings really are.

William Masters and Virginia Johnson conducted some of the first extensive research studies about sexuality in the latter half of the twentieth century. One finding is important for understanding the nature of our sexuality as men. That is that male fetuses have regular erections, as do male infants after birth. Our sexuality is as much a part of us as breathing, our need for food, our need for love. Through it, we learn one of the deepest patterns embedded within nearly all life forms on Earth. Through it, we can also experience the joy of joining with another human being in one of the most intimate and pleasurable acts ever known.

Most men who will speak of it often reveal that their careers contain a deeply sexual element. William Targ, for many years the senior editor at Putnam, revealed in his autobiography *Indecent Pleasures* (Macmillan, 1975) that he always knew a book would be good because it felt sexual to him. Rare book dealers commonly say the same thing. They can tell if a book they do not know is valuable by how sexual they feel when they hold it in their hands. The deeply ingrained sexual pattern within men expands itself outward and becomes much more than simply a form of human procreation or enjoyable sharing. Our sexual vitality flows through everything we do, infuses our work, and helps us create new forms of work and play and intimacy. It is an essential element in our response to the touch of the world upon us, and it is intimately connected to our capacity for imagination.

Testosterone, research has shown, is an important neural chemical, not just a sexual hormone. It has many effects on the central nervous system and the functioning of the brain. Men enjoy watching women because it immediately stimulates testosterone production, which stimulates the imagination, which stimulates more testosterone (stop, I'm getting excited), and so on. This increase in male vitality then infuses everything a man does throughout the day. Physical agility is enhanced, energy levels increase, and the brain, infused with tremendous amounts of testosterone (some of which is tranformed into estradiol, which enhances mental acuity and functioning) becomes more mentally alert and imaginative.

The alterations in testosterone production and the ratio of androgens to estrogens that begin in middle age have tremendous effects on male sexuality. Infertility, erectile dysfunction (or impotence), prostatitis, benign prostatic hyperplasia (BPH), and prostate cancer are all increasingly common. Fortunately, they are often easy to help using natural treatments.

INFERTILITY

Generally, infertility in men refers to either low sperm count (oligospermia) or comatose sperm—sperm whose motility, or movement, is impaired. There are a number of plants, supplements, and foods that have been found to be helpful for these conditions, many of them in clinical studies or trials. Bear in mind, though, that they are not effective in cases of ductal obstruction or certain bacterial infections. For these conditions, the vas deferens (the tubes carrying the sperm) need to be cleared or the existing infection corrected.

Natural Care for Infertility

For Two to Six Months
> Chinese dogwood tea daily
> Tribulus, 250 milligrams three times a day
> Speman, 2 tablets three times a day
> Panax and Tienchi ginseng tincture, up to ⅓ teaspoon per day
> L-arginine, 500 to 3,000 milligrams daily
> L-carnitine, 500 to 1,000 milligrams a day
> Vitamin B supplement daily
> Vitamin C, 500 to 1,000 milligrams a day
> Zinc, 20 to 40 milligrams a day
> Dietary additions and considerations

CHINESE DOGWOOD

Chinese dogwood (*Cornus officinalis, Fructus corni*), also called Japanese cornel, is an ornamental tree, much like our American dogwoods. It grows naturally throughout eastern China and Japan and has been planted throughout much of the rest of the world. When ripe, the medicinally used fruits should have a sour taste and an orange color, a bit like a cross between a cranberry and a chewy orange candy.

Chinese dogwood fruit, called *Fructus corni*, or shan zhu yu in Chinese medicine, has been used for several thousand years as a tonic/stimulant for the kidneys/urinary system and tonic for the male reproductive system. The bark is used as a fever reducer, and is often used as a treatment for malaria. The fruit is usually dried and used as a tea for impotence, lack of sexual desire, incontinence, frequent urination, tinnitus, vertigo, hair loss, arthritis, and diabetes. Interestingly, these problems are all associated with lowered or altered testosterone levels and poor blood circulation (which itself is linked to altered androgen levels).

The current interest in Chinese dogwood has been stimulated by its long-standing use as a male-fertility agent in both Japan and China. While limited, the Western-style studies that have been conducted on dogwood are highly promising.

Regular consumption of an infusion (a strong tea) of the dogwood fruit has consistently resulted in better sperm motility, generally increasing movement by 68 percent. One particular chemical constituent of the fruit (as yet identified only as C4) has been isolated and found to be the most potent enhancer, enhancing motility 120 percent. Other studies have found that cornus increases blood flow to the kidneys and spleen and that the fruit enhances the antioxidant defenses of the heart's vascular endothelial tissue.[1]

Dosage
Take a steeped decoction (an ounce of the dried fruits steeped in a pint of hot water for twenty minutes) three times a day. Begin with one cup per day and slowly increase to three per day by the end of one week. Add honey if desired as the herb is somewhat sour.

Cornus can be somewhat hard to find. The Internet and Chinese herb suppliers are the best sources. See the Resources section of the book for suppliers.

Cautions

Do not use if there is blood in the urine or painful urination.

TRIBULUS (PUNCTURE VINE)

Tribulus (*Tribulus terrestris*), also called puncture vine, is a relatively small, low, weedy, shrubby, viney plant that is widely found naturally in Asia throughout the tropics and subtropics. It has also, happily, naturalized throughout California and parts of the American West. It is a reproductive and urinary tonic, helps prevent or reduce kidney stones, lowers blood pressure, acts as a diuretic, soothes irritation, works as an aphrodisiac, stimulates the production of DHEA, and helps in the treatment of angina pectoris.

Tribulus is, not surprisingly, considered a noxious weed by many Westerners, especially Australians. Asians seem more understanding, perhaps because of their long use of the herb in traditional medicine. Called puncture vine for a reason, the spiny seeds are ferocious and nearly impossible to remove once embedded. They can puncture feet, animal paws, and bicycle tires with equal impunity.

In the traditional Ayurvedic and Unani medicinal practices of India, the plant has been used for at least three thousand years for treatment of kidney stones, to increase urine production, to increase semen production, and as an aphrodisiac. Westerners, coming along some three millennia later and using an entirely different approach, are finding the plant useful for reducing kidney stones, increasing urine production, increasing semen production and sperm motility, and increasing sexual drive and performance. The actions of tribulus on the mucous membranes of the urinary tract are toning, astringent, and antibacterial, similar in action to that of buchu and uva ursi, two other well-known urinary system tonics.

Each testicle contains some five hundred convoluted tubules, which, if laid end to end, would stretch 750 feet. Inside these tubules are the Sertoli cells that make both androgen binding protein (ABP) and sperm. Androgen binding protein calls both testosterone and DHT to it in order to concentrate androgens in a specific place. ABP concentrates in the Sertoli cells and the epididymis, the long structure at the back of each testicle.

It takes sixty-four days for the Sertoli cells to make sperm, which they do in four sixteen-day intervals. Immature sperm cells are called spermatogonia. These mature in sequence into spermatocytes, spermatids, and then into spermatozoa or sperm.

Tribulus causes the hypothalamus to release more luteinizing hormone (which stimulates the Leydig cells to produce more testosterone), increases the density of the Leydig cells (thus creating more cells to make testosterone), increases the levels of androgen binding protein (ABP), which increases the amount of testosterone and DHT in the Sertoli cells and epididymis (which increases the efficiency of the maturation of sperm), increases the numbers of spermatogonia, and increases their transformation into spermatocytes and spermatids. This results in enhanced fertility in the men who take the herb.

Clinical studies have found that from 50 to 80 percent of people using standardized preparations of tribulus experience significantly improved sperm production and motility. One study noted that 500 milligrams three times a day for sixty days significantly increased sperm production for men diagnosed with idiopathic oligozoospermia (*no* sperm in the semen from no discernible cause). Libido, erection, ejaculation, and orgasm all increased significantly for 80 percent of the men. Another, double-blind, placebo-controlled trial showed significant increases in sperm motility with corresponding decreases in immotile sperm. Numerous other studies have shown similar outcomes. Tribulus has been found to increase LH, follicle stimulating hormone (FSH), DHEA levels, and interestingly, estradiol in women and testosterone in men but not vice versa. This indicates it is a *general* reproductive system tonic, not just for men or for women. (FSH stimulates the production of testosterone in the testes and subsequently the production of sperm.)[2]

Dosage

The fruit of the tribulus vine contains a number of beneficial compounds called alkaloids and saponins, some of them steroidal in nature (e.g., beta-sitosterol, campesterol). (The fruits are also high in calcium, phosphorus, and iron.) A number of researchers and clinicians feel that the herb should be standardized for what they call furostanol saponin content (one of the active constituents of the plant), and some companies do so between 40 and 45 percent furostanols. It is available under a number of brand names and can be easily found on the Internet and in many health-food stores.

The usual dosage for infertility is between 250 and 500 milligrams three times a day for two to three months (or as directed).

The fruits themselves may also be used (as they traditionally have been for millennia) as a strong tea made from the powdered fruits (1.5 to 3 grams in 8 to 16 ounces of hot water).

Cautions

Occasionally, the plant can be infected with a fungus while in storage. This can be avoided if you harvest the plant yourself or if you buy a commercial, standardized preparation. The plant itself is not known to cause adverse reactions in people; there are no known contraindications for use.

SPEMAN

Speman is an herbal combination long used in traditional Indian (Ayurvedic) practice. It contains *Orchis mascula* (65 milligrams), *Lactuca scariola* (16 milligrams), *Hygrophila spinosa* (32 milligrams), *Mucuna pruriens* (16 milligrams), *Parmelia parlata* (16 milligrams), *Argyeia speciosa* (32 milligrams), *Tribulis terrestris* (32 milligrams), *Leptandenia reticulata* (16 milligrams), and Suvarnavang (mosaic gold—16 milligrams). A number of clinical trials have explored its use in a wide variety of conditions, including oligospermia (low sperm count), oligozoospermia (no sperm in ejaculate), asthenospermia (lack of ejaculate), necrozoospermia (dead sperm), prostatitis, and BPH. About half of the men who take speman show significant increases in sperm count and motility; many of their wives subsequently conceive. The clinical studies have included as few as twenty-one men to as many as six hundred.

In only one example, 307 men between the ages of twenty-two and forty-five were given two speman tablets three times per day for three months. After three months, half of the couples conceived. Speman has been found to be effective as well in prostatitis and benign prostatic hyperplasia in a number of clinical trials.

Speman has also been used *in vivo* and been found to stimulate mouse sexual activity and to protect mouse testes, epididymis, and adrenals from cadmium poisoning. This is interesting in that speman shows a general protective and tonic effect on the male reproductive system. It corrects imbalances but also prevents future damage.[3]

Dosage

Take two tablets three times a day for three months; repeat if necessary. Speman can be hard to find; see Resources section for sources.

Cautions

Less than 1 percent of people complain of short-term dizziness, which is the only known side effect.

ASIAN AND TIENCHI GINSENG

Both Asian and Tienchi ginseng have been found to increase sperm motility in men in a number of studies. In one trial, sixty-six men with low sperm counts and low sperm motility took 4 grams per day of Asian ginseng for three months. By the end of the study, an increase in sperm number and motility was observed as well as increases in plasma testosterone, DHT, FSH, and LH. When ½ to 1 gram of Asian ginseng (single dose) was used as an adjunct to LH analogs in 112 infertile men, Asian ginseng was found to potentiate and prolong their effects. And Tienchi ginseng, in a number of studies, has been found to consistently increase male sperm motility.[4]

Dosage

Take 1 to 4 grams daily of Asian ginseng or a tincture combination of the two, up to ⅓ teaspoon daily.

Cautions

Ginsengs may sometimes cause irritability and raise blood pressure. See Chapter 2 for more information.

L-ARGININE

L-arginine, an amino acid normally present in the body, has been found, in some cases, to significantly improve sperm motility and sperm count. Arginine is an essential amino acid, needed for the replication of cells, making it an important nutrient in sperm production. It is a natural source of nitric oxide, which is crucial for erections (see Erectile Dysfunction on page 72).

One study showed a doubling of sperm count in two weeks with the use of L-arginine, in another, 74 percent of 178 men with low sperm counts showed significant increases in sperm motility and production. The latter study used 4 grams of L-arginine per day.[5]

Dosage

Take one to two 500-milligram capsules up to three times daily. Arginine is present in large quantities in pine pollen, sunflower seeds, Brazil nuts, almonds, peanuts, lentils, kidney beans, and soybeans.

Cautions

L-arginine should be avoided in cases of shingles or herpes, as it can exacerbate the outbreak. L-arginine will not usually initiate an outbreak, but existing viruses can use arginine to enhance their replication. L-arginine can also affect blood sugar levels and diabetics should take it only under the supervision of a health-care provider.

L-CARNITINE

The epididymis, the oblong structure connected to the back of the testicles, is the first part of the excretory ducts of the testicles and contains extremely concentrated amounts of L-carnitine—so do sperm. Low L-carnitine levels directly cause low sperm motility and production. Increasing L-carnitine levels immediately increases sperm motility—the higher the levels the higher the motility. In one study, 1,000 milligrams of L-carnitine three times daily for three months was found to increase sperm count and mobility in thirty-seven of forty-seven men who used it.[6]

Dosage

Take 500 to 1,000 milligrams three times a day.

VITAMIN B COMPLEX

A number of B vitamins have been shown to play a role in both sexuality and sperm counts. B_{12} deficiency, for example, leads to reduced sperm counts and motility. Studies have shown significant increases in sperm count and motility when men were given from 1,000 to 6,000 micrograms of B_{12} daily.[7]

Niacin, another B vitamin, can produce a flush to the skin very similar to the sexual flush many people experience during sex. There is a dilation of capillaries and blood vessels and an increase of blood flow throughout the body. *In vivo* studies with stallions have shown that niacin increases their capacity to reach orgasm. Many people taking it also report increased enjoyment of sex. Vitamin B_5 has been shown to increase stamina and endurance and has strong effects on maintaining healthy adrenal glands, the source of most of the body's DHEA. Choline, another member of the B vitamin family, has been shown to exert strong effects on sex. Choline is involved in the production of acetylcholine, which is the primary neurotransmitter that sends signals from the brain to muscle systems throughout the body. There are some studies that have indicated that choline supplementation increases sexual responsiveness, interest levels, and stamina. A good B-complex formula is important; you may wish to add 1,000 to 6,000 micrograms of B_{12} as well.

Dosage
Take 1 tablet of a complex per day (as directed on the product label).

VITAMIN C

Vitamin C has been found to directly promote sperm health and motility. Dietary vitamin C plays a significant role in protecting sperm from DNA damage. In one study, dietary vitamin C was reduced to 5 milligrams per day from 250 milligrams. The number of sperm with DNA damage increased to 91 percent, while the ascorbic acid levels in seminal fluid decreased by 50 percent. Vitamin C has also been found to increase sperm motility in smokers (who tend to have lower sperm motility). Daily intake of vitamin C (from 200 to 1,000 milligrams) can increase sperm motility and production and reduce agglutination (the clumping together) of sperm. (If more than 25 percent of sperm clump, fertility is severely impaired.) In one study, by the end of twenty-one days, the amount of agglutinated sperm in men taking vitamin C had dropped to 11 percent. By the end of sixty days, all of the men taking vitamin C had impregnated their wives while none in a placebo group had done so. Vitamin C also increases testosterone production and improves the P-450 system in the liver, which eliminates excess estrogen.[8]

I prefer taking vitamin C as an effervescent, nonacidic powder in water; it's kind of like Alka-Seltzer. It is much easier to take this way, and it is assimilated into the body much faster.

Dosage
Take 500 to 1,000 milligrams per day.

Cautions
Large doses of vitamin C can cause stomach upset, flatulence, and diarrhea. It is often prescribed tbt, "to bowel tolerance" or tbd, "to bowel dose," meaning increase dosage until these bowel symptoms occur and then reduce. As soon as your body gets enough, it excretes the remainder. While vitamin C can be useful in some kidney conditions, you should not use vitamin C if you are on hemodialysis, or suffer from recurrent kidney stones, severe kidney disease, or gout.

ZINC

Every time a man ejaculates, he uses 5 milligrams of zinc. Zinc is highly concentrated in both sperm and seminal fluid, and frequent ejaculation can lead to zinc depletion, especially if the diet is poor. Deficiencies of zinc in men result in reduced libido, low testosterone levels, and low sperm counts. Zinc levels are usually found to be low in infertile men with low sperm counts; increasing zinc can have an immediate, powerful effect on sperm motility, production, and even testosterone levels in the blood. A number of studies have shown that zinc supplementation immediately and significantly affects sperm motility and production. Even in cases of long-standing infertility (more than five years), zinc can have a powerfully positive effect within two months. One study resulted in pregnancy in 40 percent of the men's wives within two months of regular zinc use.[9]

Dosage
Take 20 to 40 milligrams per day. It is generally recommended to not exceed 40 milligrams per day.

Cautions

Over time, zinc intake can cause copper depletion in the body. To counter-act this, most zinc supplements come with copper added. At very high doses, zinc can cause nausea and upset stomach, skin rashes, depression, folate deficiency, and lower tolerance to alcohol.

Dietary Additions and Considerations

GARLIC

Garlic (*Allium sativum*) has a long reputation as a sexually supportive food for men. Part of this is attributable to its reliable ability to reduce high blood pressure and improve blood flow. Garlic also stimulates the entire male hormonal system, increasing testosterone production and enhancing li-bido (see Chapter 2). There is some indication that it also improves sperm production. One *in vivo* trial with mice showed a significant increase in sperm production merely from adding garlic juice to their food.[10] For this and many other reasons, it makes sense to add garlic to the diet regularly and often.

OYSTERS

Oysters have long been considered an aphrodisiac. The reason: Oysters have high levels of zinc in their bodies. Zinc is, perhaps, the most essential trace mineral for the production of healthy sperm (and one of the most im-portant minerals to male health). One hundred grams, about four ounces, of oysters contains 150 milligrams of zinc. Eat as often as desired.

Foods and Conditions to Avoid

Taking all the Chinese dogwood tea and eating all the oysters in the world won't help your infertility problems if you continue any behavior that pro-motes infertility. Following are conditions and foods to avoid in order to achieve optimal fertility.

COTTONSEED OIL

Men who regularly use raw cottonseed oil have been found to possess low sperm counts and eventually experience, if they do not stop, a total failure of the testes to produce sperm. This is because cottonseed oil contains a powerful male antifertility compound called *gossypol,* which inhibits sperm production. Make sure that whatever you are eating does not contain cottonseed oil.[11]

ESTROGENIC PLANTS

Avoid licorice, black cohosh, and especially hops (as a supplement or in beer). All of these can interfere with the body's creation of sperm. Estrogenic substances such as hops interfere with the production of FSH and result in low sperm counts.

Erectile Dysfunction (Impotence)

Some thirty million American men—about one-third of the sexually active male population—have been estimated to suffer some form of erectile dysfunction. When Viagra was released, a million prescriptions were filled the first year—a billion dollars in sales for the pharmaceutical giant Pfizer. Continued use, however, has also brought recognition of its side effects. Within five months the FDA confirmed that sixty-nine people using Viagra had died; forty-six of the deaths were related to cardiovascular disease, exacerbated, many felt, by the drug. While there may be a place for Viagra, there are a great many natural approaches to treating impotence, the majority of which have few or no side effects. One of the advantages of natural alternatives is that, in the long run, they can correct the underlying causes of many forms of erection problems. Viagra cannot; it must be taken forever (a common problem with pharmaceuticals).

While there are a number of causes of erectile dysfunction, four of the most prevalent are estrogens/estrogen mimics in the environment or diet, pharmaceuticals (scores can cause erection problems), atherosclerosis of the penile artery (basically fat-clogged arteries), and diabetes—high blood sugar levels, which cause a narrowing of the blood vessels (see Chapters 4 and 8). It is thought by a number of researchers and clinicians that about half of erectile dysfunction problems come from atherosclerosis. Erection depends on a strong supply of blood to the penis and with poor circulation to the extremities due to clogged arteries, there is often an insufficient supply to produce an erection.

If you have erectile dysfunction, get a checkup and get tested for high cholesterol levels and diabetes. Simple tests in any physician's office can easily determine the presence of either of these conditions. Also, check to see if the side effect of any pharmaceuticals you may be taking is impotence. Sometimes, the problem is just that simple.

Natural Care for Erectile Dysfunction

For Two to Six Months
  Ginkgo, 30 to 120 milligrams twice a day of standardized herb
  Muira puama, 250 milligrams three times a day
  Tribulus, 250 milligrams twice a day
  Androgen Replacement Protocol (DHEA 50 to 100 milligrams daily, minimum)
  L-arginine, 1 to 2 500-milligram capsules to three times daily
  L-phenylalanine, 100 to 500 milligrams daily
  L-tyrosine, 100 to 500 milligrams daily
  L-choline, 1 to 3 grams daily
  Zinc, 20 to 40 milligrams daily
  Dietary additions and considerations

GINKGO

Scores of studies have been conducted on ginkgo (*Ginkgo biloba*) for use in stimulating peripheral circulation and improving blood flow in the brain, legs, and penis. All of them have shown ginkgo's effectiveness.

Ginkgo has gained its modern reputation for helping the memory problems that sometimes occur with aging. Numerous clinical trials have shown that it stimulates blood flow in the brain, helping to alleviate forgetfulness and other memory disorders. But ginkgo has a much larger range of action; it has been shown to be very effective in the treatment of heart disease and stroke, peripheral arterial insufficiency, eye disease, and impo-tence. Basically, ginkgo is effective anyplace in the body where there are problems from insufficient blood flow. This holds true as well for insuffi-cient blood flow to the penis. Half to three-fourths of the men in various clinical trials have regained the ability to have regular erections after ginkgo use. In one trial, sixty men who had not reacted to injections of papaverine (a potent erectile stimulant) were given 60 milligrams of ginkgo daily for twelve to eighteen months. Blood flow improved after six to eight weeks of use, and after six months, in 50 percent of the men, the ability to have erec-tions was restored. Another study explored the use of 80 milligrams three times a day in fifty men with dysfunction due to arterial insufficiency. The group was split into those who could achieve erection after injection of a drug (twenty men) and those who could not (thirty men). After six months of ginkgo use, the twenty men in the first group could achieve erections in-dependently, as could nineteen of the men in the second group. Another trial found that after nine months, 78 percent of the men reported signifi-cant improvement in their ability to achieve erections. Ginkgo has even been found to help restore erections when the cause of dysfunction is from antidepressant pharmaceuticals.[12] *For long-term resolution of erection prob-lems from arterial insufficiency, this is one of the primary herbs to use.* For short-term, immediate gratification, potency wood and tribulis are more effective.

Dosage

The active constituents in ginkgo that help are considered to be present in insufficient quantities in the whole plant, and standardized extracts or cap-sules that concentrate them are generally suggested for use. Fifty pounds of ginkgo are used to make one pound of standardized extract. Usually the ex-tracts contain at least 24 percent ginkgoflavonglycosides—what researchers consider to be the active constituents of the plant.

The suggested dosage is 60 to 240 milligrams per day. Improvement can usually be felt in two months, restoration of regular erection ability can often take six months of regular use. Ginkgo's effectiveness has been found to increase when used with L-arginine and magnesium.[13]

Cautions

There is sometimes sensitivity to ginkgo preparations. Caution should be used if you are taking antithrombotic (anti-blood-clotting) medications.

Uncommonly, side effects are mild gastrointestinal upset or headache and, very rarely, allergic skin reactions. In very large doses, ginkgo can cause diarrhea, irritability, and restlessness. Because ginkgo is a PAF inhibitor, it should be avoided before surgery.

MUIRA PUAMA

Muira puama, or potency wood (*Ptychopetalum olacoides, P. uncinatum, P. guyanna*), is native to Brazil and has a long history of use as an aphrodisiac and nerve stimulant in South American medicine. It was "discovered" by the Western world in the mid-nineteenth century and rose to prominence in the early twentieth. It has been a regular part of medical practice in England, France, and Germany since that time.

Muira puama seems to possess a consistently strong activity as a neuromuscular tonic, helping to alleviate muscle and joint pain. However, the primary benefits in erectile dysfunction are that it relaxes and calms the body (which reduces stress's effects on sexual arousal while promoting blood flow to the penis) while stimulating sexual arousal, erection, and central nervous system activity. These effects have been borne out in clinical use and trial.

In one clinical trial, 262 patients with low libido and the inability to maintain or have an erection were given 1 to 1.5 grams of potency wood extract. After two weeks, 62 percent of the men experienced a return of libido and 51 percent of the men noted significant help with erectile function. Another trial found positive benefits for men with sexual asthenia (fatigue, loss of strength, or lack of sexual vitality—typical signs of low testosterone levels or androgen/estrogen imbalance). One hundred men complaining of impotence, lack of libido, or both took part in the trial; ninety-four completed it. Sixty-six percent of the couples reported significantly increased frequency of intercourse, stability of erection was restored for 55 percent, 66 percent reported reduced fatigue, and 70 percent reported intensification of libido. Sleep improvement and increased morning erections were reported by many of the men.[14]

The reasons for potency wood's actions are unknown; however, the plant does contain a number of plant steroids, such as beta-sitosterol, which has a normalizing/enhancing activity on male hormone activity. The herb has shown the strongest effects when the cause of erectile dysfunction is not mental or emotional in nature and possesses a strong element of fatigue and stress.

Dosage

Muira puama has been used for hundreds of years in the Amazon as a tea for helping men with sexual dysfunction. However, a number of clinicians feel that the most effective form of the herb is as a tincture. Take 1 to 3 milliliters (¼ to ¾ teaspoons) twice daily. Suggested daily dosage of the powder is 1 to 2.5 grams per day (about ½ to 1¼ teaspoons) or 1,000 to 2,500 milligrams of the encapsulated herb.

TRIBULUS (PUNCTURE VINE)

Tribulus has been found effective in a number of studies for helping stimulate erection. In one study of seven impotent men using 1 tablet, 3 times a day, of standardized tribulus (250 milligrams) for two weeks, four experienced improved erection, including prolonged duration of erection after treatment had ceased. Another study with fifty-three men using three tablets (250 milligrams) twice a day for three months showed significant improvements in a majority of the men in sex drive, erection, ejaculation, and orgasm. Three studies on diabetic men with erectile dysfunction found increased erection and sexual intercourse in 60 percent. Treatment for as little as four weeks showed improvement in erection and duration of coitus and postcoital satisfaction in fifty-six men.

Part of the reason for tribulus's effectiveness is that it is a potent hypotensive (lowering blood pressure by relaxing the muscular coat of blood vessels), it facilitates the actions of nitric oxide and acetylcholine in the penis, and it stimulates the production of DHEA in the body.[15] More on tribulus can be found in the previous section on infertility.

Dosage

Between 250 and 500 milligrams three times a day for two to three months (or as directed) of the standardized herb as tablets or capsules.

Cautions

Occasionally, the plant can be infected with a fungus while in storage. This can be avoided if you harvest the plant yourself or if you buy a commercial, standardized preparation. The plant itself is not known to cause adverse reactions in people; there are no known contraindications for use.

L-ARGININE

L-arginine is the biological precursor for the formation of nitric oxide, which the body needs for erections to occur. The body converts arginine to nitric oxide during sexual arousal and uses it to generate an erection. The nitric oxide dilates and relaxes the blood vessels in the penis, allowing them to engorge with blood and the penis to become erect. The more sexually stimulated a man becomes, the more rapidly the body's arginine is converted to nitric oxide. If the body is low in arginine, erections can be feeble or nonexistent. Increasing arginine supplementation alone has been shown to result in better and longer-lasting erections. Arginine is often used among animal breeders to enhance erections in bulls, roosters, and horses. Expanding research is showing that men can use the supplement with equally good results.[16]

Dosage

Take one to two 500-milligram capsules up to three times daily. Some researchers have suggested using 6 to 18 grams forty-five minutes before sex.[17] Others feel that lower doses of between 1.5 and 3 grams are sufficient. Taking the supplement just before sex allows the body sufficient amounts to generate an erection in response to stimulation. Daily supplementation will bring arginine levels up over time. Arginine-containing foods should be added to the diet. (See Infertility above.) Two ounces of sunflower seeds will supply about 4 grams of arginine, the amount many naturopaths recommend for low sperm counts. Other foods high in arginine are carob, peanuts, sesame seeds, soybeans, watercress, almonds, Brazil nuts, chives, and lentils.

Cautions

L-arginine should be avoided in cases of shingles or herpes as it can exacerbate the outbreak. L-arginine will not usually initiate an outbreak, but existing viruses can use arginine to enhance their replication. L-arginine can also affect blood sugar levels and diabetics should take it only under the supervision of a health-care provider.

L-PHENYLALANINE AND L-TYROSINE

These two amino acids are precursors to L-dopa. L-dopa stimulates both erections and sexual desire in people who take it regularly. Normally, these are people with Parkinson's disease whose bodies have quit making L-dopa in sufficient quantities. The primary side effect of the supplements for male Parkinson's patients seems to be heightened sexuality and a penchant for grabbing nurses.[18]

Dosage
Take 100 to 500 milligrams each daily.

Cautions
High doses of these supplements can increase blood pressure, especially if taken along with MAO inhibitors. Use with caution or under a health-care provider's supervision in hypertension.

L-CHOLINE

A number of studies have shown that acetylcholine plays an essential role in the transmission of nerve impulses from the brain to the penis during sexual arousal. The tissue in the penis that engorges with blood is high in acetylcholine, which plays an essential role, along with nitric oxide, in erections. L-choline is now considered to be an essential nutrient, needed by the body to generate sufficient acetylcholine for neurotransmission in the brain and, importantly, is crucial for sexual arousal. Studies have found that the supplemental use of choline increases the body's ability to generate erections.[19]

Dosage
Take 1,000 to 3,000 milligrams daily.

Cautions
High doses may cause stiff or tight muscles in the neck or shoulders, tension headaches, or mild diarrhea. Some clinicians suggest taking choline with vitamin B_5, pantothenic acid. B_5 stimulates the health and activity of

the adrenal glands and the adrenal output of male hormones. A few studies have found that the combination of choline and B_5 leads to longer and more pleasurable erections. Some companies offer combinations of B_5, choline, and arginine.

ZINC

Because zinc is so intimately connected to sexual health in men, it is essential to consider adding it regularly to the diet. A significant number of men with erectile problems have been found to be deficient in zinc. Zinc is essential in the maintenance of testosterone levels in the body and the health and vitality of sperm.

Dosage
Take 20 to 40 milligrams daily. It is generally recommended to not exceed 40 milligrams of zinc per day.

Cautions
Over time, zinc intake can cause copper depletion in the body. To counteract this, most zinc supplements come with copper added. At very high doses, zinc can cause nausea and upset stomach, skin rashes, depression, folate deficiency, and lower tolerance to alcohol.

Dietary Additions and Considerations

GINGER

Ginger has a long tradition of use as an aphrodisiac; in traditional Chinese medicine it is considered a sexual tonic. Contemporary research has shown that it does have a strong effect on helping prevent or reverse atherosclerosis and it stimulates peripheral circulation as well. Since atherosclerosis of the penile artery is the cause of half the erectile dysfunction of men over fifty, any food that can reduce or reverse it has a place in the diet. Suggested serving: daily in the diet, fresh grated in food, and one to two times per day as tea.

GARLIC

Because garlic is so powerful for reducing atherosclerosis and thus helping improve blood flow to the penis, it should be liberally included in the diet (see Chapter 4).

FAVA AND OX-EYE BEANS

There are now a significant number of clinical trials that show that adding foods high in soluble fiber to the diet, especially beans, regulates blood sugar in the blood. Beans in general are important but when impotence or erectile dysfunction are also problems, fava beans are strongly indicated.

Fava and ox-eye, or velvet, beans contain significant amounts of L-dopa, an important prosexual chemical and dopamine precursor. L-dopa has the well-known side effect of increasing sexual interest and activity in anyone who takes it. It is also specific for helping create erections. Too much can cause a spontaneous persistent erection (priapism), which can sometimes be painful. Though neither bean contains enough to cause priapism by itself, healthy quantities of these beans can help stimulate erection while helping regulate blood sugar. Both have a reputation as aphrodisiacs, especially the velvet, or ox-eye, bean, which is a traditional aphrodisiac in Panamanian folk medicine.[20] The sprouts of both contain even higher levels of L-dopa and are a good addition to salads. You can find these beans at many health-food stores and they can be easily ordered over the Internet.

Suggested serving: 8 to 16 ounces three or more times per week.

THINGS TO AVOID

Again, avoid all estrogenic plants, specifically hops, black cohosh, licorice, and especially hopped beers. Examine *all* pharmaceutical medications to determine if they can cause impotence.

PROSTATITIS AND BENIGN
PROSTATIC HYPERPLASIA (BPH)

The prostate is a walnut-sized gland that sits just below the bladder and wraps around the urethra—the tube through which the urine flows. If the prostate swells, it can cut off the flow of urine, sort of like kinking a garden hose. The more it swells, the slower and more problematic the urine stream. So it takes a while to get the urine going, the urine stream is weak, the urine dribbles on for a bit afterward, it takes more push to empty the bladder, and the bladder may only partially empty, making more trips to the bathroom necessary—usually in the middle of the night (nocturia). And to top it off, the stream isn't hard enough to fully open the tiny flaps at the end of the penis and the urine stream shoots out in two directions. No matter how you aim, while one stream will go in the toilet, the other hits the wall, or the floor, or the seat. Your wife and friends begin to insist you sit down to pee. And it all used to be so easy.

Inflammation and enlargement of the prostate have both been around a long time. For hundreds of years they were lumped together in a condition called strangury—a lovely, beautifully descriptive term—the *strangling* of the urethra that causes the urine to emerge drop by drop. (It also referred to painful urination, I suppose from the expression on men's faces when they tried to go.)

Prostatitis, or inflammation of the prostate, is different from benign prostatic hyperplasia, or BPH, although both of them are treated nearly the same with natural protocols. Prostatitis means inflammation of the prostate gland, while BPH refers to a nonmalignant, abnormal growth in prostate tissue. Normally walnut-sized, during severe BPH the prostate can literally grow to the size of a grapefruit. The degree of the growth in prostate tissue and the impact on quality of life are measured from (mild) Stage I to (serious) Stage IV. Prostatitis is not usually accompanied by the same degree of prostate growth as that seen in BPH.

No one knows why most prostatitis occurs; less than 10 percent is caused by bacterial infections because it is difficult for bacteria to get into the prostate. Usually those that do are immediately killed by the body's immune system—a short-term, limited condition called acute prostatitis. Chronic bacterial prostatitis occurs when the bacteria are not killed, their population is only decreased, and they continually cause problems. Both of these are usually caused by a urinary tract infection in which, for a variety of reasons, the urine backflows into the prostate, infecting it as well. This can be helped by using BPH herbs and supplements while adding a urinary antibacterial such as uva ursi. If the bacterial infection is severe the protocol for a urinary tract infection should be followed (see Chapter 6). Other forms of prostatitis (chronic and asymptomatic prostatitis) occur from no known causes. The prostate is just mildly inflamed, with or without symptoms. These more common forms of prostatitis respond very well to the same protocols that are used for BPH.

There is currently a tremendous difference of opinion as to the cause of benign prostatic hyperplasia. Conventional medical thought is that the accumulation of dihydrotestosterone, or DHT, in the prostate is the problem. As testosterone enters the prostate, more than 95 percent of it is converted to DHT by the enzyme 5 alpha reductase. This DHT binds strongly to androgenic receptors in the prostate. Because it is the DHT that stimulates growth of the prostate when testosterone levels rise just after birth and at puberty, physicians have come to believe that DHT is the cause of its growth in middle age. There are a number of problems with this perspective, the most obvious being that this growth of the prostate is occurring as testosterone levels in the body begin to *fall,* not rise. Prostate growth earlier in life only occurred during testosterone increases.

This confusion about the prostate and its enlargement later in life is not surprising. As Dr. John Isaacs of the Johns Hopkins School of Medicine comments:

Despite the major progress that has occurred in the biological sciences during the past fifty years, it is rather remarkable that we are about to enter the twenty-first century and still the specific function of the prostate gland is unknown. Indeed the prostate is the largest organ of unknown specific function in the human body.[21]

Standard medical intervention for BPH takes a two-pronged approach. The first is to relax the smooth muscle contractions in the prostate through the use of alpha-blocker drugs. This allows the urine to flow more freely and alleviates some of the symptoms of BPH. The second intervention is to prevent the conversion of testosterone to DHT through the use of 5 alpha reductase blockers, usually the pharmaceutical Proscar (generic name finasteride).

Finasteride is usually of benefit only in men whose prostates are severely enlarged, from the size of a tomato to that of a grapefruit, generally Stage III or IV. The drug needs to be taken for at least six months before there is any indication of effectiveness and usually one year for maximum effect. It does reduce DHT concentration in the prostate by some 80 percent but the prostate only reduces its size by 18 percent in less than half of the men after one year of use. Only one-third to two-thirds of men (depending on the studies) show improvement in their symptoms.

Finasteride, in about 10 percent of men, causes impotence, decreased libido, and/or breast enlargement. It also decreases the levels of PSA, or prostate specific antigen, that circulate in the blood. Increased PSA levels indicate the presence of prostate cancer about 70 percent of the time. This allows physicians to treat it before it spreads to other parts of the body. Finasteride interferes with the creation of PSA by normal prostate cells but not PSA created by prostate cancer cells. This means that men on the drug can show low levels of PSA even when they do have cancer. BPH is also considered to be a possible early indicator of eventual prostate cancer. Yet in at least one trial, men who took finasteride were found to have an increased risk of prostate cancer.[22]

Emerging research is beginning to indicate, however, that the conversion of testosterone to DHT may not be the reason behind inflammation of the prostate. Prostate growth, which in younger life is directly dependent on testosterone, begins to increase again in middle age exactly at the point when *testosterone levels begin to fall.* This later decrease in the body's levels of free testosterone is amplified by the simultaneous increase in SHBG levels, which binds up even more free testosterone, causing testosterone levels in the body to fall even lower. For this reason alone the assumption that DHT levels are the cause of prostate enlargement seem suspect. Several studies have even shown that men with enlarged prostates do not have higher levels of DHT than men without prostate enlargement. In fact, in men with BPH, DHT levels were found to be slightly lower than in healthy men.[23] Extensive studies have also been done to see if Chinese men, who have low rates of BPH, have lower 5 alpha reductase activity in their prostates than American men. The studies, which were designed to normalize the populations for numerous factors, found that Chinese men and American men have the same levels of activity of 5 alpha reductase. The researchers commented that the studies indicate that the cause of BPH is environmental and dietary, *not* 5 alpha reductase activity.[24] Something else is causing the epidemic of prostate enlargement in men.

Estrogen and the Prostate

Very simply, the prostate contains two predominant types of tissues; stromal (which is mostly smooth muscle and connective tissues) and glandular (mostly epithelial cells). Epithelial cells secrete prostate fluid and are also the site of most prostate cancers. Stromal tissues are the tissues that usually enlarge during BPH. (The glandular tissue enlargement that occurs during prostate cancer can cause the same symptoms as BPH. Both types of enlargement cause the urethra to squeeze shut.)

What researchers are discovering is that estrogens and androgens work together in the prostate to regulate its function. New findings show that while estrogens directly affect stromal tissues, they also condition the response of epithelial tissues to androgens. When androgen and estrogen levels alter, especially estradiol, the most potent estrogen, the evidence now strongly suggests, the prostate gland's tissues begin to grow in significantly different ways.

One study in Japan examined the levels of total testosterone, free testosterone, and estradiol in men who participated in a large mass screening for prostate disease. While free testosterone and total testosterone levels were found to be irrelevant to prostate disease, the levels of estradiol and the ratio of estradiol to both types of testosterone was found to be a significant indicator of prostate disease. The higher the level of estradiol and the higher its ratio to both free testosterone and total testosterone, the larger the prostate was found to be. Another study, at Harvard Medical School, supported this when it found the most significant indicator of BPH to be the level of estradiol in the blood. Researchers have in fact found that prostate tissue from men with BPH converts androgens to estrogens (primarily estradiol) at extremely high levels compared to healthy prostate tissue. This indicates that the enzyme aromatase, which converts testosterone to estradiol, has become highly activated in their prostates.[25] This is a cause for concern in that it results not only in higher estradiol levels but in much lower concentrations of testosterone in the prostate.

Studies have found that vitamin D is actually an important steroid hormone with powerful impacts on the prostate. When testosterone levels are low, vitamin D potentiates abnormal prostate tissue growth. With sufficient testosterone levels, it promotes normal prostate growth and cellular health.[26]

Higher estradiol levels are a concern because prostate stromal cells (the cells that usually enlarge during BPH) are the primary target of estrogens in the prostate gland. As androgen levels fall in the aging male body, the activity of estrogen receptor genes increases, leading, in many men, to increased stromal cell growth. Estrogen has been found to be a specific messenger molecule for the prostate's stromal tissue, initiating its growth. The impacts of estrogen, especially estradiol, on stromal tissue have been found over and over again to be one of the primary factors in the development of BPH. During BPH, this estrogen-activated stromal tissue can increase up to two and a half times its normal ratio to other prostate tissues.[27]

Estrogen increases have also been linked with elevated levels of insulin growth factor 1 (IGF-1) in the prostate. Elevated IGF-1 causes cells to grow and prevents old cells from dying. High IGF-1 levels have been positively correlated with prostate cancer. Estradiol has been found to be the most potent estrogen that affects prostate tissues. It causes an eightfold increase of intracellular cAMP—cyclic adenosine monophosphate—in the prostate. Cyclic AMP or cAMP, is a messenger molecule that is activated by hormones. Once activated, it initiates a wide range of activity within cells, including cellular growth. Levels of cAMP are also directly correlated to the amount of PSA that the prostate cells release.[28]

Androgens, especially testosterone, are converted into either DHT or estradiol through specific chemical pathways in the prostate. Part of the potential danger in focusing on 5 alpha reductase blockers is that they force testosterone and other androgens away from DHT conversion and into estradiol conversion, thus raising estradiol levels in the prostate. DHT, rather than stimulating prostate growth, tends to decrease estradiol levels and estradiol's impacts on prostate health. The primary factor emerging as most important in prostate disease is how much estradiol is either being taken in the diet (e.g., hopped beers) or how much estradiol is being made in the body or the prostate through the action of the aromatase enzyme. (Rises in estrogenic pollutants in the environment exactly parallels the increase in prostate disease in men.) Increased DHT levels, reduced aromatization, and reduced estradiol have all been correlated to better prostate health. *Because there is such controversy about the causes of prostate enlargement, you should explore the matter carefully and make your own decisions.*

Natural Care for the Prostate

Natural protocols for prostate disease are very effective. In Europe, they are the treatment of choice in 90 to 95 percent of cases. They work as well as they do not because they interfere with the conversion of testosterone to DHT but because they relax the muscle tissue in the prostate, allowing urine to flow better, act as a prostate-specific anti-inflammatory, block the conversion of testosterone to estradiol, and normalize hormonal activity in the prostate gland. Natural protocols are much cheaper, they do not have to be taken forever, they tend to lower the risk of prostate cancer, and they have few side effects when compared to pharmaceuticals. Because they possess such strong anti-inflammatory actions, these herbs are also specific for prostatitis.

Natural Care for Prostatitis and BPH

For Three to Twelve Months
> Nettle root, 300 to 600 milligrams twice a day
> Saw palmetto, 160 milligrams standardized extract twice a day
> Rye grass pollen (Cernilton or equivalent), 60 to 120 milligrams two to three times a day (especially for prostatitis)
> Omega-3 fatty acids, 1 tablespoon flaxseed oil daily
> Zinc, 50 milligrams a day

(For severe bacterial prostatitis follow the UTI protocol in Chapter 6.)

NETTLE ROOT

Nettle root (*Urtica dioica*) has been used to treat both BPH and prostatitis in at least thirty clinical studies. Participants in the studies ranged from as few as twenty men to as many as 5,400. In men with Stage I to III BPH, nettle root consistently reduced nighttime urination (nocturia), improved urine stream, decreased urine remaining in the bladder after urination, decreased prostate size, and significantly lowered the score on the International Prostate Symptom Score (IPSS) questionnaire (this rates the degree of negative effects the prostate inflammation is causing in urination in seven areas plus overall quality of life).

Here are only a few examples: Sixty-one to 83 percent of 5,492 men who used 1,200 milligrams of nettle root daily for three to four months found significant relief from BPH symptoms. In twenty-six men who used 1,200 milligrams of nettle root daily, prostate volume decreased in 54 percent and residual volume of urine in 75 percent.

Seventy-nine men who used 600 milligrams per day for sixty-eight weeks (sixteen months) found that urine flow significantly increased and urination time significantly decreased. Twenty patients who used a nettle root/saw palmetto combination in a placebo-controlled, randomized, double-blind trial found their flow rate significantly improved over placebo. Their IPSS scores declined from 18.6 to 11.1 but with continued use continued to decline even lower, to 9.8. The study found that continued use of herbs increases prostate shrinkage *over time,* improving prostate health the longer they are used. The same study compared 489 men with others using finasteride (Proscar) over a forty-eight-week period and found that IPSS scores dropped similarly in both groups but with fewer side effects in the men using herbal extracts.

Needle biopsies were taken in a number of studies to discover exactly what was happening to the prostate in men taking nettle root. Researchers found that nettle root reduced the activity of the smooth muscle cells in the prostate, caused a shrinkage of both the smooth muscle tissue and the epithelial or glandular tissue, and increased epithelial secretions.

Nettle root has been found to be consistently anti-inflammatory (both to the prostate and other tissues), to inhibit sex-hormone-binding globulin (SHBG), to inhibit DHT binding to SHBG, and to be anti-aromatase (inhibiting the conversion of testosterone to estradiol).

The herb contains a number of powerful chemical constituents that are either unique to this plant, in these quantities, or in these combinations. Of note are histamine, formic acid, acetylcholine, 5-hydroxytryptamine, and various glucoquinones. Nettle is also exceptionally high in a number of vitamins and minerals, including zinc, and contains more protein than any other land plant.[29]

Dosage

Capsule dosage ranges from 300 to 1,200 milligrams per day for three to twelve months in the majority of the clinical trials. Tincture-dosage range is ¼ to 2 teaspoons daily of a 45 percent alcohol/water tincture for one to twelve months.

Make sure in buying capsules and tinctures that you get the root and *not* the leaves, as each is used for different conditions. The root is often combined with saw palmetto. A significant number of effective trials have been carried out on this type of combination.[30]

Cautions

Mild side effects have occasionally been reported with the root, usually mild gastrointestinal upset. With the plant, only mild side effects are noted: skin afflictions such as rashes and mild swelling. *The Physicians' Desk Reference for Herbal Medicines* lists a contraindication for the plant in cases of fluid retention from reduced cardiac or renal action. No contraindications are noted for the root.

SAW PALMETTO BERRIES

Saw palmetto (*Serenoa repens*) is listed in the German Commission E Monographs and the American *Physicians' Desk Reference for Herbal Medicines* (as well as numerous herbals) as being an anti-androgenic herb. This could easily raise concern for men wishing to restore androgenic levels in their bodies. However, those sources are incorrect. In actuality, saw palmetto is an *endocrine* agent, more specifically, one that exerts steroidogenic normalizing actions on the prostate. Saw palmetto blocks both testosterone and DHT binding to androgen receptors but *it also blocks the action of estrogen in the prostate, interfering with estradiol binding to estrogenic receptors.* More technically, the herb suppresses expression of estrogen, progesterone, and androgen receptors in the prostate. Saw palmetto, in essence, successfully competes for both androgenic and estrogenic receptors in the prostate. This makes the herb a prostate tonic—which hormonal receptors it affects depends on how the prostate is malfunctioning. By interfering with the steroid hormones that are overactive, saw palmetto normalizes hormone action within the prostate gland, reducing cell proliferation and prostate growth. And while saw palmetto (and nettle root as well) does inhibit 5 alpha reductase, it and nettle root are both some 5,600 times less powerful than Proscar (finasteride), lending considerable weight to the speculation that this action of saw palmetto is unrelated to its positive actions in the treatment of BPH. In fact, while saw palmetto has been found to lower the concentration of DHT in prostate tissue by as much as 50 percent, studies have shown that, at the same time, 5 alpha reductase activity in the prostate is unaffected.

Importantly, saw palmetto is also an anti-inflammatory through at least three different chemical mechanisms, which helps the prostate to decrease in size. Saw palmetto has been found to significantly reduce epidermal growth factor in the periurethral region of the prostate—the region of the prostate that surrounds the urethra coming down from the bladder. It is also an alpha-adrenergic receptor antagonist, which means that it relaxes smooth muscles throughout the body, including the prostate. These mechanisms alleviate the pressure of the prostate on the urethra, easing symptoms.

Saw palmetto has been used in at least twenty clinical studies ranging in size from 14 to 1,300 men and has consistently shown effectiveness in reducing prostate problems. Eighty to 90 percent of the men using saw palmetto in clinical trials report significant improvement in their prostate problems. Researchers have noted that for most men using the herb (88 percent) urinary flow increases, actual size of prostate decreases, and prostate symptom scores all decrease. In general, the herb needs to be used for from forty-five to ninety days to produce benefits. The longer it is used, the more benefit is achieved.

In one study, 505 men with Stage I to III BPH took 160 milligrams of saw palmetto twice daily for three months. Urine flow increased by 25 percent after ninety days, the amount of urine remaining in the bladder decreased by 20 percent, and the prostate reduced in size by 10 percent. IPSS scores decreased by 35 percent. Another four-month study with 1,334 men found that residual urine volume decreased by 37 percent and nighttime urination by 54 percent. Half the men experiencing painful urination before the trial reported relief.[31]

Dosage
Standardized extract/capsules are 85 to 95 percent fatty acids and sterols. Take 160 milligrams twice a day. Or take powdered/encapsulated freshly dried berries, 1 to 2 grams per day.

Cautions
Rarely, saw palmetto will produce stomach upset and nausea.

RYE GRASS POLLEN

Rye grass pollen (*Secale cereale*) has been used in Europe for prostatic, arthritic, and cholesterol problems for nearly fifty years with tremendous success. The pollen is generally sold in proprietary formulas under names like Cernilton or Cernitin. While 92 percent of the formula is rye grass pollen, 5 percent comes from timothy grass (*Phleum pratense*) and 3 percent from corn pollen (*Zea mays*). Corn pollen has been used as a longevity tonic for men and contains many of the same constituents as pine pollen.

The pollens are collected mechanically and processed through a two-stage process into pill form. Numerous clinical trials and hundreds of studies have shown this rye grass pollen combination to possess significant anti-inflammatory activity, to be a prostate tonic and normalizer, to lower cholesterol, and to be antiarthritic. Studies have consistently shown that grass pollen has a specific growth-inhibiting effect on prostatic epithelial cells and fibroblasts and that it is consistently effective in the treatment of BPH.

In one double-blind, placebo-controlled trial, fifty-seven men with BPH received either Cernilton or placebo daily. Seventy percent of the men in the Cernilton group reported significant improvement in symptoms, 60 percent of them reported improvements in bladder emptying, and most experienced a shrinkage of prostate tissues. Another double-blind, placebo-controlled trial with 103 men with Stage II or III BPH found that after taking 138 milligrams per day for twelve weeks, 69 percent of the men experienced relief of symptoms in six different categories. Another study with sixty men, 92 milligrams for six months, found similar outcomes.

Cernilton has been found to be as effective in the treatment of prostatitis as it has been for BPH. Seventy-five to 80 percent of men report relief in clinical trials of Cernilton in the treatment of nonbacterial-related prostatitis. In one trial, men taking three tablets daily of a rye grass pollen extract experienced significantly reduced symptoms.

A limited number of studies have shown that this combination of pollens is also effective in the treatment of rheumatoid arthritis.[32]

Dosage

Take 60 to 120 milligrams two to three times daily. The dosage for rye grass pollen varies considerably. From 80 milligrams a day to 500 milligrams three times a day has been used by various clinicians and in various studies. Usual dosage range in clinical studies is three to six tablets or four capsules per day. Tablets are usually 50 to 60 milligrams.

Rye grass pollen is available under several commercial names: Cernilton, Cernitin, and Prostaphil are several examples. Cernilton seems the most common. See Resources section for sources.

Cautions

This herb is contraindicated for those with pollen sensitivity.

OMEGA-3 FATTY ACIDS

In vitro studies have shown that omega-6 fatty acids actually stimulate prostate cell growth while omega-3 fatty acids inhibit it. This seems to transfer directly to people. Eskimo men who eat a lot of fish rich in omega-3 fatty acids have significantly lower risks of prostate cancer than Eskimos who do not. And one study with nineteen men found that an increase in omega-3 fatty acids for several weeks resulted in elimination of residual urine in twelve; elimination of nighttime urination for thirteen; elimination of dribbling in eighteen men; increased urine stream in all men; reduction in size of the prostate gland in all men; decreased fatigue and leg pain in all men; and increased libido and diminished residual urine in all men.[33]

Dosage

While you can buy omega-3 oil in capsules, perhaps the easiest way to take it is as flaxseed oil, 1 tablespoon daily.

Note: Coldwater fish, such as mackerel, albacore tuna, sardines, and salmon are high in omega-3 fatty acids. Eat these three times per week. If you do choose to eat salmon, try to get wild salmon. Most salmon sold in the United States is raised in pens and is nearly always treated with large quantities of antibiotics and growth enhancers.

ZINC

Zinc intake has been found to shrink the prostate and alleviate symptoms for men with BPH. Several studies have found that the use of zinc for as little as two months results in a decrease of symptoms of BPH. In one study with nineteen men, fourteen of them experienced shrinkage of the prostate as measured by palpation (touch), X ray, and endoscopy.[34]

Interestingly, high estrogen levels in the body interfere with zinc being taken up in the intestinal tract. Not only do estrogens affect male sexual functioning, but by lowering the uptake of zinc they reduce male sexual functioning even further. Androgens, on the other hand, significantly enhance zinc uptake.

Dosage

Take 20 to 40 milligrams per day. It is generally recommended to not exceed 40 milligrams of zinc per day.

Cautions

Over time, zinc intake can cause copper depletion in the body. To counteract this, most zinc supplements come with copper added. At very high doses, zinc can cause nausea and upset stomach, skin rashes, depression, folate deficiency, and lower tolerance to alcohol.

Things to Avoid

HOPS AND BEER

The potent estrogen, estradiol, found in large quantities in hops, plays a powerful role in increasing prostate size and is strongly implicated in both BPH and prostate cancer. Hopped beer should be avoided at all cost. Some studies have found that beer consumption is directly related to prostate inflammation.[35] Other estrogenic plants, such as licorice and black cohosh, should be avoided as well.

PROSTATE CANCER

Prostate cancer is unfortunately an increasingly common problem for men in this country; according to current statistics about one in nine will get it. It is now the second leading cause of cancer deaths among men in the United States. While prostate cancer is a serious problem, a few natural protocols do merit mention.

Nettle root has shown consistent ability to stop the proliferation of human prostate cancer cells *in vitro*. It is also specifically toxic to prostate cancer cells and strongly inhibits their growth. Nettle root is specifically inhibitory to the growth of epithelial cells, the cells most responsible for prostate cancer. It has been shown to specifically inhibit lymph node carcinoma of the prostate.[36] Nettle root inhibits the binding of SHBG to prostate cell membranes (helping inhibit cancer formation), blocks the conversion of testosterone to estradiol in the prostate by deactivating the aromatase enzyme, and inhibits metabolites that stimulate prostate cancer cell growth. Saw palmetto has shown activity against at least one type of prostate cancer in laboratory study. Cernilton has shown the ability to inhibit prostate cancer growth in a number of studies. Like nettle root, it is specifically inhibitory to abnormal epithelial cell growth. Milk thistle seed has shown strong anti-prostatic cancer activity. A combination of milk thistle constituents called silymarin has been found to inhibit cancer formation, promotion, and progression by interfering with cellular signaling in prostate tissue. Quercetin has been found to inhibit the mutation of the p53 suppressor gene, a malfunction connected to the development of prostate cancer. Selenium has been found in a number of studies to specifically inhibit prostate cancer growth and formation. And if taken with vitamin E, its actions are even more potent. Lycopene has been found to be highly concentrated in men's testes, adrenal glands and prostate. Low lycopene levels have been directly tied to prostate cancer. Men eating at least ten servings of tomatoes (which are high in lycopene) per week have only about half the incidence of prostate cancer as that seen in the general population. A large National Cancer Institute study found that low intake of omega-3 fatty acids was directly correlated with prostate cancer as well. *In vitro* studies have found that omega-3 oils actually inhibit the formation of prostate cancer cells. Vitamin D has been found to inhibit prostate cancer formation. A lack of vitamin D in the diet has been tied to the development of prostate cancer.

And while both testosterone and DHT have been implicated in many people's minds with the emergence of prostate cancer in men, intriguing studies, mostly in Europe, indicate that testosterone or androgen replacement therapies in fact result in less prostate cancer, not more. The highest risk for developing prostate cancer, a number of studies have found, is in those with the lowest plasma androgen levels and the highest levels of estradiol. Testosterone and androgen replacement therapies (especially DHT) have not been found to be associated with prostate cancer—quite the reverse. However, 5 alpha reductase reduction therapies, in some instances, have been found to put men at a higher risk for prostate cancer.[37]

For the most comprehensive look at natural approaches to prostate cancer treatment see Donald Yance's *Herbal Medicine, Healing, and Cancer* (Keats, 1999). For more on information about androgen replacement therapies and prostate cancer see Jonathan Wright's *Maximize Your Vitality and Potency (for Men Over 40)* (Smart Publications, 1999).

Natural Care for Prostate Cancer

For Six Months to Two Years

Nettle root, 300 to 1,200 milligrams daily

Saw palmetto seed, 160 milligrams twice daily (standardized to 85 to 95 percent fatty acids and sterols)

Rye grass pollen, 80 to 500 milligrams three times daily (Cernilton or equivalent)

Milk thistle seed, 1,000 milligrams a day standardized extract (70 percent silymarin complex)

CoQ-10, 150 to 300 milligrams daily

Omega-3 fatty acids, 1 tablespoon of flaxseed oil daily

Lycopene, 15 milligrams daily

Alpha lipoic acid, 600 milligrams daily

Vitamin E, 400 to 800 international units daily

Vitamin D, 400 international units daily

Selenium, 200 to 400 micrograms daily

Zinc, 40 milligrams daily

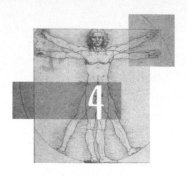

The Heart

A merry heart causeth good healing . . .

—HEBREW ADAGE

The heart has its own memory.   —BALZAC

As we age, our heart changes, both literally and metaphorically. When the world is young, the young heart is open to anything that comes its way. But the years take their toll. Loves lost, dreams unfulfilled, the betrayal of friends begin teaching the heart at a cellular level truths that the young cannot, by their nature, understand. Of course, there are also loves found, dreams fulfilled, and friends who remain. All this mixes together in a form unique to each individual and makes up the truth that the heart comes to know as its own. The heart seasons, grows scar tissue, changes. It becomes less naive. This constant impact of the world upon us causes all of us to close down parts of our heart, to become hard-hearted to some extent—to pass the beggar in the street without a second thought. We are told it is a part of maturing but I think there is a part of all of us that wonders if this is true. Unknown to most of us, through all this "maturing," the heart is storing certain memories away, and one day, unexpectedly, following some wisdom of its own, the heart begins releasing them into our consciousness. The oddest thoughts and memories seemingly forgotten all these years begin to come back to us: a comb sitting on a dresser, the look in a friend's eyes in response to an unkind word, our internal four-year-old-child memory of an injured dog by the side of the road.

Every memory of the heart contains some meaning that the heart knows we must accommodate to fulfill the maturing of our character. These memories represent some unfinished business of the soul. Only conscientious examination will reveal just what the nature of that unfinished business is. And so the heart gives us its memories to think about, until we understand them.

Each of these memories has a deeper connection to the literal heart than most of us know. Modern research is confirming ancient understandings that the heart is much more than the muscular pump that science has assumed it to be.

The heart beats 100,000 times a day, 40 million times a year, some 3 billion times in the seventy to eighty years of a human life. It pumps two gallons of blood per minute, one hundred gallons an hour, through vessels and arteries with a combined length of 60 thousand miles (more than two times the circumference of the Earth).

That is how most people think of the heart, an amazing muscular pump. But there are also more than 40,000 sensory neurons in the heart, the same kind of neurons that are found in the brain. Each individual section of the brain contains thousands to millions of neurons, several billion when all are added together. Importantly, certain crucial subcortical centers of the brain contain the same number of neurons as the heart. The heart, like those areas, possesses its own nervous system and, in essence, actually *is* a specialized brain that processes specific types of information. It is tightly interwoven into the brain, interconnected with the amygdala, thalamus, and cortex.

These three brain centers are primarily concerned with (1) emotional memories and processing; (2) sensory experience; and (3) problem solving, reasoning, and learning. What this means is that our *experience* of the world is routed first through our heart, which "thinks" about the experiences and then sends the data to the brain for further processing. When the heart receives information back from the brain about how to respond, the heart analyzes it and decides whether or not the actions the brain wants to take are going to be effective. There is a neural dialogue between the heart and brain and, in essence, the two decide together what to do. While the brain can and does do a great many things with the information it receives, the heart can override it, directing and controlling behavior if it decides, through a process no scientist understands, to do so.

While scientists are excited about the knowledge they are gleaning about the heart and its functions, none of it is really new. All of this knowledge about the heart, throughout history, has been known to the world's cultures.

Our language (as do all languages) contains wisdom about the heart that we rarely call up into our conscious minds. We have all known, at one time or another, a man who is "bighearted," a woman who is "goodhearted," or even have had friends who are "kindhearted." If we tell them so we may do it in a "heartfelt" way. We sometimes eat a "hearty" meal, share a "hearty" laugh, or even look "hearty." Our profession or our mate may become the "heart" of our life, or we may work for long years to attain our "heart's desire." And because the heart does in fact act as a specialized brain, it is actually possible to "follow your heart" or to "listen to your heart."

If we are dejected or hopeless it may be said that we have "lost heart." If a loved one rejects us we can become "brokenhearted." If we are being unkind someone may implore us to "have a heart" or not be "heartless." People can be "coldhearted" and cruel and it is literally possible to be "hardhearted"—during arteriosclerosis, or hardening of the arteries, bony calcium growths can form in the openings to the heart and occlude blood flow. These growths can become stone hard, hard enough to break saws specially designed to cut through bone.

The complex web of emotions that are processed through the heart's neural network each day literally serve as stimuli for the release of specific neural and biochemical agents by the heart, the shifting of pulse flow, changes in heart rate, and modification of the magnetic field of the heart. All these alterations communicate with the brain and body and shift physiology either directly or indirectly through responses by other organ systems. Changes can include blood vessel size, heart rate, alterations in the balance between the autonomic and parasympathetic nervous systems, enhancements in certain brain functions, and the body's blood levels of cortisol, DHEA, and Immunoglobulin A (IgA).

THE NEUROLOGICAL HEART

Over the past twenty years, researchers in an emerging specialty, neurocardiology, have discovered that the heart really is a specialized brain in its own right. It can feel, sense, learn, and remember (as Balzac said it could some 150 years ago). Much of the information we gather from the world around us is first processed by the heart, which generates emotions in response to the type of information we are receiving. Emotional complexes are the linguistics of the heart. They are sophisticated informational cues or gestalts about the world around us and can be extremely complicated. Emotional language is very different from language built around words. These latter languages tend to be handled more linearly (two-dimensional processing), while the emotional language of the heart is handled more intuitively (three-dimensional processing).

As the heart processes experiences emotionally, with each beat it sends out a burst of neurological information to the brain, which, in response, exerts a regulatory effect over multiple systems of the body. This influences physiology, thinking, and future action. The brain and the heart exist in a tightly coupled feedback loop, constantly exchanging information, each of them shifting body physiology in response.[1]

Many of the emotional experiences that flow through the heart are stored as memories within the heart much as memories are stored in the brain. The heart literally learns from the emotional experiences it has and begins to act in certain ways from what it learns. It begins producing different hormones and creating different beating patterns, depending on what experiences flow through it *and what it decides about those experiences*. A person's heart literally can become small or big, or cold, or hard. And as the heart changes, the body follows.

The heart also manufactures neurotransmitters: norepinephrine, dopamine, and (possibly) acetylcholine. Dopamine is created from the dietary precursor L-dopa (or *its* precursors, tyrosine and phenylalanine), and is an essential chemical enabling the transfer of information from neuron to neuron. In other words, the heart makes the neurotransmitter it needs as it needs it to communicate information to the brain. L-dopa is also intimately connected to sexual interest and erections in men and the ability to have orgasms for women. Low dopamine levels are at the heart of the development of Parkinson's disease.

Acetylcholine is an essential brain transmitter as well, playing a crucial role in memory. Problems with acetylcholine in the brain is one of the reasons for the loss of memory in Alzheimer's patients.

THE HORMONAL HEART

The heart actively creates a number of essential hormones, some unique to itself. Three of the most important are *atrial natriuretic factor* (ANF), *brain natriuretic factor* (BNF—because it was first found in the brain), and *calcitonin gene-related peptide* (CGRP).

ANF regulates blood pressure, body-fluid retention, smooth-muscle states, and electrolyte homeostasis. It affects the brain, adrenal glands, kidneys, and body musculature. ANF decreases aldosterone production in the adrenal glands (thus lowering the body's tendency to retain sodium and water) and also inhibits the production of cortisol, one of the body's major stress hormones. Cortisol has a strong impact on the body's androgen levels, reproductive and adrenal organ growth and function, and immune system health and vitality, among other things. Excesses of cortisol have been connected to a large number of chronic diseases. The more ANF the heart produces, the lower the cortisol levels. More poetically, the more open the heart, the less stressed the body.

CGRP acts synergistically with nitric oxide to help relax the blood vessels and protect the arteries from atherosclerosis, coronary artery disease, and stroke. A number of inflammatory agents (prostagladins, histamine, and bradykinin), and the metabolic end product lactic acid, trigger the release of CGRP so that blood vessels dilate.

Among other things, when a person is under stress, BNP activates a specific pathway in the neural cells of the brain and the heart that causes the secretion of a unique protein—beta-amyloid precursor protein. This protein protects the neurons from stressors (such as toxic levels of glutamate), especially those in the hippocampus of the brain. In other words, the heart creates a specific hormonal neuroprotector to protect brain function. (See also Alzheimer's Disease, Chapter 10.)

Like dopamine, norepinephrine (and also epinephrine—aka adrenaline) is made from the precursors L-dopa, tyrosine, and phenylalanine. Norepinephrine regulates the movement of fats in the bloodstream and the contraction of arterioles and plays an essential role in regulating arterial health, fat processing, and atherosclerosis.

When we are cared for, or care for others, the heart releases an entirely different cascade of hormonal and neurotransmitter substances than in other, less hopeful, circumstances. Falling in love causes a tremendous expansion of the heart, a flood of both DHEA and testosterone through-out the heart and body, and a flow of other hormonal chemistries such as dopamine, all of which affect adrenal, hypothalamus, and pituitary hormonal output. More IgA, or Immunoglobulin A, is also released, stim-ulating the health and immune action of mucous membrane systems throughout the body. IgA is commonly present in the lining of the mucosal membranes of the body and regulates the movement of foreign substances into the body through the membranes. Low IgA levels allow more penetra-tion of bacterial or viral toxins into the body and can allow disruption of in-testinal health, interfering with nutrient uptake and contributing to such conditions as irritable bowel syndrome (IBS) or inflammatory bowel dis-ease (IBD). (This is one of the reasons why lowering stress levels has been found to positively affect the health of those with IBS and IBD.)

THE BIOPHYSICAL
AND BIOENERGETIC HEART

As the heart beats, it creates a pressure wave that travels through the arter-ies, faster than the blood itself. All the cells of the body feel the heart's pres-sure waves and learn to understand the meanings encoded within them. The pressure waves change as heart hormonal balance, rhythm, and beat change and this change communicates knowledge to the cells about what types of information the heart is processing.

The pressure wave, as it travels through the system, also creates an elec-trical voltage. As these rhythmic pressure waves squeeze the cells in the body, some cells' proteins generate an electrical current in response. The pulsing of the blood literally creates an electrical dialogue between the cells and the heart.

The heart itself possesses an electromagnetic field, which is five thou-sand times stronger than the brain's. It permeates every cell of our body and strongly affects brain wave patterns. While this field can actually be mea-sured by instruments (up to ten feet beyond our bodies), it is immediately sensed by other people. We literally can feel if someone has a "good heart."

THE SEXUAL HEART

The heart is also an important sexual organ because of its processing and production of sexual hormones. There are more testosterone receptors in the heart than in any other muscle in the human body. And for good reason, testosterone is essential in creating strong muscles. So the heart possesses abundant quantities of the enzymes necessary to convert DHEA to more potent androgens such as androstenedione and testosterone. The heart makes testosterone as it needs it to keep local levels high and the heart muscle strong. Some researchers have found indications that the heart actually makes an androgen binding protein (ABP) very similar to the one made in the testes' Sertoli cells, in order to concentrate both testosterone and DHT in the heart.

Beyond the ability of testosterone and DHT to increase muscle mass, testosterone is also important in that it is a major agent in the production and release of nitric oxide in the body, making it a major stimulator of arterial dilation. The nitroglycerine that people take for heart attacks works because the body takes nitric oxide from the nitroglycerine molecule and uses it to dilate the blood vessels around the heart, providing it with more oxygen. The body's testosterone normally keeps nitric oxide high enough to provide proper arterial dilation. More nitric oxide is created and released if more dilation is needed.

CARDIOVASCULAR DISEASE

Two of the more common reasons for heart and cardiovascular disease are deterioration of the blood vessels of the body and a catabolic (breaking down) rather than an anabolic (building up) heart dynamic.

Deterioration of the blood vessels is most often caused by their inability to self-repair. Blood vessels are composed of a very thin layer of endothelial cells on the inside, then a collagen layer, then muscle, then an outer coat, or perivascular sheath. Collagen allows vessels to stretch and bend, to be flexible. As they age, somewhat like a flexible garden hose that is exposed to the sun for years on end, the blood vessels can begin to stiffen and then crack. Much of this deterioration is caused by oxidation, the same kind of process that degrades garden hoses. Normally, the body repairs oxidized collagen as fast as it degrades. But when it deteriorates faster than it is repaired, tiny cracks begin to form in the vessel walls. To repair the collagen in blood vessels the body needs vitamin C.

A vitamin C–dependent enzyme, prolyl hydroxylase, is the catalyst that enables collagen to form. Without vitamin C, prolyl hydroxylase cannot maintain activity; collagen cannot form fibers properly; and bones, cartilage, blood vessels, and skin cannot heal efficiently. Collagen itself is usually high in vitamin C.

Human beings are one of only four animals on Earth who cannot synthesize vitamin C in the body. (The others are our close relatives the gorillas, plus guinea pigs, and fruit bats.) So we must ingest enough vitamin C in our diets to prevent collagen deterioration and also ingest substances such as proanthocyanidins (OPCs) that potentiate the vitamin C, and antioxidants (OPCs, anthocyanidins, procyanidins) that can protect collagen tissues from damage. Normally, if the body has sufficient vitamin C, the collagen repair of blood vessels is an efficient, ongoing process. If there is insufficient vitamin C, OPCs, or antioxidants in the diet, over time, the blood vessels cannot be repaired efficiently and they begin to crack.

The body covers cracks in blood vessels with cholesterol and then the cholesterol with calcium as a kind of "scab." This protects the damaged blood vessel and interposes a new "wall" between the collagen and the blood. When the underlying crack heals, the body removes the calcium and cholesterol. The scab is reabsorbed into the bloodstream and carried away. But, if there is not enough vitamin C, OPCs, or antioxidants, the damage does not heal and new cracks continually occur in other parts of the circulatory system. Over time, the blood vessels are covered with cholesterol/ calcium patches and the vessels become less and less flexible. Sometimes, a spasm of a blood vessel, usually near the heart, can cause the calcium scab to crack and the softer cholesterol underneath to spurt out of the break. This causes blood platelets to congregate on the cholesterol, form fibrin, and make a blood clot. These clots usually become part of the patch on the vessel wall, but they can sometimes break off and occlude the heart (this is a heart attack) or lodge in the brain and cause a stroke.

A catabolic dynamic, the second major factor influencing heart health, is often initiated by stress, aging, or both. The more stress a person experiences, the lower the ANF production and the higher the levels of cortisol and adrenaline that are produced. This causes a narrowing of the blood vessels and a lowering of DHEA levels in the heart and throughout the body. Aging, to some extent, will produce the same effect because as DHEA levels fall, cortisol levels increase.

Low free testosterone levels, high estrogen to androgen levels, and high cortisol to DHEA levels are significant factors in heart disease in men.

High estradiol levels alone have been linked to heart disease (which is another reason why hopped beers should be avoided).[2] In fact, as free testosterone levels decrease (and the androgen to estrogen ratio changes) all the cardiovascular risk factors increase.

- Cholesterol and triglyceride levels rise

- Coronary and other major arteries constrict

- Blood pressure rises

- Insulin levels increase

- Abdominal fat and waist-to-hip ratio increases

- Lipoprotein A levels increase

- Fibrogenin levels rise

- LDL levels rise

- HDL levels decrease

- HGH output decreases

- Energy levels decrease (leading to less physical exercise)

As the physician Eugene Shippen says in his book *The Testosterone Syndrome,* "No other single factor in the male body that we know of correlates with more risk factors for heart disease than testosterone."[3]

Given all this, it is not so surprising that American men, especially as they move into middle age, suffer such high levels of heart disease. It is estimated that one in four Americans—some 50 million people—are hypertensive. Cardiovascular disease is the primary cause of death of more people than the next seven leading causes combined. We are literally dying by the millions from broken hearts every year.

Healing the Heart

Three of the most important things to do in healing the heart are (1) adjust androgen levels, (2) consume plants and supplements that support a healthy cardiovascular system, and (3) support your heart in our language's deeper sense of the word.

Adjusting Androgen Levels

One of the most effective approaches to heart disease is to make sure that the androgen/estrogen levels in the body are balanced, the DHEA/cortisol levels are balanced, and there are sufficient levels of free testosterone. A significant number of clinical studies have shown that simply increasing free testosterone levels and improving other androgenic factors in men alleviates many of the physical aspects of heart disease.[4] Some of the ways testosterone does this is that it increases the health of the heart muscle, stimulates the formation of new muscle fibers in the heart, increases heartbeat strength, dilates blood vessels throughout the body (especially around the heart), increases blood flow to the extremities, restores arterial circulation to the skin, and enhances musculature, healing, and health of the blood vessels.[5] Testosterone also maintains the health of the endothelial cells that line blood vessels. This layer of cells is only a few microns thick and they make a slick, smooth surface over which the blood can flow. The endothelial cells have the same electrical charge as blood cells and repel them to keep them from sticking (much like positive-pole batteries do when forced together). Collagen lies just under the endothelial cells and when a vessel cracks, it breaks the endothelial cells open and exposes the collagen. Collagen has the opposite electrical charge to blood and when it breaks through, the blood cells begin sticking to it. Cholesterol covers the break to allow the blood to flow as smoothly as before. The endothelial cells also, importantly, produce an anticoagulant to keep blood from clotting. When they are healthy, there are fewer clots in the circulatory system. Testosterone helps endothelial cells regenerate and stimulates their production of anticoagulants. Importantly, the anticoagulant that the endothelial cells produce also dissolves the fibrin around which blood clots form.[6] This helps break down any older clots that have formed in the cardiovascular system. Testosterone also helps maintain the structure and health of the muscle tissue that lies just under the collagen. Testosterone and collagen supporters, like vitamin C, work together to maintain all the necessary components of the vascular system.

Plants

Plants can also play a major part in the healing of the heart or in keeping it healthy (besides simply increasing testosterone levels). The source of the medicinal actions of many plants is their secondary chemistries, named such because researchers thought them unessential by-products. The primary chemistries are things like glucose and cellulose, which give the plants their energy and shape. Secondary chemistries are present in plants in tiny amounts, often parts per million, yet are able to powerfully effect biological changes in the plants and in any organism that ingests the plants. Some of the more powerful secondary constituents in plants are called *cardiac glycosides* and are highly useful for impaired heart function or arrhythmias because they increase the strength of the heart's pumping action. The most famous of these is digoxin, which is from the foxglove plant. Lily of the valley, as another example, has similar actions to foxglove but with far fewer side effects. Of more importance, however, are herbs whose effects lie in areas other than merely increasing the strength of the heart's muscular pumping. While cardiac glycoside-containing plants increase heart pumping action, other plant constituents can offer long-term tonic effects for the heart—healing and repairing the overall vascular system itself. Still others are circulatory stimulants that help warm cold extremities, or peripheral dilators that are useful in arteriosclerosis, hypotensives that help lower blood pressure, or hypertensives that help raise it. The world's healing traditions are filled with plants that have found a place in the healing of broken hearts. Perhaps the most important general cardiovascular tonic is hawthorn. It can help normalize function in atherosclerosis, cardiac arrhythmia, congestive heart failure, hypertension, and peripheral vascular disease.

Supporting the Deeper Heart

The rhythmic beating of the heart is rarely steady and uniform. It should normally go through a wide range of patterns as it responds to the information it gets from the world around it. Beating patterns are, it is now known, reliable indicators of heart disease. In other words, the more flexible the heart, the more healthy it is. Human touch, from a loved one or even massage, has been shown to improve the flexibility of heart rhythms. The messages that we receive through our heart (for instance, the caring encoded in a loved one's touch) are sent to the brain and throughout the body as the heart responds to their underlying meaning. Whatever we take into our bodies, whether it be caring or food, affects the heart. This is why so many people recommend that it is important to engage each day in something that is fun, something that has meaning, something that feels good to the heart. For people with broken hearts, this begins training the heart to a different pattern, a different beat, however measured or far away. Perhaps, one more healthy than that followed in the past. The heart can then begin to rebuild itself, actually making new muscle and blood vessels from special stem cells it calls to itself from other sites in the body—literally, it "takes heart."[7]

Natural Care for the Heart

For Twelve to Eighteen Months
  Hawthorn, 120 to 900 milligrams three times daily
  Androgen replacement protocol (pine pollen, 5 grams once or twice daily)
  DHEA, 25 to 50 milligrams once or twice daily
  Vitamin C, .5 to 3 grams daily or tbt
  Magnesium, 200 to 400 milligrams three times daily
  Coenzyme Q-10, 150 to 300 milligrams daily
  L-carnitine, 300 milligrams three times daily

HAWTHORN

Hawthorn (*Crataegus oxyacantha*) is a member of the rose family, a family of plants intimately related to the heart in many cultures' traditions. The rose is, in fact, an ancient European symbol of love and a healthy, open, and caring heart. It is still used this way for many people, the symbol of a gift from one heart to another. Red roses were commonly used in ancient medical traditions as a heart tonic, to heal broken hearts. In Belize, in Central America, they still are used much that way, though usually for babies, children, and new mothers. Most of the rest of the world uses hawthorn.

The berries of the hawthorn bush (and sometimes the leaves and flowers) have been used as a heart tonic for at least two thousand years in Western medicine and for a bit less than seven hundred in China. They are specific for nearly every manifestation of heart disease: atherosclerosis, cardiac arrhythmia, congestive heart failure, hypertension, and peripheral vascular disease. *In vivo* studies have found that the herb lowers blood pressure, increases blood vessel dilation throughout the body, lowers cholesterol levels in the blood, and is powerfully antiarrhythmic, slowing and normalizing heartbeat. Both *in vivo* and *in vitro* studies have shown that hawthorn increases both the amplitude of heart contractions and its stroke volume. Studies also show that if blood pressure is too low, hawthorn raises it; if it is too high, hawthorn lowers it. It is, in fact, a normalizer of blood pressure and a regulator of blood flow within the body. While substances like adrenaline or digoxin increase the heart's rate and beat strength in order to increase blood flow in the body, hawthorn lowers heart rate and still accomplishes the same thing. With hawthorn, muscular contractions of the heart are slower, longer, and more powerful. This particular type of beating pattern is associated with higher ANF levels, more relaxed states, and lower cortisol levels—basically an anabolic pattern. Adrenaline, on the other hand, is a catabolic heart stimulant. Hawthorn is virtually the only anabolic heart medicine known.

Dozens of clinical trials have been conducted with hawthorn extracts on thousands of people with heart disease. All have confirmed the herb's remarkable effectiveness. In one study, 300 milligrams of the dried leaf was taken daily in a placebo-controlled, double-blind trial of forty-six men with angina. After four weeks, angina had been reduced in all patients by 86 percent. In another study, seventy-eight people with chronic heart failure were given 600 milligrams daily of hawthorn for eight weeks. Exercise tolerance significantly increased; heart rate and blood pressure both significantly decreased. Another study showed that 87 percent of participants in a hawthorn trial experienced lower cholesterol levels, 80 percent had lower triglycerides. All experienced lower blood pressure and more dilation in coronary vessels. In another trial, 1,011 people were given a standardized extract, 900 milligrams, for twenty-four weeks. A significant improvement was seen in exercise tolerance, fatigue levels, palpitation, and dyspnea. Ankle edema and nocturia were reduced by 83 percent. A more stable heart rate and reductions in blood pressure were common. A significant reduction in the number of people with ST depression, arrhythmia, and ventricular extrasystole was seen.[8]

Part of the reason that hawthorn reduces cholesterol is that it literally repairs the cellular structure of blood vessel walls. Hawthorn contains procyanidins, a flavonoid complex similar to those found in bilberry (anthocyanosides) and pine bark and grape seed (proanthocyanidins—aka OPCs). Procyanidins protect collagen fibers from damage, increase their elasticity, and reinforce the cross-linking of collagen fibers to make them stronger and hence make the blood vessels less prone to cracking. Procyanidins increase intracellular vitamin C levels (which is necessary for collagen synthesis), stimulate circulation to peripheral blood vessels, are potent antioxidants, and are strongly anti-inflammatory. They also lower cell membrane permeability and help protect cellular integrity. Like OPCs, procyanidins promote insulin secretion by the pancreas and inhibit sorbitol accumulation within cells. Both sorbitol, a by-product of glucose metabolism, and glucose naturally damage blood vessel walls and cellular tissues if they are not properly processed by the body. It is, in fact, the increased sugar concentration of the blood that causes many of the circulatory problems suffered by diabetics. Hawthorn protects the vessels by increasing their strength and integrity while reducing substances in the blood that are caustic to vessel structure.

Because the circulatory channels are not cracking, the body has no need to increase blood cholesterol levels to coat the vessels in an attempt to repair them. Blood cholesterol levels then naturally drop *without* reducing cholesterol in the diet. This is why the French can eat large quantities of fat in their diets and still have low rates of heart disease. The red wines they drink contain proanthocyanidins (and polyphenols), which keep blood vessels healthy. The so-called bad cholesterol that people are so afraid of is the type of cholesterol that the body uses in blood-vessel repair, which is why its levels tend to be high in blood when there is heart disease. High cholesterol is a symptom of cardiovascular disease, *not* a cause.

Hawthorn also has a direct effect on the diameter of blood vessels and arteries, causing them to dilate. This increases the oxygen being received by the heart. Hawthorn also changes the rhythm and pattern of the heartbeat. The heart beats slower, the beats last longer, and the power is increased. The longer the herb is used, the more healing occurs in vessel walls and the more toned the muscle of the heart becomes.

How hawthorn does this is not completely understood, but part of the way it affects both blood pressure and heartbeat is that it regulates the amounts of calcium and potassium in the blood and heart (also see Hypertension). This regulatory action of hawthorn can help prevent the buildup of calcium growths in the vessels of the lower legs and in the openings to the heart. Hawthorn also inhibits *angiotensin converting enzyme* (ACE), which converts angiotensin I to angiotensin II, a potent vasoconstrictor. This helps keep the circulatory vessels dilated. Hawthorn berries are, in essence, a type of rosehip. Like rosehips, they are very high in vitamin C. Hawthorn's vitamin C and procyanidins act synergistically (as they do in pine) to produce healthy collagen tissues throughout the body. Hawthorn also contains calcium, magnesium, phosphorus, potassium, and tyramine, all of which have important actions on the heart and blood vessels.

Dosage

Take 120 to 900 milligrams of the herb daily, or ¼ to ½ teaspoon three times daily of the tincture.

The dosage range in most clinical studies has been from 120 to 900 milligrams daily. Most of these studies have used nonstandardized (i.e., raw herb) extracts, either in capsules or as an alcoholic tincture. Some practitioners are suggesting that the extracts be standardized for 1.8 percent vitexin-4'-rhamnoside or 10 percent procyanidin content. Not everyone agrees. The herb is effective in both forms and a number of people feel that the herb is most efficacious in whole form without the seemingly inevitable human tinkering.

Cautions

Hawthorn is as safe an herb as can be found. You would need to consume seventy ounces (over one gallon) of the tincture at one sitting to experience acute side effects. Although the German Commission E lists no known side effects, at very high dosages the herb may rarely cause nausea, breathing difficulty, fatigue, sweating, and rash. There are a few anecdotal, never verified reports of high dosages causing heart arrhythmia, central nervous system depression, or hypotension. There are no reports of adverse effects with normal low dosing. The herb should be used in combination with heart pharmaceuticals only under health-care supervision. Hawthorn is, in many respects, a food and can be readily consumed in the diet. The plant is extremely prolific and there are scores if not hundreds of various species growing throughout the world. Many of their berries are regularly used as foods in the diets of the people who live where it grows. Interestingly, as wild foods are being discovered by the great chefs of New York and Paris, hawthorn is being included on menus at exceptionally high prices. Whatever we cut off as part of our day-to-day life (e.g., walking or hawthorn berries) tends to come back as art (jogging or hawthorn berry pasta sauce).

ANDROGEN REPLACEMENT THERAPY
WITH PINE POLLEN

Increasing free testosterone levels, adjusting the androgen/estrogen balance (especially testosterone/estradiol), and decreasing the amount of cortisol relative to DHEA in the body have all been found to positively benefit heart health. Testosterone has been found to improve blood content and glucose uptake, relieve angina, relieve intermittent claudication, improve blood flow and vascular health, normalize blood pressure, and even cure gangrene caused by blocked blood flow to tissues.[9]

One Chinese study of sixty-two men with angina, for example, found that testosterone supplementation reduced angina in 77 percent and improved heart function (increased blood flow as measured by EKG) in 70 percent of the men. In 1984, a Danish physician, Jens Moller, published the results of his clinical work with thousands of men. Testosterone replacement, he found, commonly resulted in the reverse of heart disease and its symptoms. (Neither did it cause inflammation of the prostate in his client populations. Rather, reduction in size was the usual outcome.) An American study of testosterone replacement in the treatment of heart disease with one hundred men found similar outcomes, as have numerous other studies. Many studies have clearly shown that the lower the level of free testosterone, the *more severe* the coronary artery disease a man is likely to suffer.[10]

Pine pollen can be an important part of any androgen replacement therapy in heart disease. While pine pollen contains significant amounts of testosterone and other androgens, it also contains high levels of arginine, leucine, lysine, methionine, phenylalanine, tryptophan, tyrosine, riboflavin, nicotinic acid, pantothenic acid, pyridoxine, biotin, inositol, and folic acid. It also contains trace amounts of alanine, amino-butyric acid, aspartic acid, cystine, glutamic acid, glycine, hydroxyproline, isoleucine, proline, serine, threonine, and valine. Many of these constituents have significant activity in maintaining heart health. Arginine, for example, is used to make nitric oxide, which expands blood vessels in much the same manner as nitroglycerine tablets. And lysine causes the type of cholesterol that plugs cracked walls, lipoprotein A, to become less sticky, releasing its hold on the vessel wall and facilitating its travel back to the liver for processing.

Dosage
Take 5 grams of pine pollen one to two times daily.

Cautions
Some people are sensitive to pine products—seeds, pollen, bark, resin, and so on. Negative reactions can run from mild allergies to anaphylactic shock. **If you have a history of allergies to pollen or severe reactions to bee stings, do not use without consulting your health-care practitioner.** Adolescents should not use pine pollen.

DHEA

DHEA has been found to be consistently low in men with heart disease while DHEAS (a body-stabilized form of DHEA) levels have been found to be inversely related to both the number and degree of damaged coronary vessels. Men with aortic calcification and low pulse wave velocity have consistently been found to have low DHEA levels. Low DHEA levels have also been found in young men with myocardial infarction. DHEA has been shown to prevent both heart disease and atherosclerosis in a number of animals. And a significant number of *in vitro* studies have shown that it supports the formation and activity of healthy vascular tissue. DHEA affects vascular reactivity by affecting calcium metabolism and influences the rate of smooth muscle development in vascular tissue. DHEA helps slow down the clotting of blood (anti-platelet aggregation activity) much like aspirin. However, the data suggests that DHEA is more effective in men than in women in preventing or healing heart disease.[11]

Dosage
Take 25 to 50 milligrams daily. The dosage range has run from 25 to as much as 1,600 milligrams daily in different studies.

Note

While most of the studies showed mild to moderate positive effects for men, a few did not. Unfortunately, nearly all the studies were poorly designed. The smoking of commercial tobaccos actually increases the body's testosterone and DHEA levels even as it affects heart health negatively through other mechanisms. So even though smokers show high DHEA, they may actually have heart disease, thus throwing off a study's comparison between DHEA levels and heart disease. Alcohol consumption raises DHEA levels as well, while estrogen replacement, phytoestrogens, and estrogen mimics all lower it. The presence of these factors in the participants' lifestyles were not examined.

VITAMIN C

Because of its importance to collagen repair and synthesis, sufficient vitamin C is important in the diet. A healthy intake of vitamin C–rich foods from fruits and vegetables can help, as can vitamin C supplementation.

Dosage

Take .5 to 3 grams per day in two divided doses, or to bowel tolerance. Many people prefer vitamin C as effervescent salts (see the Resources section). (It is somewhat like an Alka-Seltzer.)

Cautions

Vitamin C will cause stomach upset, flatulence, and diarrhea at higher doses. As your body gets enough of the vitamin, the rest is excreted through the bowels. It is more effective to keep levels high through the day by dividing the doses morning and evening. Start at a low dose and work up. It can upset the stomach. While vitamin C can be useful in some kidney conditions, you should not use vitamin C if you are on hemodialysis, or suffer from recurrent kidney stones, severe kidney disease, or gout.

MAGNESIUM

Magnesium is essential for the heart to beat properly and levels are often low in people with heart disease. Increased magnesium intake has been correlated in numerous clinical studies to increased heart health in congestive heart failure (CHF), cardiac arrhythmia, mitral valve prolapse, and various cardiomyopathies. Magnesium supplementation has been shown to help atrial fibrillation, ventricular premature contraction, ventricular tachycardia, and severe ventricular arrhythmia. In some cases, magnesium alone can reverse the condition. Improvements in some instances occurred within as little as fifteen minutes (usually with intravenous use).[12]

Dosage
Take 200 to 400 milligrams three times daily.

Caution
Magnesium is normally well tolerated; however, people with certain kinds of severe heart disease, such as high-grade atrioventricular block, should only use magnesium under the supervision of a health-care provider.

COENZYME Q_{10}

Coenzyme Q_{10} (CoQ_{10}) has been used in at least twelve clinical trials for congestive heart failure (CHF) with as few as 17 patients to as many as 2,600. It has consistently shown the ability to improve cyanosis, edema, heart palpitations, shortness of breath, sweating, vertigo, enlargement of the liver area, arrythmia, and venous congestion in about 75 percent of those taking it. Mitral valve prolapse has been improved to normal in a number of studies, as have a number of other cardiomyopathies. In all studies, the longer the supplement is taken the better the outcomes. At least eighteen months of supplementation is necessary for mitral valve prolapse, twelve months for other cardiomyopathies.[13]

Dosage
Take 150 to 300 milligrams daily.

L-CARNITINE

A number of double-blind, placebo-controlled trials have shown that carnitine helps restore heart function in people with CHF. The longer the supplement was used, the better heart function became. Studies generally showed that after six months, heartbeat was more powerful, more blood was being consistently pumped, and the length of time people were able to exercise increased.[14]

Dosage
Take 300 milligrams three times daily.

FASTING

One of the most effective methods of reversing cardiovascular disease, dissolving fatty plaque accumulations from vessel walls, lowering blood pressure, and correcting angina, intermittent claudication, and even congestive heart failure, is fasting. The studies I have reviewed have consistently shown remarkable recoveries from a variety of circulatory problems through fasting even in cases that were considered untreatable by other approaches. While beyond the scope of this book, if you have high blood pressure, fasting is an option that you should explore. (See the Resources section for more information.)

HYPERTENSION

Hypertension is simply high blood pressure that occurs either from vasoconstriction or a narrowing of the vessel walls because of their occlusion by fatty plaques. About sixty million Americans are estimated to have high blood pressure, 80 percent of whom are in the borderline to moderate range. Nondrug therapies have consistently been shown to be superior to pharmaceuticals in reversing or controlling high blood pressure for most people.

Noncholesterol-related hypertension is frequently stress induced. The epinephrine (adrenaline) released by the adrenal glands when the body is under stress naturally causes a constriction of blood vessels. People who are highly driven, type A personalities (catabolic rather than anabolic) often release high levels of adrenaline into their bloodstreams regularly, which eventually can cause chronic high blood pressure. Because coffee initiates adrenaline release it can also generate high blood pressure. Other constituents in coffee and black tea also contribute to the problem. Caffeine and theophylline, strong alkaloids in coffee and tea, block the actions of adenosine, an important compound in the body that relaxes peripheral blood vessels and regulates coronary blood flow.

For noncholesterol-related hypertension, the best approach is to quit caffeine intake, relax the body, move it to a more anabolic style of functioning, balance androgen levels, and use herbs and supplements that will relax the blood vessels, thus lowering hypertension. Relaxation techniques such as meditation and biofeedback are very effective for helping with this form of hypertension.

While an excess of fats in the diet can increase blood serum levels to unacceptable degrees, many of the problems with cholesterol come from damaged blood vessels that the body is using cholesterol to repair. For cholesterol-related hypertension, it is crucial to begin repair of the blood vessels and arteries so that the body quits generating high serum cholesterol levels to repair them. And while lowering fats in the diet can help, vessel repair is much more important than merely lowering the intake of cholesterol or using cholesterol blockers. Treating the cholesterol is, in general, only treating the symptoms not the cause.

Natural Care for High Blood Pressure

For Eight to Twelve Months

 Hawthorn, 120 to 900 milligrams three times daily
 Garlic, 600 to 1,200 milligrams daily
 Motherwort tincture, ¼ to ½ teaspoon three times daily
 Pine bark or grape seed extract (OPCs), 150 to 300 milligrams daily
 Vincamine (periwinkle), 20 milligrams three times daily
 Potassium, 300 to 400 milligrams three times daily
 Coenzyme Q_{10}, 50 milligrams two to three times daily
 Omega-3 oils, 10 capsules daily (or 1 tablespoon flaxseed oil daily)
 Celery, 4 ounces fresh juice or 4 stalks per day
 Dietary additions and considerations
 Biofeedback (if low cholesterol) or other stress-reduction techniques

HAWTHORN

Because hawthorn dilates blood vessels, repairs and protects vessel walls, and lowers cholesterol in the blood, it is essential for hypertension. At least two dozen studies have found it effective in clinical trials for lowering blood pressure.[15]

Dosage
Take 120 to 900 milligrams daily.

Cautions
Hawthorn is as safe an herb as can be found. You would need to consume seventy ounces (over one gallon) of the tincture at one sitting to experience acute side effects. Although the German Commission E lists no known side effects, at very high dosages the herb may rarely cause nausea, breathing difficulty, fatigue, sweating, and rash. There are a few anecdotal, never verified reports of high dosages causing heart arrhythmia, central nervous system depression, or hypotension. There are no reports of adverse effects with normal low dosing. The herb should be used in combination with heart pharmaceuticals only under health care supervision. Hawthorn is, in many respects, a food and can be readily consumed in the diet. The plant is extremely prolific and there are scores if not hundreds of various species growing throughout the world. Many of their berries are regularly used as foods in the diets of the people who live where it grows. Interestingly, as wild foods are being discovered by the great chefs of New York and Paris, hawthorn is being included on menus at exceptionally high prices. Whatever we cut off as part of our day-to-day life (e.g., walking or hawthorn berries) tends to come back as art (jogging or hawthorn berry pasta sauce).

GARLIC

Garlic (*Allium sativum*) possesses a number of important actions that are specific for both serum cholesterol levels and high blood pressure. It tones the heart muscle, dilates blood vessels and arteries, lowers serum cholesterol levels, and reduces clotting of the blood.

As a vasodilator, garlic appears to affect the circulatory system through six different mechanisms. Garlic increases the amount of adenosine in the bloodstream, which directly increases the diameter of blood vessels and coronary arteries. It has also been found to strongly affect the potassium and calcium channels, acting somewhat like a calcium channel blocker. Garlic also inhibits ACE, the enzyme that converts angiotensin I to angiotensin II, a potent vasoconstrictor. Garlic stimulates the production of nitric oxide, the body's potent vasodilator (4 grams of garlic can double the body's nitric oxide levels within three hours). Garlic lowers the sensitivity of blood-vessel walls to adrenaline, helping reduce the impacts on blood pressure from catabolic, hyperenergetic states. And finally, garlic has been found to act as a smooth muscle relaxant, especially for the intestines and the muscle layers in peripheral blood vessels, the coronary arteries, and the blood vessels of the kidneys. The garlic compounds that cause these vasodilation effects have not been identified, though part of it does come from garlic's adenosine content. The vasodilation effects of garlic are completely unrelated to allicin—a substance garlic is often standardized for. Allicin-free garlic extracts dilated blood vessels just as effectively as allicin-containing ones.

Garlic also has profound effects on blood cholesterol levels. It lowers triglycerides and LDL cholesterol and increases HDL cholesterol. Part of the mechanism for this is that garlic is a strong antioxidant and its regular use repairs damaged blood vessels, making serum LDL cholesterol go down. It also appears to interfere with the synthesis of LDL cholesterol in the liver and with cholesterol absorption from food. The compound in garlic that appears to be mainly concerned with lowering blood cholesterol levels is allicin, for which many garlic products are standardized.

Garlic is a potent antioxidant and has strong impacts on the integrity and health of vessel walls. It stimulates the healing and integrity of vessel walls and reduces inflammation. Some garlic compounds are very similar to the flavonoids in pine bark and it is thought that they are responsible for these actions of the plant.

After cholesterol covers a crack in a vessel wall, cholesterol itself is covered with a calcium "scab" in order to allow the cellular tissue underneath to heal. If the underlying condition of the blood vessel worsens, the cholesterol and calcium covering enlarges. As blood vessels constrict or spasm, the calcium covering can crack and the liquid cholesterol squirts out. This attracts blood platelets, which attach to the cholesterol and release compounds that stimulate blood clotting. The initial stage of this is the creation of fibrin. Fibrin looks like a tangled grouping of fine threads. Red blood cells catch in the fibrin and form a clot. While the clogging of a vessel from atherosclerosis is a long, slow process, a blood clot can occlude a vein in only a few minutes, leading, in some cases, to an immediate heart attack or stroke. Often, however, these blood clots are small and do not occlude the blood vessel. They, in essence, form another scab on top of the calcium/cholesterol scab that is already there. Garlic interferes with the adhesion of these blood platelets to cholesterol and increases the body's ability to degrade the fibrin (fibrinolysis) around which blood clots form. (Decreased fibrinolysis is a common problem in people with atherosclerosis.) Garlic even acts against nonfibrin clotting agents such as the coagulase enzyme produced by staph bacteria. Garlic will usually decrease clotting of the blood by 50 percent within just a few hours of ingestion. The longer garlic is in the diet, the more sustained its anticlotting effect. Garlic also helps by lowering the viscosity of the blood. More commonly, this is referred to as "blood thinning" and aspirin is the most commonly used substance for this purpose.

In essence, garlic helps heal the underlying condition that causes atherosclerosis and promotes the resolution of the conditions that result from it—increased cholesterol in the blood, increased blood viscosity, increased platelet aggregation, and increased fibrin formation. It is not known which garlic compounds are responsible for all these actions. Allicin has been comprehensively linked to the antiplatelet aggregation action but is not responsible for the fibrinolysis or the thinning actions of garlic.

Garlic has also been found to act as a tonic on the heart muscle. Prolonged use has normalized its function, increased its tone, strengthened its beating patterns, and increased personal sense of well-being. Garlic also has direct effects on the adrenal glands, shifting adrenal production from cortisol to DHEA and normalizing adrenaline output.

These effects of garlic have been found to be consistent in hundreds of clinical trials and studies. While impacts of the plant will vary in different people, in men with cholesterol levels in the 220 to 290 milligrams per deciliter range, the daily use of garlic generally lowers LDL cholesterol levels about 15 percent and increases HDL levels by 10 percent. Blood pressure lowers an average of 11 millimeters in the systolic and 5 in the diastolic.

The longer it is used, the better and deeper the impacts on cardiovascular health. As simply one example, 308 people with high blood fats, high cholesterol, high blood pressure, coronary heart disease, diabetes, and liver ailments were given 120 milligrams of garlic oil (equivalent to 50 grams of garlic—a bit less than 2 ounces) daily for twenty to thirty days. All factors, including blood sugar levels, significantly improved.

Raw, fresh garlic is considered to be the most effective way to take garlic for cardiovascular disease. However, because of the smell, many people will not do so even if it means a continually deteriorating disease condition. As a result, a number of companies have created deodorized garlic extracts. These are as effective for high cholesterol and high platelet aggregation as fresh garlic. A number of companies have also standardized their products for the allicin content even though this is only one of the many active compounds. These standardized extracts are not as effective for high blood pressure, heart toning, and so on as raw garlic or even cooked garlic in the diet. A number of studies have shown that eating lots of cooked garlic regularly in the diet will produce the same effects as taking raw garlic or a standardized extract. Cooking deactivates the allicin but this makes little difference in outcomes. *Onions possess the same actions as garlic and should be liberally added to the diet.*[16]

Dosage
Take 1 to 4 cloves of fresh garlic daily, swallowed like a pill, or 600 to 1,200 milligrams daily of a standardized extract. Add liberally to the diet as food. *The longer any of these are used, the better the outcome.*

MOTHERWORT

Motherwort's Latin name (*Leonurus cardiaca*) means "lion heart" and has been considered a specific for heart conditions for millennia in European traditions. The herb is an exceptionally reliable nervine and helps relax nervous or overstressed conditions. This makes it especially useful for hypertension caused by excess adrenaline production and too much coffee. Though this alone will lower blood pressure, the herb has a direct vasodilation effect as well. It is also a specific remedy for heart palpitations.[17] The herb is a general cardiac tonic and exerts its actions, in part, by shifting the heart from a catabolic pattern to an anabolic one. It is an extremely reliable herb for stress.

Dosage
The tincture is usually used and can be taken up to ½ ounce at a time. The usual dose is ¼ to ½ teaspoon three to four times daily.

PINE BARK AND GRAPE SEED EXTRACT (OPCS)

The proanthocyanidins in these plants are some of the most potent substances known for protecting the integrity of collagen-dependent cellular structures. This makes them especially useful for any situation where there is deterioration of vessel walls (as there often is in atherosclerosis). (See "Hawthorn" for more on the actions of proanthocyanidins.)

Dosage
Take 150 to 300 milligrams daily.

Cautions
Some people are sensitive to pine products—seeds, pollen, bark, resin, and so on. Negative reactions can run from mild allergies to anaphylactic shock. **If you have a history of allergies to pollen or severe reactions to bee stings, do not use without consulting your health-care practitioner.** Adolescents should not take pine pollen.

PERIWINKLE (VINCAMINE)

While periwinkle (*Vinca minor, V. major*), or its extracted constituent, vincamine, is better known for treatment of stroke (see Chapter 10), it is also an effective herb for lowering blood pressure and improving the tone and health of the vascular system. Double-blind trials and ECG readings have shown that vincamine improves electrical activity in the brain; memory, concentration, behavior, and speech disorders; irritability; vertigo; headaches; tinnitus; and blood flow in the retina of the eye. Researchers comment that the supplement is of particular use in cases of stroke, arteriosclerosis, and hypertension. Improvement is normally seen after three to six weeks of use.[18]

Dosage

Take 60 milligrams of vincamine two or three times a day. Vincamine is the form used for clinical trials and is widely available on the Internet and through health-food stores.

Cautions

Extreme overdoses of vincamine extracts can cause serious drops in blood pressure. Those with brain tumors, intracranial pressure, and low blood pressure should not use it. It may occasionally cause nausea. If this happens, lower the dosage or discontinue use.

As the raw herb can lower blood pressure and is a powerful treatment for diarrhea and excess bleeding (its traditional use), avoid if you have low blood pressure or chronic constipation. Some people have reported stomach upset. The German Commission E Monographs suggest that the use of the vincamine extract is of more benefit and is more reliable than the herb itself.

POTASSIUM

Although salt (sodium chloride) intake has been associated with high blood pressure, reducing salt alone will not usually lower blood pressure. It must also be accompanied by increased potassium intake. Potassium and sodium exist in a delicate balance in the body and it is the ratio of sodium to potassium that is important. Simply having low body potassium will cause high blood pressure. The minimum recommended ratio of potassium to sodium is 5:1. In contrast, most Americans have a potassium to sodium ration of less than 1:2. Increasing vegetables and fruits in the diet while reducing salt intake will usually correct this, as most fruits and vegetables have a potassium to sodium ratio of 50:1.

A number of clinical trials have shown that simply supplementing the diet with potassium will lower high blood pressure. One double-blind, placebo-controlled, crossover study showed that 2.5 grams of potassium daily lowered systolic by an average of 12 millimeters and diastolic by 16 millimeters. This is roughly similar to the findings of other studies. Systolic declines were similar in most of them, diastolic a bit less.[19]

Dosage

Take 300 milligrams three times daily. The recommended daily allowance (RDA) is 1.9 to 5.6 grams daily. Most potassium, however, should come from food. Berries are particularly high in potassium as are any dark green leafy vegetables (especially dandelion leaves) and the following juices: celery, carrot, and beet. You can also supplement the diet with such salt substitutes as Nu-Salt or Nosalt, which are actually potassium chloride rather than sodium chloride salts. These offer a dosage of 530 milligrams per ⅙ teaspoon. OTC potassium supplements are limited to 99 milligrams per tablet.

Cautions

Do not take with kidney disease or severe heart conditions, such as high-grade atrioventricular block. Use under a physician's guidance if you are currently taking any other drugs, as there are a number of negative drug/supplement interactions on record.

COENZYME Q₁₀

Thirty-nine percent of people with high blood pressure have been found to be deficient in this enzyme. A number of studies have found that with *four to twelve* weeks of use, blood pressure will lower in a significant number of people with hypertension. Usually the drop is about 10 percent of high blood pressure values.[20]

Dosage

Take 50 milligrams two to three times daily.

OMEGA-3 OILS

Over sixty clinical studies have shown that increasing omega-3 oil intake will reduce blood pressure. Most studies used fish oil capsules (about ten per day). Flaxseed oil contains the same oils and the dose used in the trials is about equal to 1 tablespoon of flaxseed oil per day.[21]

Dosage
Take 10 capsules daily (or 1 tablespoon of flaxseed oil daily).

CELERY

Celery is a specific tonic for the adrenal glands and kidneys. Not surprisingly, it also affects blood pressure. Angiotensin, which (when converted to angiotensin II) constricts blood vessels, is made from renin in the kidneys. Besides containing constituents that increase male hormones, celery also contains the compound 3-n-butyl phthalide, which has strong blood pressure lowering effects, presumably from its effects on angiotensin production. Blood pressure can drop about 12 percent from eating four celery stalks per day (or drinking the juice of four celery stalks) and blood cholesterol can lower by about 7 percent.[22] Because of its importance in helping maintain androgen levels, any indication of coronary disease makes this an important food to add to the diet.

Dosage
Consume 4 stalks per day or 4 ounces of juiced celery (about four stalks).

Dietary Additions and Considerations

Eat plenty of potassium-containing foods (e.g., avocados, lima beans, potatoes, tomatoes, bananas, spinach, and asparagus), high fiber, and high-complex carbohydrates. Lots of celery, garlic, and onions. Other plants that can help lower blood pressure are tomato, broccoli, carrot, and saffron. Reduce caffeine and salt intake. Coldwater fish, such as tuna, mackerel, and sardines, are high in omega-3 oils.

Fasting

Oddly enough, one of the most effective methods of reducing high blood pressure is fasting. The studies I have reviewed have shown that fasting consistently lowered blood pressure even in cases that were considered untreatable by other approaches. While beyond the scope of this book, if you have high blood pressure, fasting is an option that you should explore.

Biofeedback and Stress Reduction

A significant number of clinical studies have shown that biofeedback can consistently alter blood flow throughout the body, increasing circulation to the extremities and lowering overall blood pressure.

In most instances, when learning biofeedback, you rest in a comfortable chair and are taught a number of relaxation techniques. An electrical monitor is hooked up to your body, the location changing depending on what physiological system you are working on. If it is the temperature of your hands, a sensor is hooked up to your hands and you can read the outputs on a screen in front of you. If it is blood pressure (BP), a BP cuff is used so that you can monitor your BP in the same manner. It is possible, with a little work (and not very much at that) to exert significant control over a large number of bodily functions formerly considered outside conscious control. With practice, people have even been able to control the firing of a single neuron in their hands. They can make it fire in patterns, do drum rolls, or tap in slow, single beats at will.

Other stress reduction techniques, such as transcendental meditation (TM), yoga, and even deep-breathing exercises, are beneficial as well. Biofeedback is most useful if you want control over a specific autonomic system of the body. TM is useful if you want to be able to maintain a relaxed state no matter what is happening around you. Yoga is useful if you also want to develop more flexibility in your body and joints. Deep breathing is for those of us who want a remote to get that remote off the top of the television. There is less effort involved and it still alters the overall picture.

Arterio- and Atherosclerosis

Arteriosclerosis involves both the arteries themselves and the arterial wall. From Greek roots, it literally means hard (*sclerosis*) artery (*arterio*). The term was created to describe a form of arterial hardening where large amounts of calcium are deposited in the arterial walls. This most often occurs in the leg veins and/or heart arteries of people with diabetes late in life after years of poor diet. The veins literally become stonelike over time and are so hard they can break saws during the amputations that the hardening sometimes makes necessary.

The best-known form of arteriosclerosis is called atherosclerosis and describes a condition where fatty deposits build up on the walls of blood vessels and arteries. As the fatty deposits, or plaques, build up they occlude or reduce the flow of blood. If it occurs at the openings into the heart, the reduced blood flow deprives the heart of enough oxygen and causes angina or heart pain. The constriction of the blood vessels and arteries also allows the formation of blood clots. If they do so in the heart, they can cause a heart attack. In the brain they can cause a stroke. These are, respectively, the first and third major causes of death in the United States (cancer is the second).

While cholesterol's reputation has been effectively tarnished in most people's minds, emerging research is beginning to show that that decision might have been a hasty one. Cholesterol is in fact an essential substance for the body to remain healthy. Some studies have begun to show that reducing cholesterol may in fact do more harm than good.[23] The problem is not so much the cholesterol but why it is being used to line the arteries in the first place. Curing the underlying condition that leads to cracks in the blood vessels and consuming substances that strengthen them, making them less susceptible to cracking or that hasten their healing, is essential (see above).

Arteriosclerosis can be treated by following the protocol for hypertension with a few alterations. For arteriosclerotic conditions where calcium is building up, hawthorn and garlic are essential. They will help reduce calcium buildup in the aorta and lower extremities and help restore function. Ginkgo, in cases of impairment from decreased blood flow, will help increase blood circulation in the vessels and reduce impairment by getting more oxygen to the tissues. Generally, potassium, motherwort, and biofeedback and stress reduction are not specifically indicated for high serum cholesterol problems.

Natural Care for Atherosclerosis

For Twelve to Eighteen Months
    Follow the regimen for hypertension and add:
    Guggul, standardized, 500 milligrams three times daily
    Ginkgo, 80 to 160 milligrams daily (in case of imipairment from reduced blood flow)
    Vitamin B complex, daily

Oatmeal, daily
Dietary additions and considerations

GUGGUL

Guggul (*Commiphora mukul*) is an Ayurvedic herb that has been used in India for centuries for treating circulatory disorders. A significant number of studies have shown that it is very effective in lowering blood cholesterol levels. In most studies, over a four- to twelve-week period, total serum lipid levels dropped an average of 30 percent. LDL cholesterol levels tended to drop 25 to 35 percent and HDL to rise about 20 percent. Guggul works through an entirely different mechanism than the pharmaceutical statin drugs that are used by millions of people to control cholesterol levels. Statins block the body enzyme that synthesizes cholesterol in the liver. Guggul, on the other hand, blocks the action of a specific cell receptor, called FXR, that increases the level of cholesterol in the body. This causes more cholesterol to be excreted.[24]

Dosage
Take 500 milligrams three times daily, standardized for 25 milligrams gugulsterones per 500-milligram tablet. Generally sold as *gugulipid*.

Cautions
Nonstandardized extracts have occasionally caused skin rashes and diarrhea.

GINKGO

Ginkgo (*Ginkgo biloba*) is indicated in arteriosclerosis because it increases blood flow in peripheral blood vessels. Ginkgo is specifically indicated if blood flow has been reduced to the brain, heart, or extremities. It helps keep oxygen levels in the affected tissues high while other herbs and supplements are healing the underlying condition. It is of particular benefit in erection problems, intermittent claudication, cardiac arrhythmia, macular degeneration, cold extremities, varicose veins, and stroke—basically, any condition of decreased blood flow due to arteriosclerosis.

Dosage

Normal dosage runs from 40 milligrams three times a day to 40 milligrams four times a day of an extract standardized to 24 percent ginkgoflavoglycosides.

Cautions

Sensitivity to gingko preparations can sometimes occur. Caution should be used if you are taking antithrombotic (anti-blood-clotting) medications. Uncommonly, side effects are mild gastrointestinal upset or headache, and very rarely, allergic skin reactions. In very large doses, gingko can cause diarrhea, irritability, and restlessness. Because ginkgo is a PAF inhibitor, it should be avoided before surgery.

VITAMIN B COMPLEX

Vitamin B_5, B_{12}, folic acid, and niacin have all been linked to lower serum cholesterol levels. Numerous studies have shown that increasing supplemental or dietary intake of vitamin B in its various forms can lower serum cholesterol levels.[25]

Dosage

Take a high-quality vitamin B complex once or twice daily.

Dietary Additions and Considerations

Turmeric, eggplant, fenugreek, garlic, onion, ginger, green tea, avocado, celery, carrots, salmon, sardines, shiitake mushrooms, flax, and hot peppers have all been found to reduce cholesterol levels in the blood. All these should be liberally added to the diet. However, one of the more interesting findings was that daily oatmeal (100 grams—about 3 ounces) for from three to fourteen weeks would reduce cholesterol levels in the diet by up to 20 percent.[26] The longer oatmeal was consumed, the larger the drop. Given oatmeal's application in maintaining healthy androgen levels and its ability to act as a nervine, reducing stress and lowering adrenaline levels, it makes sense if you have high cholesterol to add this food to the diet regularly.

ANGINA

Angina, or chest pain, most often occurs because of inadequate oxygen to the heart. It is usually caused by clogged arteries or atherosclerosis. Most people describe it as a squeezing or pressure-type pain radiating out from the chest to the left shoulder blade, arm, or even jaw and lasting up to twenty minutes. This kind of angina (so-called stable angina) often occurs after physical exertion: working out, a brisk walk, or even walking upstairs. In Prinzmetal's, or unstable, angina the coronary artery goes into spasm unrelated to atherosclerosis. Unstable angina generally occurs irregularly while resting and is more common in women under fifty. Magnesium supplements almost always relieve the problem.

It is crucial with angina to work with herbs and supplements that will reduce blockage in the coronary arteries. Again, hawthorn is essential (see more under "Cardiovascular Disease," above).

Natural Care for Angina

For Twelve to Eighteen Months
Follow the regimen for hypertension and atherosclerosis and add:
Khella, 250 to 300 milligrams daily
Magnesium, 200 to 400 milligrams three times daily
L-carnitine, 500 milligrams three times daily
Androgen replacement protocol (as discussed under "Heart Disease")
Dietary additions and considerations

KHELLA

Khella (*Ammi visnaga*) has been used in Egypt for some four to six thousand years for the treatment of heart disease and angina, one of the few herbs that has come out of ancient Egyptian tradition. Khella works fairly rapidly to dilate the coronary arteries, increasing blood supply to the heart. Scores of clinical trials have explored the herb and one of its constituents, *khellin;* it was even endorsed by the *New England Journal of Medicine* in 1951 as a safe and effective treatment for angina pectoris. Normally, the herb is found standardized for its khellin content, 12 percent.[27]

Dosage
Take 250 to 300 milligrams daily.

Cautions
Khellin can cause skin sensitivity to light and caution should be exercised by fair-skinned people, especially if you spend any time in the sun. In rare instances, the herb may cause mild liver inflammation or jaundice. These conditions clear when the herb is discontinued.

MAGNESIUM

Over four thousand people have participated in studies on the effects of magnesium in alleviating heart attacks. Intravenous magnesium immediately on admittance to the hospital reduces complications as well as death rates. This bears out the results of other studies showing that a majority of people with heart attacks have chronic low magnesium levels. Magnesium relaxes the coronary arteries, allowing more blood (and hence oxygen) into the heart, and improves the pumping action of the heart muscle. In Prinzmetal's, or unstable angina, magnesium supplementation alone can alleviate the problem.[28] (For more on magnesium, see Chapter 11.)

Dosage
Take 200 to 400 milligrams three times a day.

Caution
Magnesium is normally well tolerated; however, people with certain kinds of severe heart disease, such as high-grade atrioventricular block, should only use magnesium under the supervision of a health-care provider.

L-CARNITINE

In a significant number of trials, L-carnitine has been found to relieve angina, increase exercise times, improve energy levels, reduce heart disease, and protect the heart from damage. As oxygen levels to the heart fall because of occlusion, L-carnitine levels also fall. Reduced L-carnitine leads to a number of problems as it is essential in the heart muscle for healthy functioning.[29]

Dosage
Take 500 milligrams three times a day.

Dietary Additions and Considerations

The following foods have been found to help reduce angina: oatmeal, ginger, garlic, blueberries and blueberry juice, pineapple and pineapple juice, carrots, celery, fennel, parsley, and parsnips. They should be liberally added to the diet.

VARICOSE VEINS AND HEMORRHOIDS

Varicose veins occur when blood pools in the veins of the lower extremities because the valves that prevent blood from flowing backward in the veins don't work properly. The venous walls are often fragile and distend from the pressure, something like balloons filling with water. They then swell, often leaking blood into surrounding tissues. Most varicose veins form on the back of the legs; about forty million Americans have them. When they occur in and around the anus they are called hemorrhoids; about ninety million Americans have those.

Varicose veins are often caused by standing for long periods in one place. At such times, the pressure in leg veins can increase 1,000 percent. This puts constant pressure on leg veins and, over time, results in distension. When varicose veins occur deep in the leg instead of on the surface it is called phlebitis and can be exceptionally painful. Hemorrhoids, too, can be caused by standing, or long periods of sitting. For the same reasons this causes increased pressure in the veins in the rectum. (Continual straining at defecation is often a contributing cause as well.) Both these conditions occur because venous walls lose their tone under the constant pressure. This allows them to distend. The major approach in helping to resolve the problems is to strengthen and tone the venous walls. Both these conditions, with minor variations, can be helped with similar herbs and supplements. Hawthorn and pine bark extracts have been discussed above; in scores of clinical trials, they have both been found to be highly helpful.

Natural Care for Varicose Veins and Hemorrhoids

For Six to Twelve Months
Hawthorn, 120 to 900 milligrams three times daily
Pine bark or grape seed extracts, 150 to 300 milligrams daily
Horse chestnut seed, 600 milligrams daily, standardized extract
Gotu kola, standardized for 30 to 60 milligrams triterpenic acids daily
Witch hazel (for hemorrhoids), as needed
Dietary additions and considerations

HORSE CHESTNUT SEED

The effects of horse chestnut (*Aesculus hippocastanum*) seed on varicosities has been studied in over one thousand people. Many of them have been double-blind, placebo-controlled trials designed to determine the effectiveness of the herb. The herb increases the tone and strength of the veins while it also reduces their permeability. A majority of people taking the herb have reported significant improvement in symptoms, including tension, fatigue, leg pain, itching, and reduced swelling in the veins. Interestingly, for healthy people on long airflights, a prophylactic dose of horse chestnut, 600 milligrams, helped prevent many of the leg problems that commonly occur from extended sitting on airplanes.[30]

Dosage
Take 600 milligrams daily of an extract designed to supply 100 milligrams a day of aescin (aka escin).

Cautions
Be sure you buy a standardized form of the herb as the raw form is more difficult to dose safely. The standardized herb is extremely safe; however, there are a few reports of itching, nausea, and gastric complaints in those who are sensitive to the herb.

GOTU KOLA

Gotu kola (*Centella asiatica*) has been found in numerous clinical trials to alleviate venous insufficiency and varicose veins in the lower extremities.

The herb increases the integrity of the perivascular sheath that surrounds the blood vessel, increasing its strength and decreasing its tendency to balloon. Gotu kola improves blood flow, reduces sclerosis, and enhances the connective tissue.

As only one example, in one double-blind, placebo-controlled trial, eighty-seven people with chronic venous insufficiency received 60 to 120 milligrams daily of gotu kola. At the end of sixty days, blood flow in the legs, at rest and under stress, had significantly increased and symptoms had decreased.[31]

Dosage

Take enough of the standardized herb to provide 30 to 60 milligrams of triterpenic acids daily.

Cautions

Do not confuse with kola, an herb with high levels of caffeine and from which Coca-Cola gets part of its name. (The rest comes from cocaine—i.e., cocaine-kola. Neither is currently in the soda, though now I understand why my grandparents drank so much of it.)

WITCH HAZEL

Witch hazel (*Hamamelis virginiana*) is actually the active ingredient in Preparation H pads and many other hemorrhoidal preparations such as Tucks. Witch hazel is a traditional American remedy for hemorrhoids, having already been used for hundreds of years before Tuck found it. You can buy the herb already prepared in many pharmacies; it is much cheaper than commercial preparations. You probably already know how it works from having watched the commercials: it is an astringent, helps shrink swollen tissues, and relieves itching.[32]

Dosage

Witch hazel extract can be applied with cotton balls or spread on some sterile gauze and tucked in place as needed. David Hoffmann, author of *The Holistic Herbal*, suggests an excellent topical lotion for hemorrhoids: Combine 80 milliliters of witch hazel extract, 10 milliliters of horse chestnut seed tincture, and 10 milliliters of comfrey root tincture. Apply liberally to the affected area as needed or soak a sterile gauze pad with the solution and tuck it into place.

Dietary Additions and Considerations

Ginger, garlic, cayenne, onion, and pineapple have all been shown to help varicose veins and hemorrhoids. They also help to break down fibrin, the body's clotting agent that tends to form around these kinds of venous problems. These particular foods increase blood flow and strengthen capillary walls. Add liberally to the diet.

INTERMITTENT CLAUDICATION

When the arteries around the heart narrow because of arteriosclerosis it causes angina; when it happens in the legs it is called intermittent claudication. The pain can be brought on by any exercise of the legs. Even a simple walk can set it off. About a million people in the United States have this type of circulatory problem. In scores of clinical trials, hawthorn, garlic, and ginkgo (all discussed above) have shown that they will significantly improve circulation to the legs, reduce pain, and improve walking distance. They are essential in any natural care of intermittent claudication. A large number of studies have also found that androgen replacement therapies will successfully heal intermittent claudication.[33] Horse chestnut has also been found highly effective.

Natural Care for Intermittent Claudication

For Six to Twelve Months
>Follow the regimen for hypertension and atherosclerosis and add:
>Androgen replacement protocol (as discussed under "Heart Disease")
>Horse chestnut, standardized for 50-plus milligrams of escin daily.

CIRCULATORY WEAKNESS— COLD HANDS AND FEET

When the hands and feet do not get enough blood they begin to feel cold. Many people suffer from a mild form of this throughout their life and it often increases in severity as they age. Generally, it is because the capillaries are receiving insufficient blood flow.

There are three types of blood vessels in the body: (1) arteries (which carry blood away from the heart), (2) veins (which carry blood back to the heart), and (3) capillaries. Capillaries are, by many ways of thinking, the most important of all the blood vessels. They are, in fact, responsible for all the cells of the body getting the oxygen they need. While an individual capillary is incredibly tiny, only about ⅟25 of an inch long (1 millimeter), if all the body's capillaries were joined together they would stretch 62,000 miles. There are so many capillaries that one cubic inch of muscle tissue contains over 1.5 million of them. Every cell of the body has to be very close to a capillary in order to receive oxygen. When the capillaries in the extremities do not distribute enough blood, the hands and feet get cold. In many circumstances, including diabetes, arteriosclerosis can be the cause; there is simply not enough blood getting through the vessels. Another cause is chronic narrowing or vasoconstriction of the blood vessels. Hypertension is one form vasoconstriction can take. Another more extreme form of this is called Raynaud's disease. In Raynaud's, the hands (and sometimes the feet or nose) will turn a bluish white and become seriously painful. It seems to be caused by a constriction and spasming of the blood vessels in the fingers and hands. No one knows why.

Because garlic, hawthorn, and ginkgo all increase blood flow to the extremities, they are essential. They have all shown effectiveness in many clinical trials in promoting circulation to the extremities.

Natural Care for Cold Hands and Feet

For Three to Six Months
Garlic, 600 to 1,200 milligrams daily
Ginkgo, standardized extract, 80 to 160 milligrams daily
Hawthorn, 120 to 900 milligrams three times daily
Ginger, 2 to 4 grams per day
Cayenne, as much as can be taken comfortably
Biofeedback

GINGER AND CAYENNE

Anyone who has eaten these herbs knows they are spicy and that they increase the warmth of the body. They have both been shown to increase circulation to the extremities.

Dosage
Take 2 to 4 grams of ginger daily and as much cayenne as can be taken comfortably.

BIOFEEDBACK

Biofeedback has been found to be exceptionally helpful for this problem. With minor training on biofeedback machines, people can learn to warm their hands at will. This is especially helpful for people with Raynaud's disease. If you suffer from migraine headaches, this can also help. A majority of people with migraines also have cold hands. Learning to warm the hands will, in most instances, relieve the headaches as well.

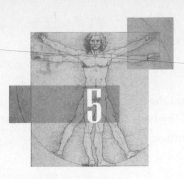

Stomach: GI Tract

The movement into middle age for many men is
marked by a greater emotionalism, just as it is with women. The older we
get the less stomach we have for life's irritations. Life's edges can be like a
meat mallet; after a certain amount of hammering, even the toughest steak
becomes tender. We start to go soft. Oddly, this tenderizing process is often
accompanied by an increased irritability—the deeper self is softened but
surrounded by an increasingly grouchy exterior. And that deeper, softer self
has become so sensitized that even the tiniest thing can set it off—much
like the digestive system later in life. The longer we live, the softer and yet
more irritated we can become.

Irritation is a mild form of anger, and anger, that much maligned and
crucial emotion, is a powerful source of energy—usually, an energy to solve
problems. Often the deeper parts of ourselves notice problems long before
the conscious mind does. Anger can erupt out of the blue, seemingly from

nowhere. The irritation gets our attention and supplies us the fuel to deal with whatever it is that has upset the status quo.

Unfortunately, there is no less welcome emotion in American society today, especially in men, than anger. Anger upsets the calm placidity of civilization, stirs the pot, and brings up things from the bottom. It also, if reflected upon, allows men to become aware of what is and is not important in their lives and supplies them the energy to bring about change. The negative side of this, of course, is that if the anger is not used to change the source of the irritation, the irritation simply continues to abrade and the problem worsens.

Our digestive systems have a lot in common with this sensitizing of the self. Able to eat anything in younger life, in middle age this begins to change. Spicy, sour, fatty, and sweet foods begin to take their toll when we eat them. We discover bloat (formerly a female condition), have more gas (beyond bonding levels), and often experience stomach distress.

The digestive system is one of the primary surfaces through which we absorb things into ourselves. Just as we change emotionally as we age, so too do our digestive systems. They become more sensitive to what they are touched by, to what they are willing to absorb. And if the wrong food enters, an irritation begins that gets our attention. If we do not take care of it, it increases the irritation, until it becomes the central focus of our life.

The Digestive System

People do not generally understand how complex the digestive system is, or even its size. The entire digestive system, which runs from the mouth to the anus, is a complex, mucus-lined, muscular tube some thirty feet long with a combined surface area of from 900 to 1,200 square feet. Twenty feet of this length is the small intestine, which removes many important nutrients from food and transfers them across their mucous membranes into the bloodstream (where they are then taken to the liver for further processing). The final five to six feet of the intestinal tract is the large intestine, or colon, where most of the remaining water is removed and any final processing that can be done is done. What remains is feces.

Saliva begins the conversion of food into usable nutrients through the action of the enzyme *amylase*, which mixes with the food as we chew.

Plants, in order to protect their sugars from foraging bacteria and yeasts, convert sugars to starch. They have an enzyme they use when they want to reconvert starch back to sugars (in barley, for example, it is called diastase). The amylase in our saliva is extremely close in structure to diastase and other starch-converting plant enzymes.

Once the food is chewed and thoroughly mixed with saliva, it moves through the esophagus into the stomach. There, the food is mixed with hydrochloric acid and stomach enzymes such as pepsin to convert the food into a thick liquid called *chyme*. While most nutrients are extracted from food in the small intestine, some of them move across the stomach membrane and even that of the esophagus into the blood that flows to the liver for nutrient processing.

At the bottom of the stomach is a sphincter, or muscular valve, that, when opened, allows food to travel into the first part of the small intestine, the *duodenum*. The ten to twelve inches of the duodenum are where most of the minerals we get from food are extracted (e.g., calcium and zinc). Once extracted they are transported across the duodenal membrane into the blood flowing into the liver through the portal vein, where they are used to maintain and regenerate the body's structure. The next section of the small intestine is the eight-foot-long *jejunum*, which extracts water-soluble vitamins, carbohydrates, and proteins. The *ileum*, the final twelve feet or so of the tract, absorbs fat-soluble vitamins like B_{12}, fat, cholesterol, and bile salts.

The small intestine uses *proteases* created in the pancreas and bile salts from the liver to help in this process. Proteases, or the pancreatic enzymes that convert food into more usable nutrients, are carried to the small intestine from the pancreas in pancreatic juice. Each day, about one and a half quarts are secreted for use. Bile is produced in the liver (stored in the gall bladder) and is an extremely caustic substance used to dissolve fat-soluble substances (fats, oils, and fat-soluble vitamins). The liver produces about one quart per day of bile and most of that is reabsorbed for future use as the food moves through the ileum.

The upper portion of the small intestine (duodenum and jejunum) is normally low in bacteria and yeasts. Both bile and pancreatic enzymes help keep it that way. The ileum has a much larger bacterial community, but the colon, which lies just below the ileum (on the other side of the ileocecal valve), is high density housing for microbes.

The colon contains over four hundred different types of bacteria and other organisms living in a complex community. These organisms help with the final breakdown of what remains of our food, secrete compounds that we need to remain healthy, and keep bowel health high. Interestingly, the community of the bowel is nearly identical with the bacterial communities that form around plant roots in an area called the rhizosphere. When a seed begins to sprout, it sends out chemical cues that call coevolutionary bacteria, fungi, yeasts, and nematodes to it. Many of these attach themselves to the exterior of the root or penetrate it slightly; others live in close proximity in the soil. This complex community processes substances that pass into and out of the roots. As parts of plants die, this community breaks down that material into soil. The bacterial community in the colon does the same thing in exactly the same way. It is no accident that human feces is sometimes called night soil. Like plant communities, the bacterial community that lives in our colon is a coevolutionary one, at least a million years old. We, like plants, send out chemical cues the day we are born calling them to our bodies. Most of them come from our mothers as we nurse and lay on her stomach. They cover our skin and the interior of our mouth, nose, and the colon and form smaller communities throughout the digestive tract. We cannot, in fact, be healthy without them.

Hormones of the Digestive System

The digestive system creates and releases a variety of hormones to carry out its functions. There are at least eight primary intestinal hormones that work together to regulate the pH of the intestinal tract, control the rate of digestion, the rate of nutrient transmission across the intestinal membranes, and the release of substances such as bile from the liver, gastrin from the stomach, and pancreatic juice and glucagon from the pancreas. Gastrin, produced in the stomach, stimulates stomach acid production. Four of the intestinal hormones are specifically designed to control the level of acidity in the stomach and the acidity of the chyme that moves through the intestinal tract. Two of them control the amount of water in feces. A relatively newly discovered hormone, *uroguanylin,* is created and released by the GI tract to maintain both salt and water balance in the body. Higher levels of salt in the diet result in more uroguanylin being sent to the kidneys, which then begin excreting more salt in the urine.

Some of the most common problems that affect men as they age are ulcers, irritable bowel syndrome, inflammatory bowel disease, diarrhea, and constipation.

IRRITABLE BOWEL SYNDROME, CROHN'S DISEASE, ULCERATIVE COLITIS

Somewhere between 5 and 15 percent of American men are thought to suffer with irritable bowel syndrome (IBS), about a million others suffer from inflammatory bowel disease (IBD). (IBD can refer either to Crohn's disease or ulcerative colitis.)

Synthetic pharmaceuticals have been linked to the rise of these diseases in the Western world, primarily the use of antibiotics and synthetic steroids such as prednisone. Diet is also a contributing factor. The increase in inflammatory bowel disorders such as ulcerative colitis exactly parallels the introduction of antibiotics into Western medical practice. The more they are used, the higher the incidence of the disease. The primary reason is that the intestinal community, with the ingestion of an antibiotic, experiences an entirely unique evolutionary event—a substance that kills off large segments of the bowel community. Especially harmful are broad spectrum antibiotics that indiscriminately kill off much of the intestinal bacteria. Once that happens, the intestinal community has to rebuild itself and it often finds it difficult to restructure as it had been. In essence, the makeup of the bacterial community changes and this causes significant changes in the health of the mucosal lining of the GI tract (and subsequently, overall health).

Newer research has shown that the coevolutionary bacteria in our bowels and on our bodies consistently act to protect their home. They provide substances necessary for their host organism to be healthy and create and release antibiotics that are organism specific. As an example, the coevolutionary streptococcal bacteria that live in the human throat create antibiotics that are specifically active against the strep bacteria that cause strep throat. The older we get, the more effective they become at preventing strep incursions. However, the use of antibiotics also kills off these beneficial organisms and, it is now being recognized, can lead to continual, and often more severe, throat infections. This same type of bacterial dynamic also exists in the colon, though the beneficial organisms are not limited to bacteria.

Some physicians that specialize in IBD, recognizing that the disease is almost nonexistent in the third world, examined the intestinal tracts of third world peoples. They found that there are commonly several species of coevolutionary worms in non-Western GI tracts. Just as with the rhizosphere around plant roots, human GI tracts have long been used to the presence of these beneficial worms in the gut. Deeper examination of the worms found that they engage in an intricate maintenance of the immune system of the GI tract (suppressing Th1 response and enhancing Th2), release substances necessary for bowel health, and help prevent pathological worm infections in the gut. Researchers who thought that these worms might be of benefit in inflammatory bowel disease used them to treat people with Crohn's disease and ulcerative colitis. With their patients' permission, the researchers gave them a single dose of microscopic worm eggs. All but one of the people experienced complete remission of the disease and he (already suffering permanent bowel damage) experienced significant alleviation of symptoms. Complete remission occurred within three weeks of administration of the eggs and they stayed symptom free for five months when, for some of them, symptoms began to recur (suggesting that treatment may need to be ongoing).[1]

In Western populations, these types of worms are generally considered an infectious agent and treated with pharmaceuticals to cleanse them from the gut. This lends more weight to some research findings that many of our Western problems come from being too clean. Children that are allowed to get very dirty in childhood have actually been found to have fewer infections as they grow. The immune system of the human species is evolutionarily designed to be activated by close contact with microbial agents through childhood.

While few people in the United States would be excited about ingesting worm eggs, the important point is that the GI tract community has formed for a reason through long evolutionary time and when we disturb it through pharmaceuticals (because there is incomplete understanding of the importance of bowel organisms), long-term problems can occur.

Once the bowel organisms are disturbed, the type of diet most people in the United States consume contributes to the problem. Sugar, refined carbohydrates, and low dietary fiber support the growth of a less healthy community of organisms. If antibiotics are avoided and a healthier diet instituted, in many instances, the bowels, will, over time, begin to correct.

This is much less likely, however, if steroids are used to combat inflammation in the GI tract. People with inflammatory bowel disease who never use anti-inflammatories are much more likely to experience remission of the disease and to have far fewer incidences of recurrence.[2]

During IBD, the lining of the intestinal tract inflames. This causes continual digestive upset, chronic (often bloody) diarrhea, painful cramping, fever, fatigue, and weight loss. Because of the inflammation in the intestinal lining, nutrients cannot transfer across the membrane, and chronic deficiency diseases can occur. Over time, the lining of the intestinal tract ulcerates, and there can be severe bleeding, even complete rupture of the bowel.

IBS, or irritable bowel syndrome, is the mildest form of the disease. The most common symptoms are bloating, abdominal cramping, and mild diarrhea, loose or frequent painful bowel movements. The more severe ulcerative colitis occurs in the colon, and Crohn's disease is a serious inflammation (with ulceration) that can occur anywhere in the GI tract (though it is most often in the ileum of the small intestine).

Oddly, given the prevalence of these diseases, there have been few clinical trials with natural substances. Possibly this is because the diseases primarily occur in antibiotic-prone Western nations and Western nations usually do not perform a lot of clinical trials with herbs. One interesting trial was, however, conducted in Japan using a traditional European remedy—malted barley—and it was found to cure people with ulcerative colitis when used as food daily.[3] This is not surprising. During ulcerative colitis, mucins or the *glycoproteins* that keep the colon elastic and viscous are disturbed. The colon produces far less mucus than it should to protect the bowel and keep it healthy. Barley, which is highly mucilaginous, recoats the membranes, soothes and protects, and acts as a general anti-inflammatory.

Mucin deficiency has been linked to a colon suffering an overgrowth of a particular bacteria, *Bacteroides vulgatus*. This bacteria, when it encounters carrageenan, a substance used to stabilize milk proteins in most milk products, degrades the carrageenan into a substance that is harmful to the bowels. For this reason, anyone with IBD, especially ulcerative colitis, should not consume dairy products or any product containing carrageenan.

Crohn's disease occurs most often in the ileum of the small intestine, just after the duodenum and jejunum. Interestingly, most sucrose and glucose are absorbed through both the duodenum and jejunum. High sugar absorption through these membranes interferes with the motility of the intestinal tract. It causes the peristalsis or muscular movements of the tract to slow down. Constant high sugar levels can eventually cause this part of the intestine to paralyze or become atonic. This has been linked to the eruption of irritable bowel syndrome and small intestinal bacterial overgrowth (SIBO). The small intestine normally has a much smaller bacterial community than the colon, especially the duodenum and jejunum, but under certain circumstances, bacterial populations bloom there. Usually the causes are antibiotic overuse, a poor diet—high in sugars and low in fibers—and ileocecal valve atrophy (usually from poor bowels caused by a long-term low fiber, high-sugar diet). A poorly functioning immune system can also allow the flow of bacterial pathogens into the small intestine (which is partly where the worms come in). The treatment for these three bowel conditions is similar with several slight variations.

Natural Care for IBS, Crohn's, and Ulcerative Colitis

For Three to Twelve Months
Malted barley, prepared, 1 to 4 ounces daily
Slippery elm bark, ½ to 1 cup prepared bark three times daily
Oats, as oatmeal, daily
Psyllium seed, once a day
Applesauce, once a day
Licorice root/marshmallow root powders in apple juice, once a day
Ginger/chamomile tea, 4 to 6 cups daily
Glutamine, 500 to 1,000 milligrams three times a day
Folic Acid, 400 milligrams daily
EPA, 600 to 2,400 milligrams daily
DHA, 240 to 960 milligrams daily
Zinc picolinate, 30 to 50 milligrams daily
Pancreatin (for IBD), [8 to 10x] 350 to 700 milligrams three times a day between meals
Boswellia (for ulcerative colitis), 550 milligrams three times a day
Enteric-coated peppermint oil capsules (for IBS), 0.2 to 0.4 milliliters twice a day between meals
Dietary additions and considerations

BARLEY

Both barley (*Hordeum vulgare*) and barley water have been used in the treatment of severe intestinal disorders for centuries. Barley is highly mucilaginous, like psyllium seed, and coats and soothes the intestinal tract as it
moves through the bowels. The type of barley used in the Japanese trial
mentioned earlier is a unique form of barley—it is malted. This is a very old
European remedy for intestinal diseases. Malted barley is simply the barley
seed allowed to germinate. The tiny barley plant grows perhaps two or three
inches long, germination is then stopped, and the seeds dried and lightly
crushed.

When barley begins to germinate, the seedling releases an enzyme, diastase, which it uses to convert its carbohydrates to a sugar (maltose in this
instance) to fuel its growth. People with inflammatory bowel diseases often
have insufficient digestive enzymes and the diastase in the malted barley is
used by the human body to help it convert the starches present in food to
sugars. The sweet sugars in the malt enter the bloodstream quickly, giving
strength with less digestive work. They are also better for the body than the
sucrose that makes up common table sugar. The barley is highly nutritive
as well; these nutritive levels increase during malting.

When any grain is malted, its nutritional aspects are considerably enhanced. It becomes high in ascorbic acid, niacin, biotin, pantothenic acid,
folic acid, inositol, and so on, generally double to triple the quantities before malting. The nutrients in barley are specifically the ones that most
people with IBD are most deficient in. As well, barley is highly medicinal
for the intestinal tract. It is mucilaginous, so it coats and soothes the intestinal tract; it is a mild nervine, so it helps reduce pain and cramping in the
tract while helping relax strained nerves; and it is a mild anti-inflammatory.
The barley's constituents are readily absorbed across the intestinal membrane even in IBD.

As noted earlier, malted barley has been used in some clinical studies
to successfully treat ulcerative colitis. An interesting aspect of this is that
malted barley is high in S-methylmethionine (SMM). SMM is also exceptionally high in cabbage and cabbage juice. Cabbage juice has been successfully used in a number of trials to heal ulceration of the GI tract, including
those occurring as far down as the jejunum. In fact, SMM has been found

to be specific for both healing and protecting the GI tract from ulceration. SMM is present in most barleys but during malting SMM levels double. Barleys that are malted at lower temperatures, e.g., pale and pale amber malts, contain the most SMM, while those malted at higher temperatures (dark malts) contain little. (At higher temperatures SMM degrades into di-methylsulfoxide—DMSO). The presence of SMM explains, in part, the powerful effects of both malted and unmalted barley on healing intestinal ulceration.[4]

Dosage

One bowl of pearl barley cooked in malted barley water. To prepare barley for inflammatory bowel disease, the best approach is to use a combination of barley and barley malt. First you need to buy some malted barley and some pearl barley. The malted barley can be most readily had from home-brewing supply stores. Buy either pale malt or pale-amber malt. Slowly boil 2 to 4 ounces of the malt in a quart of (nonchlorinated) water for one hour. Then strain and use this liquid to cook the pearl barley. Use the amount of liquid called for on the directions that come with the pearl barley. Generally it needs to slowly boil for about thirty minutes.

Note: This may be combined with the following slippery elm bark preparation.

SLIPPERY ELM BARK

Slippery elm bark (*Ulmus fulva*) is also a very old European remedy for healing intestinal diseases. It is generally prepared like a gruel and is considered specific for any condition where there is intestinal inflammation and digestive weakness. The herb is harvested from the inner bark of one specific type of elm tree (though most of them will work similarly) and it is then powdered. It should be a light pinkish tan in color.

The herb coats and soothes the intestinal tract, provides easily absorbable nutrients, is mildly anti-inflammatory, and has shown antimicrobial actions as well. The bark contains starches, sugars, vitamins A, B complex, C, K, and P. It also has high levels of calcium, magnesium, and sodium and moderate amounts of chromium, selenium, phosphorus, silicon, and zinc.

Dosage

Drink 4 ounces three times a day. Use one and a half ounces of powdered bark per 12 ounces of water. Mix the powdered bark with a tiny amount of (nonchlorinated) water to make a thick paste (you should treat it much like wheat flour), slowly add the rest of the water and bring to a gentle boil. Simmer gently for ten to fifteen minutes. Remove from the heat.

Note: This may be combined with the barley preparation.

OATS

Oats (*Avena sativa*) provide many of the actions of both barley and slippery elm. They are highly nutritive, mucilaginous, and also act as a reliable nervine helping relax the tension that often accompanies chronic bowel disease. Because they are high in fiber, they help normalize the bowel.

Dosage

Have at least one bowl of oatmeal daily.

PSYLLIUM SEED

Psyllium seed (*Plantago ovata*) is a bowel tonic. If you are suffering constipation it will loosen the bowels. If diarrhea, it will firm them up. Regular intake of psyllium is indicated if you have problems with normal bowel movements. People with IBD often have chronic diarrhea and those with IBS sometimes have chronic constipation. Psyllium can be used as a bowel normalizer. The seeds absorb water and swell and press on the intestine, signaling peristalsis to begin. Because they are slippery as they absorb water, they can move through the gut with surprising ease. The slipperiness comes from mucilage, which tones, soothes, and heals the GI tract as the seeds move through. Because they contain so much fiber, they help heal and normalize the bowel. Their mucilage is important in IBD because the mucous membranes are often so inflamed and irritated.

You might want to try some applesauce with your psyllium. Both applesauce and apple juice act similarly to psyllium in normalizing and healing the bowel. Have a serving daily.

Dosage

Take 3 to 10 tablespoons of psyllium in water. Take lots of water, as they swell.

Cautions

Psyllium has produced allergic reactions in some people and caused asthma attacks in some asthmatics who breathed the dust.

LICORICE ROOT AND MARSHMALLOW ROOT

Both licorice (*Glyurrhiza glabra*) and marshmallow root (*Althea officinalis*) are discussed in more detail under gastric and duodenal ulcers. Basically, they provide the same kinds of mucilaginous actions as the herbs discussed above, as well as anti-inflammatory and antibacterial actions. They have been used for centuries in the healing of intestinal diseases.

Dosage

Use only the finely powdered roots. Mix equal parts of the powders together. Take one tablespoon of the mix in apple juice once a day. The best way to mix them in juice is to put the juice in a blender, turn it on, then add the powder. Otherwise the powder clumps.

    Note: Limit use of licorice to thirty days. Continue with marshmallow if desired.

GINGER/CHAMOMILE TEA

Ginger (*Zingiber officinale*) contains a number of substances that act like digestive enzymes in the human gut. It is highly anti-inflammatory and antibacterial and helps with nausea and cramping. Chamomile (*Matricaria chamomilla*) is considered specific for intestinal cramping. Further, it possesses mild antimicrobial actions and is a reliable nervine, helping relax high levels of tension.

    You might consider eating as much ginger as you can stand in your diet. It may, in some instances, be anti-inflammatory enough to completely reduce the inflammation in the GI tract. The best minimum dosage is 2 ounces per day, eaten lightly cooked in food, or 2 to 4 grams powdered ginger per day in capsules. Ginger has five different compounds that inhibit leukotriene inflammation in the intestines.[5]

Dosage
Take 4 to 6 cups daily.

GLUTAMINE

Glutamine is a primary amino acid used for the growth, repair, and maintenance of tissues. It is an essential nutrient source for the cells of the intestinal tract, improves their integrity, and has been shown to help in healing ulceration in the gastrointestinal tract.[6]

Dosage
Take 500 to 1,000 milligrams three times a day.

FOLIC ACID

Folic acid deficiencies are common in people with inflammatory bowel disease; up to 64 percent of those with the disease have them. Folate deficiency contributes to the problems of IBD by increasing malabsorption of nutrients and diarrhea. Folic acid is crucial to the health of intestinal mucosal cells. Folic acid has been found to reduce the risk of colon cancer in those with chronic ulcerative colitis.[7]

Dosage
Take 400 milligrams daily.

EPA AND DHA

EPA (eicosapentaenoic acid) and DHA (docosahexaenoic acid) are two omega-3 oils common in cold-water fish. They have been shown to be highly effective in reducing the recurrence of IBD, especially Crohn's. These fish oil components act to limit the production of the inflammatory leukotrienes in the gut. Leukotrienes increase GI tract inflammation and cause cramping and pain.[8]

Dosage

Take 600 to 2,400 milligrams daily of EPA and 240 to 960 milligrams of DHA daily.

Note: You can also take flaxseed oil, one tablespoon per day. It is converted by the body into EPA.

ZINC PICOLINATE

There is usually a significant depletion of zinc in people with IBD. The nature of the disease makes it hard for zinc to be absorbed across the intestinal membrane. The more zinc levels decline, the harder it is for the body to heal the ulceration in the GI tract, the worse the deficiency gets, and so on. A vicious circle.[9] Picolinate is a zinc-binding molecule produced in the pancreas. Supplementing the diet with zinc picolinate rather than zinc may be more effective, as zinc in this form appears to be more easily absorbed by the body during IBD.

Dosage

Take 30 to 50 milligrams daily.

Note: It is hard for the IBD body to absorb zinc supplements. This form is apparently the easiest. Note, too, that the barley and slippery elm will provide some of this necessary mineral.

Cautions

Over time, zinc intake can cause copper depletion in the body. To counteract this, most zinc supplements come with copper added. At very high doses, zinc can cause nausea and upset stomach, skin rashes, depression, folate deficiency, and lower tolerance to alcohol.

PANCREATIN

For those with IBD, the use of pancreatic enzymes can help digestion and also help reduce inflammation. While the malted barley and the ginger will often be sufficient, this extra step may be necessary for some.[10]

Dosage

[8 to 10x] Take 350 to 700 milligrams three times daily between meals.

BOSWELLIA

For those with ulcerative colitis, the gum resin of Boswellia (*Boswellia caterii*), better known as frankincense, has been found in some clinical trials to effectively heal the disease. Frankincense is highly mucilaginous and antibacterial while at the same time being highly astringent. This coats and soothes the intestinal tract while at the same time drying up secretions and so limiting diarrhea.[11]

Dosage

Take 550 milligrams three times daily.

ENTERIC-COATED PEPPERMINT OIL CAPSULES

For those with IBS, enteric-coated peppermint capsules have been found to help tremendously. The coating on the capsule or tablet allows the peppermint to drop into the duodenum without being digested in the stomach. The bile and pancreatic juices (stronger than stomach acid) dissolve the enteric coating and allow the oil to spread. Peppermint oil is highly antispasmodic and can reduce even the strongest spasms in the GI tract. It is also highly antibacterial and active against a number of bacteria that sometimes invade the small intestine.

Dosage

Take 0.2- to 0.4-milliliter capsules twice daily between meals.

Dietary Additions and Considerations

Diet in these conditions must be altered. Of primary importance is to avoid milk and wheat products as allergies to them and constituents in milk have both been linked to the conditions. You should also avoid sucrose, alcohol, and caffeine if you suffer from any of these conditions.

Cabbage juice, like barley, contains SMM (see "Barley," above) and has been used to heal ulceration in the stomach, duodenum, and jejunum. While no clinical trials have been conducted, it may possibly be of benefit in Crohn's disease occurring in the ileum.[12] The usual dose is one quart per day. While canned is available in grocery stores, freshly juiced is the best form to use. Asparagus is also high in SMM.

If you have not yet taken any corticosteroids you should consider avoiding them entirely. A number of studies have shown that long-term outcomes are significantly better for those who have never used them.[13]

ULCERS

For many years, it was assumed that ulcers were caused by stress and poor diet. I have met many people who have spent years eating boring food and muttering "*Om*" to themselves daily in an attempt to carry out their physician's regimen of healing. All to no avail. Then, not too long ago, a researcher discovered that ulceration in many instances is caused by a bacteria, *Helicobacter pylori,* which can live in the stomach, an organ formerly presumed to be bacteria free. Ninety to 100 percent of duodenal ulcers and at least 70 percent of gastric ulcers are now believed to be caused by *H. pylori.* (Many of the remaining gastric ulcers are caused by aspirin, other NSAIDs, or other pharmaceuticals.) Treatment for this bacteria and a regimen designed to heal the mucosa of the stomach lining will clear up the majority of ulcers within thirty to ninety days. I have even seen it help people who have had most of their stomach removed and whose remaining stomach more resembled swiss cheese than an organ of digestion. The following regimen will also work for most other types of stomach ulcers. While it will heal the stomach lining for those whose ulceration has been caused through prescription or over-the-counter drugs, the ulceration will recur if drug use continues. The advantage of this type of approach is that the herbs will help heal the stomach itself and promote regeneration of the tissues. Most pharmaceutical regimens will not.

For serious gastric ulcers it is important that the herbs be powdered and *not* encapsulated. Mixed with liquid and consumed, this allows the herb to make contact with the entire stomach lining. If the ulceration is in the duodenum, which lies just below the stomach, capsules should be used. The capsules tend to sit at the bottom of the stomach while the gelatin dissolves and then the whole sticky mass drops into the duodenum where it is needed. Duodenal ulcers are often accompanied by painful cramping or spasming. This can be alleviated by the addition of a few drops of peppermint essential oil to the herbal mixture before encapsulating it.

Natural Care for Mild to Moderate Gastric and Duodenal Ulcers

For Thirty to Sixty Days

DGL (deglycyrrhizinated licorice), 1 to 4 tablets daily (between meals) for 60 days

Gotu kola, 30 milligrams twice daily (between meals) for 60 days

Bismuth, 300 milligrams daily for 60 days

Enteric-coated peppermint oil (for duodenal ulceration) 0.2 to 0.4 milliliter, as needed, twice daily between meals

Cabbage juice, 1 quart daily

Natural Care for Severe Gastric or Duodenal Ulcers

For Three Months

Ingredients

4 ounces dried and powdered (as fine as possible) licorice root

4 ounces dried and powdered (as fine as possible) comfrey root

4 ounces dried and powdered marshmallow root

90- to 300-milligram bismuth capsules

1 ounce grapefruit seed extract

Directions

1. Mix powdered licorice and comfrey root together. Take 2 tablespoons twice a day (morning and evening), mixed in any liquid of choice (e.g., apple juice), for thirty days. For the next sixty days use 1 tablespoon marshmallow root mornings only. The herbs should not be in capsules in order to allow them to fully coat the stomach lining. (For duodenal ulcers, take in capsules and add 8 to 10 drops of peppermint oil to the powdered herbs before encapsulating.) You can also find these herbs already encapsulated and you can also buy enteric-coated peppermint capsules to take with them (see "Irritable Bowel Syndrome" for dosage and directions).

2. Take 300 milligrams bismuth, three times a day for thirty days (or Pepto-Bismol in similar quantities). It has been found to facilitate ulcer healing time.

3. Take 6 drops of grapefruit seed extract three times a day for fifteen days. Place the extract in a small glass of orange or grapefruit juice—it is too bitter for anything else.

LICORICE ROOT

Licorice (*Glycyrrhiza glabra*) has been found in numerous clinical trials to be effective for healing gastric and duodenal ulcers, even those of long duration. The herb is specifically antibacterial against *H. pylori* and a number of other organisms, stimulates the immune system (both white blood cells and interferon production), and coats and soothes the mucous membranes of the stomach and intestinal tract.

While extracts of licorice can possess a number of side effects (including high blood pressure and loss of potassium from the body), the whole powdered root has not been associated with them.

Many people favor the use of deglycyrrhizinated licorice (DGL), basically a licorice with some of its components removed, essentially the ones associated with the negative side effects of licorice extracts. DGL chewable tablets have been found exceptionally effective in clinical trials in the healing of ulcers. DGL does result in ulcer healing, and while there is a recurrence rate for DGL (about 8 percent) that is much lower than synthetic drugs (13 percent), a more comprehensive herbal protocol can produce an even lower recurrence rate.[14]

Dosage
Take 1 to 4 chewable DGL tablets (depending on severity of ulceration) twenty minutes prior to meals for sixty days.

COMFREY ROOT

Comfrey root (*Symphytum officinale*) possesses two primary attributes that make it an important herb to consider when treating ulcers. It is exceptionally soothing to the mucous membranes of the stomach and intestinal tract and, more importantly, it initiates a rapid healing and rebinding of the cell walls of the stomach and duodenal membranes. I have found no other herb that can rival it for actually *healing* the damage from ulcers, especially in serious ulceration.

Cautions

There is some controversy regarding this herb. It contains pyrrolizidine alkaloids, which some people have linked to a few instances of liver disease. While no studies have definitely confirmed this, it is best to be prudent. I usually reserve this herb for situations where the ulceration is severe, surgery is being offered as the only option, and limit its use to thirty days. Do not use if you have liver disease.

MARSHMALLOW ROOT

Marshmallow (*Althaea officinalis*) is the primary herb for use in inflammations of the intestinal tract. It soothes, protects, and helps reduce inflammation.

GRAPEFRUIT SEED EXTRACT (GSE)

Grapefruit seed extract is perhaps the closest there is to an herbal antibiotic. Grapefruit itself is highly antibacterial and, through a number of mechanisms, has potent impacts on bacterial integrity. GSE is produced from grapefruit juice, pulp, and seeds through a proprietary process much like pharmaceuticals. It is coming into more use as an organic antibacterial for things like swimming pools, public water systems, and even finding use as a hospital cleanser more potent than alcohol and other medical antiseptics. GSE is specifically active against *H. pylori* bacteria. However, GSE is strong. Do not exceed recommended dosage, and be sure to add it to citrus juice as it is very bitter.

GOTU KOLA

Gotu kola (*Centella asiatica*), a prominent herb in traditional Chinese medicine, has been found highly effective in a number of clinical trials in the treatment of both duodenal and gastric ulceration. In one trial of nineteen people with gastric ulcers and thirteen with duodenal ulcers, all but one were completely healed by eight weeks of treatment with 30 milligrams twice daily of the herb. In other trials, the use of bismuth with gotu kola produced even better results. In numerous trials, gotu kola has been found to be exceptionally good for all kinds of wound healing. Whether the wounds are external or internal, from ulceration, trauma, surgery, or disease, seems irrelevant.[15]

Dosage

Take 60 to 120 milligrams daily, usually in two divided doses. Some clinicians feel that the herb is better if standardized for triterpenoid acid content. This standardized extract is normally referred to as a titrated extract of *Centella asiatica* or TECA. Some of the studies have used this form of the herb.

Cautions

Do not confuse with kola, an herb with high levels of caffeine and from which Coca-Cola gets part of its name. (The rest comes from cocaine—i.e., cocaine-kola. Neither is currently in the soda, though now I understand why my grandparents drank so much of it.)

CABBAGE JUICE

In at least four studies, cabbage juice has been found to heal ulcers of the GI tract. Cabbage is high in S-methylmethionine, or SMM, formerly known as vitamin U. In one trial, fifty-five people with either gastric, duodenal, or jejunal ulcers were given one liter of cabbage juice daily. All but three experienced symptom relief within two to five days; ulcer healing in the GI tract took from eight to twenty-three days. Other trials reported similar outcomes.

Cabbage juice, oddly enough, is available in many grocery stores in the canned food section. Fresh juiced daily is better. Other foods that have shown strong anti-ulcer activity are ginger, banana, pineapple, hot red peppers, blueberry, broccoli, and turmeric.[16]

Dosage
Take 1 quart daily.

BISMUTH CAPSULES OR TABLETS

Bismuth, normally bismuth subcitrate, is a natural mineral that has been shown to produce highly beneficial effects when included in the treatment of *H. pylori*. Clinical trials have shown that outcomes are better whenever bismuth is added to the protocol.

Bismuth can, unfortunately, be hard to find. Pepto-Bismol does contain bismuth and can be substituted; however, pure bismuth is the preferred form. It can be most easily located through compounding pharmacists (call 1-800-927-4227 for one in your area) or on the Internet.

IN CASE OF BLEEDING ULCERS

A number of studies have found that rhubarb extract can alleviate the gastric and duodenal bleeding that sometimes occurs from ulceration in the GI tract. One study with 312 people found that rhubarb extracts could stop the bleeding in 90 percent of cases. In the studies, the herb took a bit over two days (about fifty hours) to stop the bleeding. Rhubarb ingestion shortens coagulation time and reduces capillary fragility and permeability.[17]

Dosage
Rhubarb tablets generally run about 5 milligrams each. They are most often used for constipation, 3 to 4 tablets for an adult daily dose. However, as they can strongly stimulate peristalsis, cramping can sometimes be a problem. Start with one tablet and work up to make sure there are no complications.

Cautions
In spite of these clinical trials, rhubarb is generally listed as being contraindicated for inflammatory bowel diseases, probably because of the stimulation on peristalsis. Michael Murray and Joseph Pizzorno, in their *Encyclopedia of Natural Medicine*, suggest drinking 1 quart of aloe vera juice

daily as a more readily available alternative. However, aloe is also contraindicated in inflammatory bowel diseases, presumably for the same reasons. The waxy outer coat of the aloe plant contains emudin, which can act as a powerful laxative. No matter what your choice, *use with care*. If side effects or discomfort develop, cease use.

OF POSSIBLE BENEFIT

Any astringent herb as a tea in copious quantities could help. The blackberry/slippery elm tea described under Diarrhea works because it dries up secretions in the GI tract. It could easily prove beneficial for bleeding ulcers.

Dosage
Take 1 quart to 1 gallon daily, until the bleeding stops.

DIARRHEA

The commonest cause of diarrhea is a disturbance of the intestinal community. This can occur from a number of causes; the two most common are pharmaceutical drugs (especially antibiotics, which kill off much of the intestinal community) and mild pathogenic bacteria, generally from food. The activist group Public Campaign estimates (from Centers for Disease Control data) that thirty-three million people become ill each year from food-borne pathogens, with some nine thousand deaths. Most stomach flu is generally a form of mild to moderate bacterial food poisoning. Diarrhea occurs because the bowel is trying to get rid of the bacterial pathogen by flushing water through the system. Normally, the body flushes natural antibacterials through the system as well (substances that do not harm the intestinal community). The reason that people often get diarrhea when they travel is that exotic food and water contain a very different mix of local bacteria and these upset the intestinal community. Our bowel community is strongly affected by what we eat and drink.

Diarrhea can be easily helped with natural remedies through both treating the pathogenic bacteria (if you know that is the problem) or simply using substances that will cause normalization of the bowel. Most antidiarrheal herbs are best used as a tea. This replaces lost water and gets the herb in quantity into the intestinal tract where it is needed. Any kind of astringent tea can be used: sage, blackberry leaf or root, or raspberry are all good teas for diarrhea and can be easily purchased in health-food stores.

Natural Care for Diarrhea

Blackberry/slippery elm tea (as needed)
Goldenseal/echinacea tincture (if necessary)
Yogurt, 1 cup daily
Psyllium seed and husk, daily
Apple juice or sauce, daily

DIARRHEA TEA

The blackberry root is very astringent and the slippery elm bark will coat and soothe the interior of the irritated intestinal tract and, like psyllium and apple, normalizes and tonifies the bowel.

Take 3 ounces of dried blackberry root and 2 ounces of dried slippery elm bark and mix well. Simmer one teaspoon of the mix in a cup of water for fifteen minutes, cool slightly, and drink as often as needed.

DIARRHEA TINCTURE

If you know that the source of the upset is bacteria in the bowel, one of the best herbs to use is goldenseal (especially mixed with echinacea). Goldenseal is specifically antibacterial for most of the types of pathogenic bacteria that affect the GI tract, including the potentially deadly *E. coli,* increasingly found in infected hamburger. Echinacea can help stimulate the production and activity of white blood cells to help clear out any infection and stimulates protection of mucous membranes from bacteria. Goldenseal can be easily found combined with echinacea in tincture form.

Dosage
Take ¼ teaspoon in water (or diarrhea tea) three to four times daily.

YOGURT

One of the best ways to help restore bowel community integrity is with any yogurt that includes live lactobacillus cultures. These bacteria are natural coevolutionary partners of the human species and are one of the first colonizers of an infant's intestines. Lactobacillus bacteria, as part of their coevolutionary role, produce a wide range of B vitamins (including B_{12} and folic acid) that are essential to our health. They also produce acidophilin, various peroxides, and other substances that are strongly antibacterial to many of the most common intestinal pathogens that affect human beings.

Dosage
Take 1 cup daily until bowel problems normalize.

PSYLLIUM AND APPLES

See page 160.

CONSTIPATION

Constipation occurs when too much water is removed from the feces as it moves through the colon. It is usually the result of a poor diet—too much meat and dairy with too few plants and liquids on a regular basis. Simply adding half a cup of bran flakes or a bowl of oatmeal daily to the diet is often enough to end constipation problems. Black tea can make constipation problems worse because the tea is highly astringent (drying to tissues). Increasing water intake will help liquefy the feces and move it through the system more efficiently.

Natural Care for Constipation

> Prunes or prune juice, daily as needed
> Cascara sagrada (if necessary)
> Oatmeal or bran flakes, daily
> Psyllium, daily
> Apple juice or sauce, daily
> 4 to 6 glasses of water, daily

PRUNES

Prunes (*Prunus americana*), or dried plums, contrary to FDA pronounce-ments, are a reliable laxative, as millions of Americans know. The prunes themselves are slightly better than the juice as they add more fiber.

Dosage
Three to four prunes or a glass of prune juice a day is often enough to regu-larize the bowels.

CASCARA SAGRADA

Cascara sagrada is a reliable laxative. Because constipation is essentially an overly dry feces, I believe the best way to use it is as a tea. It is readily avail-able at most health-food stores. Cascara can be quite strong in its impacts, causing a certain amount of cramping and a "shot from guns" experience that is only moderately enjoyable.

Dosage
Take 20 to 40 drops (1 to 2 milliliters) of the tincture in tea at bedtime.

Cautions
Used long term, cascara can result in laxative dependence. The best ap-proach is to reduce meat and dairy products and increase vegetable, fiber, and liquid intake. Cascara is really best only for short-term use.

APPLES AND PSYLLIUM

Both apples and psyllium are bowel tonics. If you are suffering constipa-tion, they will loosen the bowels. If diarrhea, they will firm them up. Regu-lar intake of apple (sauce or juice) and/or psyllium is indicated if you have problems with normal bowel movements. Psyllium seeds absorb water and swell and press on the intestine, signaling peristalsis to begin. Because they are slippery, as they absorb water they can move through the gut with sur-prising ease. The slipperiness comes from mucilage, which tones, soothes, and heals the GI tract as the seeds move through. They are official for constipation in the German Commission E Monographs and in regular medical practice in Germany.[18]

Dosage

Take 3 to 10 tablespoons of psyllium daily in water. Take lots of water as they swell. Too little water and they will absorb even more water from the GI tract and make things worse. Have applesauce or juice once a day.

Cautions

Psyllium seeds have produced allergic reactions in some people and initiated asthma attacks in some asthmatics who breathed the dust.

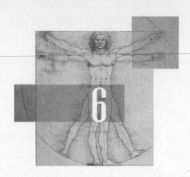

Balance: The Kidneys, Urinary Tract, and Adrenal Glands

*To dream on without waking seems not to be what
aging physiology wants. Not only do the bladder, the
sphincter, and the enlarged prostate play their roles in
getting men out of bed at night, but so does a strange,
newly discovered change in circadian rhythm.
Research on men in Denmark and Japan shows that
something happens to the younger, habitual patterns
of urine production. "Healthy young adults produce
urine three times faster during the day than at night."
Although the older men in these studies produced the
same total of urine as younger men in any twenty-four
hour period, older men were no longer retaining salt
and water during the night, and thus voiding more
frequently. . . . Men are being forced to learn another
rhythm. . . . The biological clock "intends" to rouse us
elders from sleep and awaken us to the darkness
around us.*   —JAMES HILLMAN

For Pete's sake! Hold your water!

                              —MARY BURNEY HARROD

I rarely thought about my kidneys, bladder, or blad-
der control as a young man. They just *were*, like the sun and the rain. But
suddenly in middle age, as for many men, things began to change. My

urine stream became weak and diverged into two streams, neither of which would reliably hit the target. I had to go more often and it took longer to get things moving. Suddenly the kidneys and bladder took on an importance I didn't want them to have.

Over time, I found that this was not unusual; it was happening to many men I knew as they aged. And of course, all of us were awakened in the night by the urgings of our bladders, often around three A.M., the lowest ebb of the human soul.

Once awakened at that time of the night, the mind begins to move in its own patterns, according to needs it alone seems to perceive. It is not unusual to lie silent in the dark, to endlessly replay the past, the problems of the present, or think of all the things that have been done and not done. The mind seems driven to work toward an accommodation, a completion with problems it (or the heart) has stored in memory. It is as if the human soul has to reconcile the incompletenesses of the past so that we can fully let go of one way of being and enter another.

The movement into middle age is deeply concerned with the loss of what we were and the (often unwilling) struggle to understand this new and unexpected territory that is now our home. Our kidneys and bladders awaken us, force us to grapple with the darkness inside us and the darkness around us—to engage in an introspection we would otherwise prefer to avoid. Through this deeper knowing of the self, the unresolved actions of our younger selves can be completed. We can let go of the past and find our balance once more.

That the kidneys are so intimately connected to the disturbance of the status quo, our former state of balance, is not surprising. For the kidneys are more than anything else concerned with balance.

THE KIDNEYS

The kidneys are tiny actually, only about four and a half inches long, two to three inches wide, and an inch thick. But they filter some 190 quarts of water and scores of other substances out of the blood each day. (Though after age forty this begins decreasing about 10 percent per decade.) Most of these filtered substances are reabsorbed. Ninety-nine percent of the water is reabsorbed back into the blood—only about three pints are excreted; of the 270 grams of glucose (except in diabetes), all is reabsorbed; of the

1,100 grams of chloride, only 10 grams is excreted; and of the 48 grams of urea, only 15 grams is excreted. The kidneys constantly monitor the amount of electrolytic salts: sodium, potassium, and chloride; the nitrogen; and the water coming into the body and excrete just enough to keep the balance the same. They monitor the body's acid/alkali balance and through altering urine composition maintain the pH of the body. To accomplish all this, the kidneys make and release enzymes and hormones that maintain the body's water, red blood cells, calcium and phosphorus, the mineral content of the bones, and the diameter of capillaries, among other things. The adrenal glands that make so many important androgens for men, sit just on top of the kidneys and are, in many respects, part of them.

The kidneys monitor blood pressure constantly and raise and lower it through creating and releasing a hormone called *renin*, which the liver uses to make *angiotensin*. Renin also increases the size of that portion of the adrenal gland that produces aldosterone, while angiotensin stimulates its production. (Aldosterone causes the kidneys to reabsorb more water and sodium.) Angiotensin also constricts the walls of arterioles, increases the strength of the heartbeat, and stimulates the pituitary gland to release ADH—antidiuretic hormone—which lowers the amount of water being excreted. These actions increase the blood pressure and intimately affect the levels of sodium and salt in the body.

The kidneys constantly monitor oxygen levels in the body's cells and when they are too low produce a hormone called *erythropoietin* (EPO). EPO stimulates the bone marrow to make and release more red blood cells; when oxygen levels return to optimum, the kidneys quit making EPO. Through this process the kidneys maintain the balance of red blood cells in the body.

The kidneys also make another hormone, called *calcitriol*, a unique form of vitamin D. Vitamin D is in actuality not a vitamin but a type of steroidal hormone that is synthesized in a unique endocrine system in the body. During sunlight exposure the human skin converts a form of cholesterol to vitamin D_3, the liver alters or metabolizes this again (into 25-hydroxycholecalciferol, aka 25-OHD3), and then the kidneys use that altered substance to make two highly biologically active hormones. One of them, calcitriol, acts on the cells of the intestine to increase absorption of calcium from the diet and direct it to the bones for bone formation. (Some of this calcium is also used to patch damaged blood vessels, contributing to arteriosclerosis.) Calcitriol also regulates certain parathyroid hormones that maintain the body's levels of phosphorus. The kidneys constantly monitor the levels of calcium and phosphorus in the body and increase or decrease them as needed. Through calcitriol the kidneys regulate bone mineralization and maintain the transfer of calcium to the bones to make them stronger. Thus they affect not only the bone marrow in the creation of red blood cells but also the bone itself.

Newer research has revealed that the kidneys also create arginine-synthesizing enzymes.[1] Arginine is an important precursor of nitric oxide (an erection stimulant), stimulates sperm production and motility, boosts growth hormone release, and possesses wound-healing and immune-enhancing functions.

The kidneys are also highly responsive to steroidal hormones and possess a large number of estrogenic receptor sites. Estrogens can bind to the sites in the kidneys, especially when estrogen levels in the body are high. This causes increases in body water levels, sodium content, and blood pressure. Researchers have found that high estrogen levels, especially in women using hormonal replacement for extended periods during menopause, increase the risks of both kidney and heart disease.

Low androgen levels in men also have an impact on kidney function. Research has shown that a healthy renin/angiotensin cycle is regulated by androgens through the action of a protein, the kidney androgen-regulated protein (Kap). This takes place in the part of the kidney that also produces the calcitriol that regulates bone mineralization and density. High estrogen/low androgen levels produce different actions than normal estrogen/androgen levels, especially in this part of the kidney. This possibly explains why men suffer from osteoporosis at much higher levels as they move into middle age and their androgen and testosterone levels change. It also explains to some extent the significant alteration for middle-aged men in how their bodies maintain water and sodium levels during sleep. Research has shown that healthy kidneys in men are highly dependent on testosterone—men with kidney disease have far higher levels of estrogens in their body and much lower levels of testosterone.[2] Estrogens, it is now known, also stimulate the production of epidermal growth factor (EGF) in the kidneys (which testosterone does not do). EGF has been linked to some types of prostate cancer and the estrogen-initiated EGF production in the kidneys is a potential contributing factor.

THE ADRENAL GLANDS

The adrenal glands, the two tiny pyramid-shaped organs that sit on top of the kidneys, are named for their location. *Ad* means near, *renal* is the Latin for kidney. The outer layer of the adrenal gland, the cortex, and the inner, the medulla, produce nearly 150 different hormones essential for health. The cortex itself produces more than two dozen important *corticosteroid* hormones, for example: cortisol, cortisone, aldosterone, DHEA, DHEAS, DHT, androstenedione, and testosterone. The adrenal medulla produces the most famous of the adrenal hormones, adrenaline (generally called epinephrine in the United States, adrenaline in the United Kingdom and Australia), and its close relative noradrenaline (norepinephrine). The adrenals are, in actuality, responsible for nearly 50 percent of all the androgens in a man's body. They produce significant quantities of male hormones, 90 percent of the body's DHEA, powerful anti-inflammatories such as cortisol, and fright-flight-or-fight hormones like adrenaline. They are closely tied to the testes, heart, lungs, and kidneys through intricate biofeedback loops and hormonal exchange systems. All those organs modify their creation and release of hormones as a result of the information they receive from the kidneys.

Stress has powerful effects on this hormonal exchange system. Under continued stress, the body will release high, constant levels of stress hormones such as cortisol and epinephrine. Cortisol blocks inflammation, regulates the water content of blood, and modifies blood sugar levels by releasing glucose from fats and proteins when it is needed. It also interferes with the conversion of tryptophan to serotonin. This causes an increase in wakefulness. Over time, chronic high cortisol levels can cause insomnia and constant poor sleep. In early morning, cortisol levels are high, in the evening they are low. Of significant importance is that as cortisol levels rise, DHEA levels decrease. The shift to cortisol metabolism inhibits DHEA production.

Epinephrine is used by the body as a short-burst, high-alert response to danger. It stimulates heart action, increases the diameter of air passages to stimulate oxygen uptake, and speeds up the liver's glucose production. Constant stress results in high levels of both cortisol and epinephrine and such physical symptoms as increased metabolism, hyper-wakefulness, rapid heartbeat, increased blood pressure, nervousness, increased stomach acid, increased muscle tension, and higher levels of emotional aggressiveness. Caffeine, especially at the levels found in coffee, stimulates the production of epinephrine and prevents its breakdown, which is why coffee drinking produces so many of the same symptoms.

The adrenal glands can become exhausted or suffer overstimulation after years of high cortisol production. This is especially serious in men with decreased androgen levels. Once the adrenals become overtaxed or exhausted, energy levels decline both from lack of normal adrenaline/cortisol levels and from low androgen levels.

THE KIDNEYS AND ADRENAL GLANDS IN CHINESE MEDICINE

While many of the actions of the kidney/adrenal system are new to Western science, they are not to the Chinese. Chinese physicians have long understood the close connection of the kidneys to the heart and intestines. Within their system, disharmony between the heart and kidney or kidney and intestines was known to be the cause of numerous diseases, including kidney stones, urinary gravel, and certain blood circulation problems. Chinese physicians also understood the connection of the kidney to low androgen levels. They call it "empty kidney-glands," meaning there is insufficient vital hormone production. This is especially perceptive in that the term for this condition occurred many thousands of years before any Western scientist knew that the adrenals, glands located on the kidneys, produce many of the essential hormones and androgens for male health. The kidneys are considered to be an organ of balance and do, within the Chinese system, affect the functioning of the inner ear. Vertigo (and even tinnitus) can be a sign of a disordered kidney, the imbalance in the kidney causing a literal inability to balance.

GENERAL TONICS FOR THE KIDNEYS/ADRENALS

Western understanding of the kidney/adrenal system is in its infancy. Most natural treatments are designed to treat specific conditions, not the whole system. The kidneys are, perhaps, the most neglected area of natural medicine in the Western world.

Daily Tonic Regimen for Exhausted Kidneys/Adrenals

Corn, 2 to 4 ounces of juice daily
Celery, 3 juiced stalks daily
Asian (or Siberian) ginseng, 100 to 200 milligrams daily
Nettles, 300 to 1,200 milligrams daily
Vitamin B_5 (pantothenic acid), 100 to 500 milligrams daily
Zinc, 20 to 40 milligrams daily

CORN

Although most people do not realize it, corn (*Zea mays*) is a specific tonic for the whole urinary tract, including the adrenals. The corn kernels, corn silk, and pollen are all kidney/adrenal specific though the pollen is somewhat difficult to find.

Corn pollen has been used similarly to pine pollen in a number of cultures as a restorative of male vitality and contains many of the same amino acids and vitamins that are found in pine pollen. Corn pollen is included in Cernilton, the rye grass pollen mixture that is so successful in treating prostate disease. Corn juice has been found to stimulate the production and release of luteinizing hormone (LH), which promotes the production of testosterone and its release into the bloodstream.[3] And corn silk is highly effective for cystitis, acute and chronic inflammations of the bladder, urethritis, and prostatitis.

Corn is an anodyne (pain soother), a diuretic (increasing urine output), demulcent (soothing to mucous membranes), anti-inflammatory, antispasmodic, and tonic. The Spanish writer Garcilaso de la Vega (1539–1616) commented that he was highly impressed

> with the remarkable curative properties of corn, which is not only the principal article of food in America, but is also of benefit in the treatment of diseases of the kidney and bladder, among which are calculus and retention of urine. And the best proof I can give of this is that the Indians, whose usual drink is made of corn, are afflicted with none of these diseases.[4]

While most people don't think of drinking corn, it has been used for some ten thousand years to make *chicha,* a special kind of beer unique to the Americas. While chicha is difficult to find in the northern United States, you can easily run corn kernels through a juicer each morning to obtain the juice. As the corn juice is a bit thick, I blend it with 4 ounces of celery juice, a really delicious combination. There is no better overall tonic for the kidney/adrenal system than this combination.

Dosage

Take 2 to 4 ounces of juiced organic corn kernels daily (about 2 to 4 ounces of kernels).

A Note on Corn Silk

Corn silk is most often used for inflammation in the urinary tract. In a number of clinical trials it has been found to be especially effective in reducing excess water retention, swelling, and edema. The stigmas—the four- to eight-inch-long fine, silky threads that you pull off corn on the cob as you shuck it—are what is normally used for urinary tract problems. They are best used fresh. A tea or tincture of corn silk can be added to the juice daily if you are experiencing specific urinary tract problems.

Dosage

Steep 2 teaspoons of the silk in 8 ounces of hot water for fifteen minutes and drink three times per day. The tincture may be purchased in health-food stores: Take 3 to 6 milliters (¾ to 1½ teaspoons) three times daily.

CELERY

Celery (*Apium graveolens*) is a specific for the kidneys and a tonic equal in power to corn. As with corn silk, celery is better known through its use as celery seed for specific urinary complaints. However, the whole plant is an exceptional kidney tonic.

Celery is high in *apigenin,* which expands (dilates) blood vessels and helps prevent high blood pressure. It also contains over a dozen compounds that act much like the calcium channel blockers used for treating angina and arrythmia. Celery seed has been found to be effective for gout (helping eliminate uric acid from the body), reducing kidney stone formation, increasing urine flow, as a mild antimicrobial for the urinary tract, as an anti-inflammatory and antispasmodic for the urinary and digestive tract, and (in Chinese medicine) for helping dizziness. And finally, celery contains a number of compounds that are very similar to both androstenedione and testosterone, which is why it has been used since antiquity as a sexual tonic for men.

In short, celery affects the entire urinary network and most of the bodily systems that the kidneys do: heart, digestive system, adrenals, and blood vessels.

Dosage

Three celery stalks juiced daily (makes 3 to 4 ounces of juice), best if blended with the corn as a general tonic.

A Note on Celery Seed

If you have specific urinary system complaints you might try adding a squirt of celery seed tincture (or a cup of celery seed tea) to your juice each morning.

Dosage

Take 1 to 2 milliters (¼ to ½ teaspoon) tincture up to three times a day or 1 to 2 teaspoons of the crushed seeds steeped fifteen to twenty minutes in water as a tea up to three times daily.

ASIAN GINSENG

Asian ginseng (*Panax ginseng*) acts as a general adaptogenic tonic for the whole body and exerts specific actions on the adrenal glands. In many traditions it is considered to be a specific tonic for the adrenals. Asian ginseng counteracts many of the effects of excessive cortisol and adrenaline production, reduces stress, enhances well-being, and balances androgen levels in the body.[5]

Note: Siberian ginseng has many of the same actions and acts as a more long-term tonic for stressed adrenals. If Asian ginseng is too energetic for you, you may wish to use Siberian ginseng instead (see Chapter 3 for details).

Dosage

Take 100 to 200 milligrams up to 1 to 9 grams daily. Start low and work up. At higher doses, ginseng may cause many of the same problems it alleviates.

Cautions

Ginseng can be quite stimulating and should be used in small doses initially and increased once you are used to it. It can sometimes cause hypertension, especially with large, sustained doses, and is contraindicated in those with high blood pressure. Under a health practitioner's supervision, it can be used with care if you have moderate hypertension. Sustained overuse can cause insomnia, heart palpitations, muscle tension, and headache. It may cause difficulty in sleeping if taken before bedtime. Because it affects androgen and testosterone levels, it should not be used by adolescent males.

NETTLES

Nettles (*Urtica dioica*) are an ancient tonic for the body, including the kidneys and adrenals. The plants are high in many nutrients that are necessary for kidney health, including magnesium and potassium. Nettles are listed in the German Commission E Monographs as both a preventative and treatment for kidney stones and inflammation of the lower urinary tract.[6] The root and fresh plant are both diuretics, and nettles have been found to exert powerful effects on prostate health and to keep androgen levels higher by interfering with their conversion into estrogens. The fresh plant is best used either as a tea, in soup, or as a cooked green. Because of their sting, nettles should *not* be eaten fresh—cooking inactivates the sting. Due to the sting and general unavailability of nettles, most people take an encapsulated freeze-dried extract. This preserves the activity of many of the most active principles of the plant.

Dosage

Take 300 to 1,200 milligrams of the freeze-dried extract of the plant (not the root).

Cautions

Mild side effects have occasionally been reported with the root, usually mild gastrointestinal upset. With the plant, only mild side effects are noted: skin afflictions such as rashes and mild swelling. *The Physicians' Desk Reference for Herbal Medicines* lists a contraindication for the plant in cases of fluid retention from reduced cardiac or renal action. No contraindications are noted for the root.

VITAMIN B₅ (PANTOTHENIC ACID)

Vitamin B_5 deficiency shows as adrenal atrophy accompanied by fatigue, headache, sleep irregularity, nausea, and abdominal problems. The vitamin is used by the body to keep the adrenals healthy and is often low in people suffering from exhausted or overworked adrenals.[7]

Dosage
Take 100 to 500 milligrams daily.

ZINC

Zinc promotes the conversion of androstenedione to testosterone and is crucial throughout the androgen system. Levels in adrenal-exhausted people are often very low.

Dosage
Take 20 to 40 milligrams daily. It is generally recommended to not exceed 40 milligrams of zinc per day.

Cautions
Over time, zinc intake can cause copper depletion in the body. To counteract this, most zinc supplements come with copper added. At very high doses, zinc can cause nausea and upset stomach, skin rashes, depression, folate deficiency, and lower tolerance to alcohol.

Herbs to Avoid

COFFEE

Coffee is a strong diuretic, increases sweating, and stimulates adrenaline production and release by the adrenals. It strongly impacts both the kidneys and adrenals and, over time, works them to exhaustion. Coffee, especially by men with androgen or adrenal deficiencies or kidney disease, should be consumed only in moderation. The herb, with long, heavy use, overstimulates both the kidneys and adrenals, often producing chronic anxiety, depression, insomnia, and irritability.

In spite of this, caffeine is often an important element of a healthy diet (it is a potent anticarcinogenic compound in moderation) and is found in many plants in much lower quantities than in coffee, the cocaine of caffeine-containing plants. Black and green tea are much better choices for daily consumption. If you are reducing coffee intake, go first to black tea, then to green. Stopping cold turkey will usually produce one of the truly great one- or two-day headaches of all time.

Coffee, for those of us who are unrepentant lovers of the smell and taste, can best be enjoyed as an occasional treat—espresso, cappuccino, or latte so strong the little hairs on the back of the neck stand up.

LICORICE

Licorice affects many of the hormonal actions of the kidneys. In high doses it can cause a specific kind of anemia, an insufficiency of red blood cells in the muscles—myoglobinemia—possibly by interfering with the kidneys' creation of EPO. Too much licorice for extended periods can result in higher cortisol levels in the body because licorice inhibits 11-beta hydroxysteroid dehydrogenase, an enzyme that is involved in the conversion of cortisol to cortisone in the adrenal glands. Licorice also causes increased water retention in the body (edema), increases in sodium retention, hypokalemia (loss of potassium from the body), high blood pressure, and cardiac problems (from potassium loss). Plasma renin levels, ADH, and aldosterone levels all decrease when licorice is taken. Licorice is a specific herb for reducing renin levels in the body; the area of the kidney where renin is produced is one of its major sites of action. While licorice reduces renin (and as a result aldosterone) levels, it also acts as a renin and aldosterone mimic by increasing water and sodium in the body, raising blood pressure, and so on. If these functions of the kidneys are not working well, licorice can temporarily be used as a substitute. For that reason it has been used as an aid in low blood pressure. Licorice is contraindicated in kidney disease except under the supervision of a health-care provider.

VITAMIN C

While vitamin C can be useful in some kidney conditions, you should not use vitamin C if you are on hemodialysis, or suffer from recurrent kidney stones, severe kidney disease, or gout.

CYSTITIS AND URINARY TRACT INFECTIONS (UTIs)

After processing by the kidneys, urine collects in a lower section of the kidney, an area called the *pelvis,* and then drops down through the *ureters* and into the bladder for storage. (Structurally, the ureters are made of an outer fibrous coat, two middle layers of smooth muscle, and an inner, mucous membrane layer.) The bladder is simply a collapsible bag, lined with mucous membranes, composed of three layers of smooth muscle. The *urethra* leads from the floor of the bladder out into the world. In women it is only about one and a half inches long, while in men the urethra is at least seven inches longer (depending on your math). In a man's body, the urethra has to travel down from the bladder, through the prostate, through the pubic bones, then through the entire length of the penis. For this reason (and because prostatic fluid is highly antibacterial) men have far fewer urinary tract infections than women. Women are more prone to UTIs because their urine is chemically somewhat different than men's (making it better suited to fostering bacterial growth), because of the shorter length of the female urethra, and because of its location inside the vagina.

Normally the urine is acidic and it becomes more so depending on the amount of protein that is eaten in the diet. Vegetarians, in consequence, can sometimes have alkaline urine—the more vegetables they eat the more alkaline the urine can be. Urine is usually highly antibacterial (which is why many military organizations suggest peeing on the feet to cure athlete's foot during extended duty in the field). However, some bacteria have learned to live in the urinary tract (often because of improper medical procedures in hospitals or improper use of antibiotics) and others take advantage of chemical changes in urine because of illness or a change in diet.

A urinary tract infection (UTI) is usually an infection of the urinary passages—the tract. Cystitis, on the other hand, generally refers to an inflammation of the walls and lining of the bladder only, most commonly from a bacterial infection. The treatment for both is very similar—usually, three types of herbs are used, depending on the symptoms: antibacterial herbs, herbs that soothe spasms in the muscle layers in the tract and bladder, and demulcent herbs that soothe the mucous membranes that line the tract and bladder. Sometimes, diuretic herbs will be added to promote urine flow through the whole system.

Many herbs are especially effective for urinary tract infections because the body excretes the plants' active chemistries through the kidneys. This takes the antibacterials directly to the areas where they are needed. It is often beneficial to drink a fair amount of water to help things along.

Natural Care for UTI and Cystitis

For One Week to One Month
>Uva ursi, 2 to 4 milliliters tincture (½ to 1 teaspoon), three times a day.
>Juniper berry (see "Cautions")
>Corn silk, 2 milliliters tincture (½ teaspoon), three times a day
>Black haw, 5 milliliters tincture (1¼ teaspoons), three times a day
>Cranberry or blueberry juice (naturally sweetened), 16 ounces a day
>Yogurt, 3 (1-cup) servings weekly
>6 glasses water (12 ounces each) daily

UVA URSI

The Latin for uva ursi—*Arcostaphylos uva-ursi*—translates as bearberry, which the herb is sometimes called. Uva ursi, a sprawling, pervasive forest groundcover with small, leathery, dark green leaves, is common throughout the world. It is high enough in tannins that some cultures have regularly used it for tanning leather. It also contains arbutin, a chemical that is broken down in the kidneys into glucose and hydroquinone. The body uses the glucose for energy and excretes the hydroquinone in the urine. Hydroquinone is highly antimicrobial and is powerfully effective against most of the bacteria that can infect the urinary tract. Uva ursi (at least as far as is known) contains more arbutin than any plant (about 10 percent); however, its close relatives, cranberry and blueberry, contain arbutin as well. The German Commission E Monographs considers uva ursi standard medical protocol for urinary tract infections[8] and except in stubborn cases I have found the herb exceptionally reliable. Usually infections clear within a week. Uva ursi is only a feeble diuretic and often works better when taken with diuretics such as dandelion leaf or corn silk, or massive amounts of water.

Dosage

Take 2 to 6 milliliters of the tincture (½ to 1½ teaspoons) three times a day.

Cautions

The herb, because of its high tannin content, can upset the stomach.

JUNIPER BERRY

Junipers (*Juniperus communis*) grow throughout the world—both wild and domesticated—and, along with most evergreens (such as pine), have long been used for urinary tract infections. With most evergreen species, the needles are usually used. Although juniper needles will work, the berries are more concentrated and are the preferred part of the plant. The berries contain an exceptionally antibacterial volatile oil (composed of a complex blend of chemical terpenes) that is excreted through the kidneys. If you have a truly stubborn urinary tract infection that does not respond to uva ursi, this can be an especially effective herb. It is, however, a strong herb and can irritate the kidneys if taken too long or in too strong a dose. Juniper berries possess two benefits over uva ursi: They are a reliable diuretic, increasing the output of urine, and they have distinct relaxant actions on the smooth muscle tissue of the urinary system and bladder. Like uva ursi, juniper berries are official in the German Commission E Monographs as a part of that country's standard practice medicine.[9]

Dosage

Take 10 to 20 drops of the tincture (⅛ to ¼ teaspoon) up to three times a day, up to seven days.

Usually the tincture is used, though the berries themselves can be swallowed whole (1 to 3 per day, up to seven days) or a tea of the powdered berries can be prepared (1 teaspoon of powdered berries in a cup of water, 1 to 3 times a day, up to seven days).

Cautions

Juniper is *not* to be used in serious kidney disease. Overuse or overdose will cause kidney inflammation and/or irritation. If side effects (kidney pain or irritation) occur, reduce dose or eliminate the herb.

CORN SILK

Corn silk (*Zea mays*) is a wonderful herb for urinary tract infections in that it coats and soothes the mucous membranes in the bladder and the urinary passages; relaxes the muscle layers lining the ureters, bladder, and urethra; increases urine flow; and gently tones and heals the urinary tract. It is especially indicated if you are experiencing pain on urination.

Dosage

Take ½ teaspoon of the tincture three times a day.

BLACK HAW

Like many of the viburnums, black haw (*Viburnum prunifolium*) is an antispasmodic and mild pain-dampening nervine. It will be of help if the pain on urination is severe—it relaxes the urethral passages and diminishes pain. It should only be added to the protocol for UTI and cystitis if you are experiencing strong pain.

Dosage

Take 1¼ teaspoons three times a day.

CRANBERRY OR BLUEBERRY JUICES

Cranberry and blueberry juices contain arbutin, though in lesser amounts than uva ursi, and like uva ursi, will help in urinary tract infections. They also contain hippuric acid, an effective antibacterial. One study in the *Journal of the American Medical Association* revealed that both cranberry and blueberry juice interfere with the ability of bacteria to adhere to the walls of the urinary tract. As a result, infectious bacteria are simply flushed out of the body during urination.[10]

Note: Many of the more common commercial cranberry juices are sweetened with sugar; they should not be used. As many people find unsweetened juice too sour, try one sweetened with apple or grape juice.

Dosage
Drink 16 ounces per day.

YOGURT

Jim Duke, in his *Green Pharmacy*, notes that a number of studies have shown regular consumption of yogurt in the diet can prevent bladder and urinary tract infections. The yogurt needs to have live cultures (most do) and the package will list them.

Dosage
Eat three 1-cup servings weekly if you have a history of urinary tract infections.

WATER

It is necessary in urinary tract infections to make sure you drink enough water to keep the urinary passages well irrigated. This will, in addition, increase the effectiveness of the herbs.

Dosage
Drink five to six 12-ounce glasses per day.

KIDNEY STONES

Kidney stones are one of the all-time "I wish I were dead" experiences. The stones, especially oxalate stones, are sharp, and when they drop from the kidney down into the ureter they take their long, slow time scraping along the entire length of the system. Temporary relief occurs when they drop into the bladder, but if they then move on into the urethra it all begins again until, with a final agonizing yelp, the stone exits the penis. The pain is often debilitating and major painkillers are usually necessary. (Basically, you fall on the floor, curl into a ball, and pray for God to kill you. If God does not kill you, there are some anger problems that have to be resolved later.) As the stone moves through the system, the tract tends to spasm; they call it a colic, which is putting it mildly. You may both vomit and sweat profusely; you will feel weak and noodlelike for some time as each spasm passes.

Prior to 1920, stones generally formed in the bladder, now they tend to begin in the kidney. In fact, since the 1920s, both the frequency of stones and their formation in the kidney has increased to the point that some 10 to 12 percent of American men are projected to experience them at least once. This trend corresponds both to the change in diet and the alteration of androgen levels in men that have taken place in the past eighty years. Changes in estrogen/androgen ratios and increased levels of estrogens in the kidney interfere with kidney hormone activity, especially that concerned with calcitriol, the hormone that governs calcium and phosphorus balance, kidney filtering, and excretion. This is tremendously exacerbated by the modern diet.

Most people who get kidney stones tend to consume a low-fiber, refined-carbohydrate diet high in alcohols, meats, fats, and enriched milk products—basically, meat-and-potatoes diet with a glass of milk and a couple of scotches after dinner. For most of us, our parents' (and—at one time or another—our) meals.

Both factors, estrogens and diet, seem to enhance each other in the creation of stones.

Kidney stones form around substances in the urine, somewhat like making crystal sugar candy by suspending a string in sugar-saturated water and waiting as the crystals "grow" on the string. After larger urinary crystals form, pieces can sometimes break off and be carried slowly through the tiresomely long system. Most of the stones, about 75 percent, form from

---

BLADDER STONES AND PROSTATE DISEASE

Bladder stone formation is sometimes exacerbated if you have an enlarged prostate. Because the swollen prostate does not allow the bladder to completely empty, dissolved crystals can build up in the bladder and precipitate out as stones. The stones then have a hard time flushing out of the bladder—it is difficult for them to make it over the hump in the floor of the bladder caused by the swollen prostate. In such cases, reducing prostate inflammation is extremely important (see Chapter 3). Otherwise, they can be treated much like kidney stones.

---

some type of calcium salt (calcium phosphate or calcium oxalate). About 15 percent come from a noncalcium salt (magnesium ammonium phosphate), uric acid stones make up about 5 percent of stones, and a tiny fraction are cystine crystals.

Although vegetarians generally have lower stone formation, those that do form tend to be calcium phosphate stones, which have a liking for the alkaline urine of vegetarians (or those with bacterial infections). Calcium oxalate stones tend to form around oxalates, chemicals found in certain types of foods such as spinach and beets. Both types of calcium stones are aggravated by the consumption of high-calcium, low-magnesium, vitamin D–enriched milk in the diet. Magnesium is necessary in the diet to make sure that the calcium is kept in solution in the urine and does not precipitate out and solidify. Uric acid stones are usually found in a heavy meat eater's acidic urine. Cystine stones usually occur because there is an abnormal increase of cystine in the urine.

The only sure way to find out the exact composition of the stone is to pee into a container each time you go. Eventually the stone will move through the whole system and there will be a definite "plink" as it hits the bottom of the container. You can retrieve it, take it in, and have it analyzed. Unfortunately, this does no good when the first attack hits. More positively, some naturopathic physicians have begun developing protocols to help identify stones before they are expelled. This includes hair analysis, examination of the diet, and analysis of the urine and its constituents.

Once you know you have a tendency to kidney stones, they can often be

---

KIDNEY STONE PREVENTION TEA

Take 3 ounces each of (dried) dandelion leaf, couch grass, beggar's-lice, java tea, goldenrod, and peppermint leaf. Mix well. Add one ounce of the mixture to a half quart of boiling water. Immediately remove from heat and cover. Let steep twenty to thirty minutes, then strain. Add one additional quart of water to the strained tea and drink all of the one and a half quarts of tea (warm) within thirty minutes.

This is best done on a weekend, or whenever you do not need to work, as you will be going to the bathroom much of the day.

Caution: This tea mixture should not be used in cases of severe gallstones, where there is a chance of bile duct obstruction, or in cases of edema due to impaired heart or kidney function.

---

prevented by following a protocol that helps prevent their formation or flushes them out when they are tiny—before they get large enough to be a problem. Especially important is to drink a lot of water to keep the urine diluted. Concentrated urine (which is generally darker in color) contains more of the particles around which stones can form. And as noted earlier, regular nettle consumption is considered specific for the prevention of kidney stones. (See page 171.)

Natural Care for Preventing Kidney Stones

For Six to Twelve Months
    Nettle leaf, freeze-dried extract, 300 to 1,200 milligrams daily
    Kidney stone prevention tea, 1½ quarts once a week
    Magnesium, 600 milligrams daily *or* magnesium citrate, daily in water
    Vitamin B$_6$, 25 milligrams daily
    Vitamin K, 2 milligrams daily
    Radishes, liberally in the diet
    Lemonade, mildly sweetened, daily (see magnesium citrate)
    Water, 48 ounces per day
    Dietary additions and considerations

KIDNEY STONE PREVENTION TEA

Caution
This tea mixture should not be used in cases of severe gallstones where there is a chance of bile duct obstruction, or in cases of edema due to impaired heart or kidney function.

DANDELION LEAF

Dandelion (*Taraxacum officinale*) is perhaps America's most recognized plant; Americans spend millions each year trying to permanently uproot them from their yards. Once considered to be an important food and medicinal plant (my great-grandparents ate it regularly), for most people it is now relegated to the dust heap of herbal history. That is unfortunate because it is one of the most potent of medicinal plants. While the root is one of the prime herbs for the liver, the leaf is a strong kidney remedy, primarily a diuretic. Dandelion is in fact one of the all-time great diuretics. One common French name, *pissenlit* (piss-the-bed), indicates why it should never be taken at night.

Dandelion contains a surprising number of essential minerals. Those of us guilty of trying to kill it generally do not recognize that dandelion brings up minerals from the deeper soil, stores them in its cells, and releases them into the upper soil to maintain soil-mineral balance. It does much the same thing for the kidneys when used medicinally. Although it provokes a tremendous amount of urine, it also supplies high levels of potassium, an important mineral that all diuretics remove from the body. While synthetic diuretics deplete potassium, dandelion adds back more potassium than it removes. Dandelion supplies a generally tonic action for the kidneys, increasing their action, and is especially useful in keeping the kidneys and urinary tract flushed, helping to prevent stone formation.[11]

COUCH GRASS

Couch grass (*Agropyron repens*) is a common lawn-invading weed, and like dandelion is not much respected in the United States. In Europe—England, and Germany especially—it is esteemed as a primary urinary tonic. The plant is a diuretic, demulcent, and antimicrobial. It increases urine flow, coats and soothes the mucous membranes of the urinary tract, and disinfects. It is in fact a useful herb for mild urinary tract infections. It has also been found to be useful in increasing urine flow in those with inflamed prostates. Couch grass is especially good for helping prevent kidney and bladder stones. It is official in Germany for this purpose and as a preventative for lower urinary tract inflammations.[12] The root (more accurately, a creeping rhizome) is used.

BEGGAR'S-LICE

Beggar's-lice (*Desmodium styracifolium*), long used in Chinese medicine for kidney stones, substantially increases urine volume, decreases the amount of calcium in the urine, and increases the excretion of citrates. Higher citrate levels in the urine have been found to substantially inhibit stone formation. *In vivo* studies with chemically induced stone formation in rats found that beggar's-lice reduced stone formation by two-thirds. In clinical studies, stone formation has been lowered by 50 percent. The plant also affects kidney and adrenal actions on vasoconstriction and lowers blood pressure. Related *Desmodiums* have been found to possess specific activity on calcium and potassium activity in the body, especially the lungs, to relax smooth muscle tissue, and to be antibacterial and anti-inflammatory.[13]

JAVA TEA

Java tea (*Orthosiphon stamineus*), sometimes called Indian kidney tea, or even cat's whiskers (from its very long flower stamens), while a native of the Sunda Islands and Australia, has been naturalized throughout the world as an ornamental. Many people in the United States grow it, unaware of its tremendous medicinal qualities. The leaves are usually used and the plant is an official medicinal in the pharmacopoeias of Germany, France, Indonesia, the Netherlands, and Switzerland. Java tea possesses a number of complex functions, acting as a unique kidney herb in ways that are not completely understood. The plant is an antibacterial diuretic but also increases elimination of nitrogenous wastes and excessive sodium chloride from the urine. It will also lower nonprotein nitrogen levels in the blood. Limited clinical trials in Malaysia and Singapore have shown that the plant is effective in helping prevent the recurrence of kidney stones. Additional clinical work in Thailand has found that java tea will prevent the formation of uric acid stones while promoting the excretion of both uric and oxalic acid from the body. The complex flavonoids in java tea have been found to be powerfully protective against oxidative free radicals, while also stabilizing the enzymes of the kidney and protecting them from breakdown. This enzyme-stabilizing effect helps protect the kidneys and promote their more efficient action. There is some research showing that the plant helps relax the ureters that lead from the kidney to the bladder, thus helping kidney stones, gravel, and urine pass more easily.[14]

GOLDENROD

Goldenrod species (*Solidago* species) are common throughout the world. In the United States, they are mostly known for their contribution to hay fever season and its symptoms. In spite of this, goldenrod is a very effective medicinal plant for healing the urinary system. It is a reliable diuretic but is also a tonic for the kidneys, for example reducing the amount of albumin excreted in the urine. The herb seems to potentiate the efficiency of the kidneys, even in serious kidney disease, and corrects underlying pathology such as the presence of albumin in urine. It also can tone and strengthen capillary walls, helping to enhance the capillary filtering action of the blood vessels of the kidney. The herb is especially good if there is an underlying inflammatory condition of the kidneys, where it acts as a powerful anti-inflammatory. It is an official plant in German medical practice and the German Commission E Monographs for the prevention of kidney and bladder stones.[15]

PEPPERMINT LEAF

Peppermint (*Mentha piperita*) is well known to just about everyone. A native of Europe, it now grows everywhere. The leaf is a reliable antispasmodic for smooth muscle systems of the body (mostly of the gastrointestinal tract but also the urinary system), a mild diuretic, and just generally tastes good (which some of these herbs do not), which is why it is a part of this tea mixture.

MAGNESIUM

Magnesium increases the solubility of calcium and keeps it from forming stones. A significant drop in dietary magnesium can, by itself, produce kidney stones. A number of studies have shown that magnesium inhibits both calcium oxalate and calcium phosphate stone formation. Other studies have shown that magnesium supplements in the diet help prevent recurrences of kidney stones. And low magnesium/high calcium in the urine has been found to be an indicator of kidney stone formation.[16]

Dosage
Take 600 milligrams a day.

Cautions
Magnesium is normally well tolerated; however, people with certain kinds of severe heart disease, such as high-grade atrioventricular block, should only use magnesium under the supervision of a health-care provider.

POTASSIUM (OR MAGNESIUM) CITRATE

Citrate, or citric acid, is a major constituent in citrus fruits and has been found highly effective in preventing stone formation. Citrate binds with calcium in the urine, preventing it from precipitating out as stones. It has also been found to prevent oxalate crystals from clumping together into larger formations. A number of double-blind studies have found magnesium and potassium citrates effective for preventing stone formation when compared with placebo. In one study, only 13 percent of the citrate group had a recurrence of stones while 64 percent of the placebo group did. Lemon juice has been found to be an acceptable source of citrate in helping prevent stone formation.[17] (Don't use grapefruit juice.) While many people use potassium citrate and magnesium supplements, a more effective approach may be to simply use a magnesium citrate.

Dosage
Use as directed on the label.

VITAMIN B$_6$

When vitamin B$_6$ is added to the diet along with magnesium, the inhibiting action of magnesium is increased substantially. Vitamin B$_6$ deficiency itself can cause kidney stones. B$_6$ is especially effective in preventing the formation of calcium oxalate stones as it interferes with the production and excretion of oxalates. B$_6$ is used by the body to convert oxalates into other substances and has been found to reduce the incidence of kidney stones.[18]

Dosage
Take 25 milligrams per day.

VITAMIN K

The kidneys, as a part of their normal functioning, regularly produce substances that are powerful kidney stone inhibitors. At least one of them has been found to need vitamin K as an essential part of its synthesis.[19]

Dosage
Take 2 milligrams per day.

RADISH

A number of clinical trials in Malaysia have found the common radish (*Raphanus sativus*) to be a powerful inhibitor of kidney stone recurrence in prior sufferers.[20]

Dosage
Eat as much as desired in your diet—at least four radishes twice weekly.

Cautions
Radishes may irritate mucous membranes of the gastrointestinal tract and are contraindicated in gallstones.

WATER

The more fluids you drink, the more urinary gravel can be flushed out before it has a chance to serve as a focus for crystal formation.

Dosage

Drink 48 ounces, minimum, per day of noncity, nonchemically enhanced water.

DIETARY ADDITIONS AND CONSIDERATIONS

If you have calcium phosphate or magnesium ammonium phosphate stones (alkaline urine), eat more acidic foods, meats, fish, and eggs. If you have calcium oxalate stones avoid oxalates in your food. Oxalate-containing foods that have been shown to increase stone formation are spinach, rhubarb, beet greens, black tea, sorrel, nuts, chocolate, peanuts, almonds, bran, and strawberries. For both types of calcium stones, increase magnesium intake to increase the solubility of calcium. If you have uric acid stones (acid urine), decrease meat, especially beef, liver, kidneys, roe, and sardines. Eat a more vegetarian diet: potatoes, green vegetables, fruit. If you have cystine stones, avoid wheat, soy, fish, meat, mushrooms, and lima and garbanzo beans.

High-calcium foods have been shown to reduce the recurrence of stones because the calcium binds the oxalates in the foods and prevents them being excreted in the urine. However, *supplementation* with calcium has been associated with an increased risk of stone formation in a number of studies. If you have a history of stones, it is a good idea to avoid calcium supplements unless you are working with a health-care provider.

Foods to Avoid

Grapefruits and grapefruit juice have been found in a number of studies to increase stone formation, possibly from increasing estrogen levels at kidney-receptor sites. One large-scale study found a 44 percent stone increase in women drinking eight ounces of grapefruit juice daily.[21]

Help for Existing Kidney Stones

Some herbs and herbal combinations have been found to help break up stones, diminish their size, or help them pass more easily. Most of the effective clinical trials have been with formulas using a combination of herbs.

Western approaches tend to focus on surgery, the use of opiates until the stone passes, or some sort of vibration to break up the stones. Eastern medicine, while still occasionally utilizing opiates, tends to focus on herbal interventions. The only long-term clinical trials with herbs have occurred in China, India, and Japan.

In one trial of an Ayurvedic herbal formula, three hundred people with kidney stones were given an extract of a combination of eight herbs. Sixty-seven percent of the people passed stones and 11 percent of the remaining sufferers' stones reduced in size. Ninety-eight percent of the people reported relief from colic.[22] The formula contained cantaloupe melon seeds, caraway seeds, anise seeds, corn silk, fennel seeds, cherry bark, bay leaf, and tribulus terrestris. The combination is centered around the use of anti-spasmodic/soothing herbs (anise, fennel, caraway, corn silk) and antilithic herbs (cantaloupe seed and tribulus).

Chinese medicine tends to utilize formulas built around the herb *Lysi-machia christinae,* the primary stone-reducing and stone-preventative herb in Chinese medicine. Most of the combinations also contain the herbs *Pyrrosia lingua* (deer's tongue fern), *Plantago asiatica* (Asian psyllium) seed, and talc (hydrated magnesium silicate). Clinical trials with anywhere from thirty-two to one thousand people have been conducted. About two-thirds of the people expel stones, 10 percent have stone-sized reduction, most report relief from colic. Most of the studies found that relief occurred within one to three months, for some in as few as four days. The average time for relief was about one month.[23] Most of the Chinese trials also required the participants to do jumping exercises for fifteen minutes, thirty minutes after drinking the teas. An odd image but it seemed to help pass the stones.

The following kidney stone tea combines herbs from both approaches. (Once the stones pass, use the prevention care outlined above to help prevent their recurrence.)

Natural Care for Existing Kidney Stones

For One to Six Months
　　Kidney stone tea, 3 to 4 cups daily
　　Kidney stone tincture mix: gravel root, stone root, pellitory of the wall,
　　　　1½ teaspoons three times a day

Wild yam, 1.5 to 3 milliliters (¼ to ¾ teaspoon) three times a day
Black cohosh (see listing)
Water, 2.5 quarts daily
Hot bath and compresses

KIDNEY STONE TEA

The seeds in this formula all are reliable antispasmodics, especially for abdominal cramping. Though usually used for intestinal colic, they have a history of use in calming the spasms from kidney stones and relaxing the ureters and urethras. They are also strong antimicrobials with powerful effects on smooth muscle tissue. Celery seed is also a diuretic, antimicrobial, antispasmodic, and anti-inflammatory for the urinary passages.

To make, take 2 ounces each anise seed, fennel seed, corn silk, tribulus, pumpkin seed, Asian psyllium seed, and pyrrosia. Add 4 ounces lysimachia and 1 ounce each of caraway and celery seed. Mix well and grind finely. Add two teaspoons of the mixture to 8 ounces of hot water and steep, covered, for 20 minutes. Drink three to four cups daily, sweetened with honey if desired.

Cautions
Not for use in cases of obstructed bile duct or edema from cardiac or renal insufficiency.

Corn Silk
Discussed earlier, corn silk is a mild pain reliever, a relaxant to smooth muscle fibers, a diuretic, and a tonic for the urinary system.

Tribulus Terrestris
Tribulus, discussed in detail in Chapter 3, has been found effective in a number of clinical trials for the treatment of kidney stones.

Pumpkin Seed
A number of different melon seeds have been found effective for kidney stones. Besides cantaloupe, pumpkin seeds have been found to be especially effective. Two clinical studies in Thailand have found pumpkin to re-

duce substances that promote stone formation and increase those that in-hibit stone formation.[24] Pumpkin seeds contain high levels of zinc, free fatty acids, vitamin E, and sterols that have been found to play a role in re-ducing BPH.

Asian Psyllium Seed

All plantains (American or Asian), seeds or otherwise, are diuretic, demul-cent, anti-inflammatory, and antimicrobial. They help relax and soothe mu-cous membrane systems and help flush stones from the body.

Pyrrosia

Pyrrosia, deer's tongue fern, is also called stone reed in some Chinese com-munities for its historical use in reducing kidney and urethral stones. It is also a diuretic and helps flush out stones.

Lysimachia

Lysimachia has been found to be specific for inhibiting stone formation, es-pecially calcium oxalate stones. It reduces the formation of stone nuclei and has been found in numerous studies to reduce stone size and promote passage from the body.[25]

KIDNEY STONE TINCTURE MIX

This tincture is a mixture of gravel root, stone root, and pellitory of the wall. If you have trouble finding this mixture, you may simply buy an ounce tinc-ture of each, mix together, and use as directed. If you cannot find pellitory of the wall, substitute corn silk.

Gravel root

Gravel root (*Eupatorium purpureum*) has been used in American botanical medicine for three hundred years and by Native Americans long before that. It helps break up kidney stones and promote their removal from the system.

Stone root

Stone root (*Collinsonia canadensis*) is considered to be an antilithic. That is, it both prevents and breaks down stones in the kidneys and urinary tract. It is a diuretic, helping move liquids through the system. It has been used in American botanical medicine for centuries.

Pellitory of the wall

Pellitory of the wall (*Parietaria diffusa*) is an herb long used in English botanical medicine for soothing and relaxing the urinary system. It is a diuretic and a demulcent, helping promote water excretion and soothing mucous membrane systems.

Dosage of the tincture mixture

Take 1.5 teaspoons three times a day.

WILD YAM

Wild yam (*Dioscorea villosa*) is a tremendously effective herb for calming muscle spasms in smooth-muscle systems. It helps calm the urinary passages, allowing the stone to pass more easily with less pain.

Dosage

Take 1 to 2 milliliters (¼ to ½ teaspoon) three times a day.

BLACK COHOSH

Black cohosh (*Cimicifuga racemosa*) may be of benefit if you are experiencing extreme pain and cannot get to a physician or hospital. Some people feel it is as effective as opiates, others find it has only a minor impact, similar to a beer. Given its strong impacts on estrogen levels, it should be used for only a limited duration.

Dosage

Take ¼ to 1 teaspoon as needed for pain, up to four times a day.

WATER

The more water you drink, the faster the stones will pass, especially if you are drinking diuretic teas as well.

HOT BATHS AND COMPRESSES

Baths, as hot as you can stand them, and hot compresses applied to the painful area have been found to help both the pain and the passage of stones. A few drops of lavender oil in the water can help calm things as well.[26]

INCONTINENCE

Incontinence, or the inability to hold urine, can take a number of forms— from mild dribbling to the uncontrolled, spontaneous release of urine when the bladder is full.

Mild dribbling is often a sign of prostate problems or a weak sphincter. Complete release, on the other hand, usually occurs when control over the sphincter is lost. Whenever the bladder contains 250 milliliters (8 ounces) or more of urine, the brain is told the bladder is full and the urge to urinate enters the conscious mind. During extreme incontinence the sphincters simply relax, and that is that.

Overall, the best herb for this condition is mullein root. For those in middle age, or even the very old, it increases both sphincter tone and control.

Natural Care for Incontinence

For One to Six Months
    Mullein root, ¼ to 1 teaspoon, up to four times a day
    Corn, 4 ounces of juice (including the silk) daily as a tonic

MULLEIN ROOT

Mullein (*Verbascum* species), originally a European native, has hitchhiked throughout the world and is now thoroughly naturalized almost everywhere. It is a biannual plant—that is, it lives two years. The first year it grows close to the ground in what is called a basal rosette—a flat circular whorl of leaves. The second year it sends a stalk, depending on the species, up to ten feet tall. The stalk is topped with a sort of corncoblike flowering head, a flower for each "kernel" of the cob. Each developed kernel is filled with millions of tiny black seeds, all seeking out disturbed ground with European insistence. The leaves are soft and fuzzy and well deserve their common name of Indian toilet paper, though of course anyone can (and does) use them. The flowers, steeped in oil, are a reliable, externally applied medicinal for children's ear infections and the leaves are highly effective for bronchitis and other lung problems. The root of the plant, however, is one of the best remedies for improving tone and control of the sphincter muscles of the bladder. It seems equally useful for the mild problems associated with dribbling and the severe incontinence of aged relatives in nursing homes. The only problem I have found with the herb is convincing a nursing home staff to allow its use.

Irritatingly, given the usefulness of the plant, the root, in any form, can be hard to find. See the Resources section. Chinese dogwood may be of some benefit here as well. It has been found effective for this for centuries in traditional Chinese medicine (see "Infertility").

Dosage
Take ¼ to 1 teaspoon of the tincture up to four times day.

WEAK URINE STREAM

This often occurs from an inflamed prostate or weak sphincter. An inflamed prostate creates a condition known in previous times as strangury. The prostate has inflamed and is crushing, or "strangling," the urethra where it passes through the prostate. So you strain and push and very little comes out in the end. For this condition, see Chapter 3 under Inflamed Prostate. If your prostate is fine then try mullein root as discussed under incontinence.

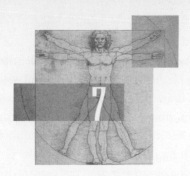

Flexibility: Bones, Joints, Muscles, and Tendons

It's only when we are relaxed that the thing way down deep in all of us—call it the subconscious mind, the spirit, what you will—has a chance to well up and tell us how we shall go. —FRANCES PERKINS

The only two known forms of life whose eyes and necks move at the same time are German generals and owls. —PETER USTINOV

Most of us do not know where we are going when we are young and so we end up in the places that fate deposits us. We find jobs, careers, and families in those places; we buy homes and fill them with the accumulation of years of human living. It becomes harder to move with each passing decade, harder to let go of the accumulated material of life, harder to box it up, cart it around, take it with us. At the same time, our interior worlds have filled up as well. Habits, beliefs, perspectives, attitudes, and thoughts accumulate by the thousands. Our minds and emotions are less flexible; we begin to suffer from hardening of the opinions. We stiffen, become less flexible, begin to dry out. James Hillman makes an interesting point when he says that perhaps some of the aging process is a kind of boiling. We are moist in early life, then like a chemical solution, we are heated by life, the water evaporates and what is left is the essential us, concentrated. The bare bones. Our character revealed.

This stiffening and drying process can become an irritant and like all irritations can cause inflammation. It is not unusual in middle age to one day look around at all the stuff our younger selves accumulated and wonder what the hell we were thinking. It is not unusual to discover that that particular couch or chair, while lovely fifteen years ago, no longer reflects who we have now become. So, a purging process begins. We begin to lighten up—to drop some of our load. Some habits of mind, ruts of character may begin to go as well. And we may begin to notice that this stiffness and inflexibility has not been limited to habits of living, mind, and emotion but has spilled over into our bodies as well. We may have garbage cluttering up our joints or our ability to move may have become impaired. Sometimes we decide to do something about it.

THE BONES

Our bones are not that different from the other cellular structures of our bodies—there are cells and there are spaces between the cells. The primary difference is that in bones collagen is laid down in fibers throughout the intercellular fluid and calcium salts harden around the collagen like a cement. The collagen fibers perform much the same function as the metal reinforcing rods in concrete walls; they strengthen the bones tremendously and still allow a certain amount of flex.

Cartilage is also collagen dependent and is very similar to bone except that calcium salts are not used. Instead, *glycosaminoglycans,* substances that become more like a firm gel, are laid down around the collagen. A particular substance in the gel, *hyaluronic acid,* gives it its unique viscous quality. The result is a much more flexible, and cushioning, substance—usually it is used to cushion the places where bones connect, such as finger joints or the vertebrae in the back.

Our human bones are very similar to the wood in trees (which use lignin instead of calcium between cells) and our bones also possesses concentric layers or rings. Just like trees, our bones are alive and like trees they possess channels through which blood (human sap) flows. All the thousands of living bone cells embedded within the calcified intercellular matrix need to have a constant supply of blood to remain healthy.

If you have ever seen the interior of an old bone you might have noticed that it looks something like a sponge. (When living, this part of a bone actually is somewhat spongy and flexible.) There is a seemingly fragile network of lacey-looking bone—bone with thousands of tiny holes throughout. Normally, in living bone, the spaces between the lace would be filled with vital, living cells. The hard, lacey, spongelike material is the calcified intercellular matrix. This is all that is left when the living cells die and decompose.

This "sponge" is surrounded by a harder, denser layer of exterior bone and often, with certain kinds of bones (so-called *long bones*), there will be a hollow interior as well. The hollow interior is filled with bone marrow, the substance from which all red and some white blood cells are made. The white blood cells that are made are called *stem* cells and are the basic immune cells of the body. These are altered in different organ systems into other types of immune cells depending on what is needed. (Some of these stem cells also flow to damaged hearts and are made into new heart muscle.) The red blood cells, the calcium salts that make up the intercellular matrix, and the hard exterior of bones are all managed by the kidneys. The kidneys release hormones that are designed to maintain the density and composition of bones and the number of red blood cells the bone marrow makes.

Besides strengthening our bodies, the bones act as a mineral storage system. Calcium, manganese, potassium, and magnesium are stored in the bone and can be withdrawn when needed elsewhere in our bodies. Each week the body cycles about 7 percent of this bone mass—bone material is constantly being removed and replaced, mostly through hormonal action of the kidneys and the parathyroid and thyroid glands. Cells called *osteoclasts* constantly travel through bone tissue, monitoring its level of health. When they encounter old bone, they dissolve and reabsorb it, which leaves a tiny cavity in its place. Other cells, *osteoblasts*, come along later, enter these spaces, and make new bone tissue.

OSTEOPOROSIS

If the amount of bone being reabsorbed exceeds the amount of bone being made, a well-known condition called osteoporosis (porous bone) occurs. The bones become less dense and weaker because there is less "cement" between the living cellular tissue. If the bone becomes weak enough, it can fracture from even a simple stress. The bones that tend to become weakest, because of their structure, are the hips, wrists, shoulders, neck, and spine. About twenty million people in the United States have some form of osteoporosis; about one-third of them are men.

While women and men both begin losing bone mass at about the same age (forty), women, because their bones are smaller to begin with, experience breakage much sooner. However, by age eighty men's bones begin breaking much more frequently and with much more serious consequences. Death for men over age seventy-five from hip fractures is nearly 30 percent, in women it is only 8 percent. There are about 1,500,000 breaks from osteoporosis each year, 250,000 of them of the hip.

While decreased estrogen in women has been tied to bone loss, in men, decreases in androgen levels are one of the primary causes. In fact, decreased androgen levels are the primary indicator in men of osteoporosis. Studies have shown that increasing androgen levels (especially free testosterone) increases bone density and decreases the chances of fracture.[1] Higher levels of DHEA, a mild androgen, increase osteoblast formation and activity, thus supporting new bone formation. The stromal cells of the bone marrow where osteoblasts are made, in fact, contain a large number of testosterone receptors. Not only does free testosterone increase osteoblast production but DHEA is converted at that cellular site into testosterone in order to keep osteoblast/osteoclast activity balanced.

While DHEA is most often made in the adrenals that sit on top of the kidneys, calcitriol, another important bone hormone, is made in the kidneys themselves. Calcitriol is a kidney-converted form of vitamin D that is fifty times more powerful than vitamin D in affecting the body's uptake of calcium and its transport to the bones for bone formation. A significant number of people with osteoporosis have been found to be deficient in calcitriol.[2] Usually these people also show increased levels of cortisol.

High cortisol levels decrease testosterone and stimulate the loss of bone mass from the body. Cortisol decreases the formation and activity of osteoblasts and increases osteoclast activity. Prescription use of corticosteroids, basically synthetic cortisones, often initiates severe bone loss and significantly reduced adrenal androgen levels.

Normally, in women, estrogen supplementation is the treatment that is used to slow osteoporosis. Estrogen slows down bone loss by interfering with osteoclast activity. It seems to regulate the sensitivity of osteoclasts to *parathyroid hormone* (PTH), which is made in the parathyroid glands (two paired glands within the thyroid gland in the neck). PTH is a hormone that increases the activity of osteoclasts, the bone-scavenging cells of the body. Estrogen, by inhibiting PTH sensitivity, slows them down considerably. Still, this is only part of the solution. Androgens are needed to stimulate osteoblast activity and hence the formation of new bone so that bones continue to be dense and strong. Testosterone supplementation in women (as well as men) has been found to significantly increase bone mass and density.

Natural Care for Osteoporosis

For Four to Twelve Months

Androgen supplementation, 25 to 50 milligrams of DHEA minimum daily

Nettle, 300 to 1,200 milligrams daily

Calcium, 250 to 500 milligrams daily

Magnesium, 200 to 600 milligrams daily

Manganese, 5 to 20 milligrams daily

Vitamin K, 100 micrograms to 2 milligrams daily

Vitamin B complex (especially B_6, B_{12}, folic acid), 1 to 2 tablets daily

Boron, 1 to 3 milligrams daily

Vitamin D_3, 400 international units daily

Resistance exercise (e.g., weight lifting)

Dietary additions and considerations

ANDROGEN SUPPLEMENTATION

An androgen replacement/balancing protocol is important for men who are showing signs of osteoporosis. Increases in free testosterone levels have consistently been linked to greater bone density in both men and women.[3] At the very least, DHEA should be added to the diet regularly. Studies have shown that the amount of serum osteocalcin doubles during DHEA supplementation, bone density at the hip increases, and plasma bone alkaline phosphatase and hydroxyproline all decrease. A number of studies have found that DHEA levels are low in people with osteoporosis and that DHEA supplementation increases bone density and mass. Because DHEA is converted by the body into either testosterone or estrogen, depending on bodily needs, it can slow down bone loss while at the same time stimulating bone formation.[4]

Dosage
Take 25 to 50 milligrams daily.

Nettle
Nettles are high in silicon, calcium, magnesium, phosphorus, potassium, zinc, manganese, selenium, and vitamins D, K, and B—in short, nearly everything needed for healthy bones. Nettle, as an additional bonus, helps keep testosterone levels from falling, thus enhancing bone formation.

Dosage
Take 300 to 1,200 milligrams of nettles daily.

CALCIUM

Calcium is needed for bone calcification. However, studies indicate that vitamin D, calcium-enriched milk does not help bone mineralization, density, and strength. One particularly large study showed that women who drank milk suffered higher levels of osteoporosis and broken bones. Of 77,661 nurses, those who drank two or more glasses of milk per day had a 45 percent higher risk of hip fracture. (Everybody does not need milk.)[5]

Calcium is better assimilated from natural food sources; the body seems to take it in more efficiently. Green leafy vegetables that contain calcium and vitamin K are best: kale, spinach, turnip greens, spirulina, chlorella, nettles, and (not green) tofu. If you do wish to use a supplement, consider calcium/magnesium citrate. It supplies both magnesium and calcium (both good for bones) and citrate, which has been found to help in preventing kidney stones.

Dosage
Take 250 to 500 milligrams daily.

MAGNESIUM

Magnesium intake increases bone mass and reduces abnormal bone formation and is essential in the formation of healthy bones. A number of studies have found that people with osteoporosis generally have lower levels of magnesium in their bodies. Increasing supplemental magnesium has been found to increase bone formation and density.[6]

Dosage
Take 200 to 600 milligrams daily.

Cautions
Magnesium is usually well tolerated; however, people with certain kinds of severe heart disease, such as high-grade atrioventricular block, should only use magnesium under the supervision of a health-care provider.

MANGANESE

Bones have relatively high concentrations of manganese and need this element for strong formation.

Dosage
Take 5 to 20 milligrams daily.

VITAMIN K

Vitamin K is needed to manufacture osteocalcin, a bone protein that attracts calcium to bone tissue. K deficiency has been found to impair the body's ability to mineralize bone.

Dosage
Take 100 micrograms to 2 milligrams daily.

VITAMIN B COMPLEX

Vitamin B complex, especially vitamins B_6, B_{12}, and folic acid, prevents the buildup of homocysteine, a triggering factor for osteoporosis (and a risk factor for heart disease) and, possibly, Alzheimer's disease.

Dosage
Take 1 to 2 tablets daily.

BORON

Boron enhances production of bone tissue and the compounds that support healthy bone formation: DHEA, testosterone, estrogen, and vitamin D. Osteoporosis is generally unknown in areas of the world where high boron levels exist in the soil.

Dosage
Take 1 to 3 milligrams daily.

VITAMIN D$_3$

Vitamin D$_3$, also called cholecalciferol, is a member of the vitamin D family that enables the body to utilize calcium and phosphorus and to assimilate vitamin A. Several studies have found that vitamin D$_3$ reduces the rate of osteoporosis and that supplementation actually increases bone density.

Dosage
Take 400 international units daily.

Cautions
Too much vitamin D$_3$ (more than 1,300 international units per day) can lead to an overabsorption of calcium and may adversely affect liver and kidney function.

EXERCISE

Bones form, in part, in response to pressure. The bones in any area of the body that experience increased pressure will become more dense in response. Gravity itself provides some of this pressure, any kind of exercise creates more. This is why weight lifting has been found to help counteract osteoporosis. In one study, seventy-year-old infirm men who engaged in powerlifting three times per week (for only *fifteen* minutes each time) showed significant improvement in mobility, balance, bone density, and flexibility. Men who had formerly only been able to walk with canes no longer needed them. Outcomes were even better if androgen supplements were also taken regularly. One of the best things about this study is that it shows how very little exercise is needed to produce benefits.[7]

DIETARY ADDITIONS AND CONSIDERATIONS

Again, eat a good diet with lots of calcium-containing foods. Especially important are green leafy vegetables, which also contain vitamin K: kale, spinach, turnip greens, spirulina and chlorella, and nettles, as well as tofu.

Avoid sugar, corticosteroids, high protein, and cola drinks. All have been shown to promote bone loss. The body buffers the increased acidity that occurs from high protein intake by pulling calcium out of the bones. This becomes a problem if there is too little calcium in the diet and osteoblast activity is low. Phosphorus, which is very high in cola drinks, has been found to cause bone loss as well by causing calcium to leach out of the bones. Several studies have shown correlations between bone breaks and high cola (and other soft) drink consumption.[8]

ARTHRITIS

Arthritis means "joint inflammation" but is more often used to refer to over one hundred different types of inflammatory or degenerative diseases of joints and connective tissue. The two most common types are rheumatoid and osteoarthritis.

Osteoarthritis is a degenerative joint disease and the most common form of arthritis, affecting 80 percent of all people over seventy years of age. In the disease, a variety of factors cause damage to both the cartilage and the joints and begin a degenerative process accompanied by pain, stiffness, and deformation of the joints. Rheumatoid arthritis results from an inflammation of the synovia, a thin, smooth membrane that lines the joints. A persistent inflammation, from unknown causes, occurs in the synovia leading, eventually, to permanent damage to the cartilage, bones, ligaments, and tendons. Some forty million people in the United States suffer from osteoarthritis, about three million from rheumatoid arthritis.

Osteoarthritis is intimately connected to the same types of processes that cause osteoporosis. This is because cartilage, just like bone, is regularly reprocessed. Old cartilage is constantly being dismantled and replaced utilizing a very similar process to that which occurs in the bones.

Cartilage, over time, becomes somewhat like a rubber band that has gotten old and begun to lose its elasticity. It cannot stretch as well, does not return to its original shape as quickly, and small cracks begin appearing throughout its length. When cartilage weakens in such a way, it is removed and replaced. When new cartilage is not created as quickly as the old is wearing out, problems begin to occur.

When the tears and nicks in old cartilage are not repaired they can become inflamed. The inflammation signals the body that the cartilage needs attention and so chemicals such as *elastase* are released to speed up the breakdown of the old cartilage, preparing the site for new cartilage to form. However, if new cartilage does not form fast enough, the problem gets even worse. While the old cartilage is broken down more quickly there is less and less healthy cartilage in the joints. This puts even more wear on the cartilage, leading to more inflammation and more breakdown. Eventually, the affected joint can become locked, incapable of movement.

Until recently most people have used nonsteroidal anti-inflammatory drugs (NSAIDs) for arthritis pain. One hundred million pounds of aspirin are ingested worldwide each year; one billion aspirin tablets are taken yearly in the United States. Aspirin and other NSAIDs can often have severe side effects; over one hundred thousand people are admitted to hospitals each year from complications of using NSAIDs; twenty thousand people are estimated to die from their use. NSAIDs such as aspirin work because they decrease the body's *prostaglandin* production, the substance primarily responsible for joint inflammation, by decreasing the activity of the body's *cyclooxygenase* (COX) enzymes. Unfortunately, prostaglandins are also essential in maintaining the health of the stomach lining and kidneys. The kidneys need prostaglandins for dilating their internal blood vessels. This boosts their ability to filter blood and maintain bodily homeostasis. NSAIDs lower the effectiveness of the kidneys and as a result, in the long run, can exacerbate a number of pathological conditions. NSAIDs commonly damage the lining of the stomach and cause serious gastric bleeding.

Another reason that aspirin has so many negative actions is that COX is not simply a single enzyme. There is a COX-1, a COX-2, and, researchers now think, many others. COX-1 is essential to kidney function and to the health of the digestive system while COX-2 is concerned more with prostaglandin production. Aspirin affects both COX enzymes. The newest medications for arthritis are COX-2 inhibitors. They are thought to just affect prostaglandin inflammatory processes without having the same negative effects on the stomach lining and kidneys that aspirins do. Unfortunately, newer findings are revealing that COX-2, like COX-1, is an essential enzyme in the body. It is needed to maintain healthy homeostasis in the brain, reproductive system, and kidneys. COX-2 has crucial roles in regulating the bodily levels of salt and water, body temperature, and immune function. COX-2 inhibitors, by generally decreasing COX-2 activity throughout the body, are now known to have widespread impacts throughout the body, including slowing the healing of gastric ulcers and exacerbating colitis and dyspepsia (severe gastric indigestion).[9] In response to emerging research, Sandor Szabo, M.D., of the University of California Irvine commented that, "[Synthetic COX-2 inhibitors (such as Celebrex and Vioxx)] definitely aren't as clean as they were promised to be."[10]

Natural treatment of osteoarthritis approaches the problem from three perspectives: (1) reducing inflammation, (2) repairing the cartilage, and (3) rebalancing the cartilage removal/replacement process. Aspirin and the more specific COX-2 inhibitors do nothing to address numbers 2 or 3, they simply reduce inflammation. Natural care alternatives for OA can reduce inflammation and alleviate pain just as well as COX-2 inhibitors or NSAIDs but they also will stimulate collagen renewal and rebalance the collagen maintenance process.

A Note About Rheumatoid Arthritis

During the progression of rheumatoid arthritis (RA) a general, COX-2-initiated inflammation occurs in the joints from no known cause. This chronic inflammation, over time, can, because of the constant irritation, turn into osteoarthritis as the cartilage begins to break down. Natural treatment of RA can reduce inflammation, protect cartilage from breakdown, and work to rebalance the body. Some common factors that have been found in most people with RA are: low DHEA levels, abnormal bowel permeability (leaky gut syndrome), unhealthy microbial community in the bowel, and abnormal immune function. Treatment for both osteoarthritis and rheumatoid arthritis is very similar. However, adding DHEA and selenium and altering the structure of the diet are exceptionally important for RA.

Natural Care for Arthritis

For Three to Twelve Months

Ginger (capsules), 3 to 7 grams (3,000 to 7,000 milligrams) daily
(or a curcumin/bromelain combination [on an empty stomach]
400 to 500 milligrams, three times daily)

Devil's claw, 1,000 to 2,000 milligrams, three times a day

Nettle (freeze-dried extract), 1,200 milligrams daily

Capsaicin cream (topical), four times daily as needed

Pregnenolone, 50 to 200 milligrams daily

DHEA, 50 to 200 milligrams daily (especially for RA)

Glucosamine sulfate, 500 milligrams three times a day

SAM-e (*S-adenosyl-methionine*), 200 to 400 milligrams daily (*Note:* Must
be taken with vitamin B complex)

Alpha lipoic acid, 600 milligrams daily (especially for RA)

Selenium, 200 micrograms daily (especially for RA)

Vitamin B complex, daily, should include B_5, B_6, B_{12}, and folic acid)

Vitamin C, 1,000 to 3,000 milligrams daily

Vitamin E, 400 to 800 international units daily

Water, 4 to 6 glasses per day

Arthritis tea if desired daily

GINGER

Ginger (*Zingiber officinale*) has been found to be a very useful anti-inflammatory for arthritis. In one trial in India, researchers gave people with osteoarthritis or rheumatoid arthritis 3 to 7 grams (1½ to 3½ teaspoons) of ginger per day. Seventy-five percent of those taking it reported relief from arthritis symptoms and a reduction in swelling. Another study with people with RA found that no matter how the herb was prepared (fresh, dried, or partly cooked) and no matter the dosage, all people reported substantial pain relief, joint mobility, swelling relief, and less morning stiffness.

Ginger has consistently demonstrated a minimum of a 56 percent inhibition of inflammatory prostaglandins and also inhibits other inflammatory compounds such as thromboxanes and leukotrienes (which makes it useful for both irritable bowel and inflammatory bowel disease). Because it stimulates microcirculation, it helps increase blood flow to the joints, enhancing repair of the cartilage. Ginger also contains melatonin, a natural hormone made in the brain, which helps regulate the body's circadian rhythms and promotes sleep. And it has been found to act as a natural COX-2 inhibitor. Irrespective of the amounts ingested, no side effects have been found.[11]

Dosage
Take 3 to 7 grams daily.

A CURCUMIN/BROMELAIN COMBINATION

Curcumin is a compound isolated from turmeric; bromelain is a complex of enzymes isolated from pineapple. Both have shown significant anti-inflammatory activity in the treatment of RA and osteoarthritis in numerous clinical trials. Hundreds of articles have appeared exploring their use.[12] Both have been found to be superior to the pharmaceutical phenylbutazone and they are exceptionally safe even in large doses. If you prefer to use these isolated compounds, they can be purchased as a combination or separately.

Some of the more interesting combinations that are available include curcumin, bromelain, ginger, and guggul (or gugulipid extract). Guggul (*Comiphora mukul*) is one of the primary herbs used for the treatment of arthritis in Indian Ayurvedic medicine. It also has been found to be effective in numerous clinical trials and several thousand years of traditional Indian practice.

You can also add liberal amounts of turmeric and pineapple to the diet. The anti-inflammatory juice drink listed under "Bursitis and Tendinitis" is a good way to take them both.

Dosage
Take 400 to 600 milligrams of curcumin three times daily. Take 250 to 750 milligrams of bromelain three times daily. Take twenty minutes or so before meals. Combination dosages depend on the particular formulation. As examples: One widely available formulation contains 350 milligrams cur-

cumin and 50 milligrams bromelain (suggested dosage 2 capsules three times a day); another contains 250 milligrams curcumin (standardized turmeric), bromelain 250 milligrams, ginger root powder 500 milligrams, and gugulipid 35 milligrams (suggested dosage 2 capsules, three times daily). See Resource section for sources.

DEVIL'S CLAW

Devil's claw (*Harpagophytum procumbens*) is an African herb used for centuries in the treatment of arthritis. A number of clinical trials have found the herb to be as powerful as the pharmaceutical phenylbutazone. The herb contains a compound, harpagoside, that is specific for joint inflammation. For some types of arthritis and at lower doses the herb has only minimal effectiveness. I have found it of most benefit for osteoarthritis.[13]

Dosage
Take 1,000 to 2,000 milligrams (1 to 2 grams), three times a day.

NETTLE

Nettle (*Urtica dioica*) is high in calcium and silicon. It possesses specific actions on the male reproductive system and kidneys. Numerous studies have found that not only does nettle possess powerful nutrients and compounds for joint and bone health, it possesses specific anti-inflammatory actions as well. Historically, its use entailed running the hands or affected area through living nettles, allowing the body to be "stung." Each hairlike "sting" of a nettle plant is actually a pressure-filled botanical hypodermic. Touching the sting breaks off the tip and allows the contents of the sting to be forcibly injected under the skin. The compounds in the nettle sting are exceptionally similar to that in bee venom (which has been successfully used in scores of clinical trials in Europe for arthritis). These nettle compounds are strongly anti-inflammatory.

Most people are not willing to sting themselves these days, but the compounds can be had just as well by taking a freeze-dried nettle extract (or drinking nettle beer, for millennia a common spring tonic or "diet" beer in

Europe). When boiling the plant, most of the sting compounds dissolve into the water, which is why nettle beer was so strongly beneficial for arthritic complaints.

Another reason for nettle's effectiveness in arthritic diseases is that it inhibits elastase.[14] Elastase, a natural substance in the body, is used to degrade elastin, cartilage, collagen, and fibronectin. This can cause serious problems in the joints, skin, and lungs if elastase activity becomes elevated, which it does during osteoarthritis.

The herb also contains high levels of boron, which the Rheumatoid Arthritis Foundation recommends (3 milligrams daily) for those with RA or OA.

Dosage

Take 1,200 milligrams of freeze-dried extract daily. The plant, if you have access to it fresh, can be steamed and eaten like spinach. It loses its sting on steaming or boiling. Wear gloves when harvesting. The steamed juice can be saved and used as a daily tea.

Cautions

Mild side effects have occasionally been reported with the root, usually mild gastrointestinal upset. With the plant, only mild side effects are noted: skin afflictions such as rashes and mild swelling. *The Physicians' Desk Reference for Herbal Medicines* lists a contraindication for the plant in cases of fluid retention from reduced cardiac or renal action. No contraindications are noted for the root.

CAPSAICIN CREAM

Capsaicin is a compound found in hot peppers (*Capsicum* species). Capsaicin stimulates the body to release its natural pain-relieving compounds, endorphins. Several over-the-counter (OTC) creams are available that contain capsaicin (Zostrix or Capzasin-P, for example). These kinds of creams have been found to be effective in reducing arthritic pain. One study showed a reduction in RA pain by one-half and in OA pain by one-third.[15]

Dosage

Topical application up to four times daily if needed.

Cautions

Don't rub your eyes or touch other sensitive mucous membranes after applying these creams. Wash your hands thoroughly. If you don't, the first thing you know you will be reading a book, unconsciously rubbing an eyelid, and a few minutes later, find yourself racing for the bathroom.

PREGNENOLONE

Pregnenolone was one of the earliest medical treatments for both OA and RA and was commonly prescribed by physicians in the 1950s. After the arrival of synthetic cortisones, the exploration into pregnenolone's benefits on arthritis unfortunately ceased. Pregnenolone has shown specific beneficial activity for a wide range of connective tissue disorders: ankolysing spondylitis, systemic lupus, OA and RA, and scleroderma. All these diseases are concerned with improper collagen formation, deterioration, or inflammation. Because DHEA (made in the body from pregnenolone) has also been found effective in treatment of collagen or connective tissue diseases (and gout) and because these diseases are so closely connected to kidney maintenance of bones and body homeostasis, there seems to be support for recognizing that osteoporosis, OA, and possibly RA are connected to hormonal (estrogen/androgen) imbalances in the body.

Numerous studies in the 1950s commonly found that people who take pregnenolone can experience significant alleviation of arthritic symptoms, generally less pain, more mobility, and less stiffness. In the five studies I have reviewed, about one-third of the people experienced a near complete remission of symptoms, one-third had marked improvement, and one-third showed no benefit. Improvement was generally seen within sixty days. The longer pregnenolone was taken in the studies, the longer benefits lasted after supplementation ceased. Pregnenolone exerts direct effects on the body's capillaries, skin, collagen formation, and mucous membranes. In treatment of scleroderma (a hardening of the skin), pregnenolone was found to soften the skin, increasing elasticity and texture. Pregnenolone also tends to produce an increased sense of well-being, more energy, better appetite, and enhanced memory.[16]

Dosage
Take 50 to 500 milligrams daily.

Cautions
At higher doses, pregnenolone can cause agitation and overstimulation. The best average dosing for arthritic complaints seems to be 100 to 200 milligrams daily.

DHEA

DHEA has been found to be especially low in people with rheumatoid arthritis. In clinical trials with people suffering lupus (a collagen, connective tissue disease), 200 milligrams daily of DHEA was found to decrease symptoms, pain, progression of the disease, and need for corticosteroids. There were far fewer flare-ups in those taking DHEA than in the placebo group. If you have RA, then DHEA is something you should definitely consider.[17]

Dosage
Take 50 to 200 milligrams daily.

Cautions
Higher dosage levels are contraindicated for adolescent males.

Cautions
Some clinicians think DHEA can exacerbate the mania stage of manic depression, others believe it is contraindicated for men whose PSA (prostate-specific antigen—an indicator for prostate disease level) is high. The only literature-noted side effect is masculinization (facial hair, etc.) in some women and the case of one woman who developed jaundice and liver problems after one week of use. It is not known if the latter side effect was related to the use of DHEA. Women seem most at risk of side effects.

GLUCOSAMINE SULFATE (GS)

Glucosamine, naturally produced by the body, is used to stimulate the body's production of glycosaminoglycans. These are the compounds that give cartilage its rubberlike nature. As people age they tend to produce less GS, which results in poorer cartilage formation. This becomes especially problematic in joints that receive a lot of wear and tear: hips, knees, hands, neck, and back. The great strength of GS is that it promotes the regeneration and replacement of cartilage. A number of controlled, double-blind trials (with up to 1,500 people at a time) have been conducted and GS has been found to be highly effective in the treatment of osteoarthritis. While those who were taking strong analgesics experienced relief more quickly, those who were taking GS pulled ahead after four weeks. The longer GS was taken, the better the results. The trial results indicated that GS appears to address the underlying symptoms and actually cures the condition, something pain medications do not do.[18] Those taking the supplement found (after four weeks) less pain, better mobility, less stiffness, and an expanded sense of well-being. Ninety-five percent of those taking GS report benefits. Normally, GS needs to be taken at least four weeks to show benefit; the longer it is taken, the longer benefits last after ceasing use.

Dosage
Take 500 milligrams three times a day.

About Chondroitin Sulfate and Echinacea
Although chondroitin sulfate (CS) has been touted for this same use, evidence indicates it is not very effective. Some research has shown that while GS absorption into the body is generally higher than 90 percent, CS is often 13 percent or less. A majority of practitioners now recommend GS over CS for that reason.

Echinacea, while rarely prescribed for either RA or OA, may in fact be a good herb to use in the treatment of both conditions. Because it interferes with the breakdown of hyaluronic acid by inhibiting the enzyme *hyaluronidase,* it keeps the cartilage between joints viscous. At least five published studies in Europe have supported its effectiveness in the treatment of RA.[19] Echinacea's effectiveness presumably comes from three different actions: its support of hyaluronic acid, its anti-inflammatory activity, and its impacts on stimulating immune function. Up to half an ounce of tincture per day is normally used in acute conditions. (See also "Bursitis and Tendinitis," below.)

SAM-E

SAM-e (*S-adenosyl-methionine*), like GS, has been found to specifically help generate the formation of new cartilage. Magnetic resonance imaging (MRI) scans have actually shown that SAM-e increases the amount of cartilage in the joints of people with osteoarthritis of the hands. SAM-e is made by the body from the essential amino acid methionine (obtained from protein-rich foods) and adenosyl-triphosphate (ATP). The body uses SAM-e to increase the production of chondrocytes, cartilage producing cells in the joints. SAM-e also helps prevent the breakdown of proteoglycans, molecules in cartilage that retain water, keeping the cartilage moist and flexible.

SAM-e is also exceptionally active in methylation, an ongoing process in the body intimately connected to brain, bone, and heart health. During methylation, one compound gives up a "methyl group" (four connected atoms) to another. SAM-e is the most active methyl donor yet discovered in the body. During this breakdown process, SAM-e metabolizes into homocysteine, a potentially harmful substance to the heart (and possibly the brain) if allowed to build up in tissues. However, in the presence of B vitamins (especially B_6, B_{12}, and folic acid) homocysteine remethylates into methionine again or is converted to glutathione (see "Alpha Lipoic Acid").

SAM-e has been successfully used in Europe for the past twenty years in the treatment of arthritic conditions. Scores of studies with over twenty thousand people have shown that it is highly effective in helping reverse OA and RA and in protecting cartilage. Because of its impacts on methylation, it has also been found to affect brain function—its first use was as an antidepressant. It was only after physicians noticed that their depressed arthritis patients were getting better that research turned to degenerative joint diseases. Most people who use SAM-e report enhanced feelings of well-being.[20]

Dosage
Take 200 to 400 milligrams daily.

Cautions
SAM-e must be taken with B-vitamin complex. Some people have reported nausea and vomiting at higher doses (400 milligrams three times daily) so start at 200 milligrams a day to see how you respond.

ALPHA LIPOIC ACID (ALA)

Alpha lipoic acid (ALA) is a powerful antioxidant, chelation agent, radioprotective agent, enzymatic catalyst, glutathione production stimulant, normalizer of blood sugar levels, neurotonic, and antiviral. It is exceptionally
potent in the liver as a protector and regenerator of liver tissue. It has also
been found to enhance energy, increase memory and mental clarity, and reduce joint inflammation.

ALA was isolated in 1951 from liver tissue. It turns out that human
cells, especially in the liver, naturally produce ALA, though as we grow
older we make less and less of it. In general, ALA does two things. It acts as
a helper, a co-enzyme, to our body's cells in utilizing energy—glucose. It
also is one of the most powerful antioxidants known that actually helps prevent damage to cells at the genetic level. Antioxidants protect our bodies
from the effects of free radicals. Vitamin C, a well-known antioxidant, is
very large and can only protect the cells from the outside. Because ALA is so
small, it can pass inside the cells and protect both the inside and outside
from the oxidative stress effects of free radicals. People with RA have been
found to consistently have lower levels of antioxidants in their bodies.

In a number of studies, German researchers have found ALA to be effective in the treatment of AIDS patients. After fourteen days of use they
found that plasma ascorbate and glutathione levels both increased. The
higher the level of glutathione, the lower the level of HIV. While ALA is itself directly antiviral against a number of viruses, glutathione is even more
effective. Research is indicating that glutathione is a powerful antiviral in
the body and is produced, in part, for that reason. It is highly synergistic
with selenium (its mineral cofactor) in carrying out antiviral actions. Interestingly, the majority of people with RA consistently have been found to
have low levels of both glutathione and selenium. This lends some cre-
dence to the persistent perspective that RA is initiated by viral factors. Many
people who have increased their glutathione levels through the use of ALA
or other glutathione enhancers have found that as body levels of glutathione (and selenium) rise, their symptoms disappear. For this reason, it
makes sense to use ALA (or another glutathione enhancer such as N-acetyl
cysteine) if you have RA. Glutathione also reduces the production of inflammatory prostaglandins and leukotrienes, which is one reason ALA has
been found to be directly effective in some cases of joint inflammation.[21]

Dosage

Take 600 milligrams daily.

Cautions

Diabetics should use only after review with their physician. ALA strongly affects blood sugar levels and will affect medical protocols. N-acetyl cysteine (NAC) is an effective substitute for ALA at 1,200 milligrams daily.

SELENIUM

Selenium is the cofactor of glutathione; it must be present for glutathione to be created in the body. It has also been found to be a powerful antiviral.

It is now known that a significant number of viruses (HIV, Epstein-Barr, influenza, and hepatitis C, for example) have developed strategies to destroy the body's selenium. As selenium levels fall, the natural antiviral actions of the body's selenium and glutathione decrease, allowing viral blooms to occur. People with RA generally have low levels of selenium and one study has shown that supplementation with selenium and vitamin E relieved symptoms of RA.[22]

Dosage

Take 200 micrograms daily.

Cautions

Selenium can be highly toxic. Although dosages can range as high as 400 micrograms per day, this may become toxic over the long run. The dosage range for safety should be between 50 and 200 micrograms daily. Signs of toxicity are nausea and vomiting and emotional instability. The metabolism of N-acetyl cysteine can deplete the body's zinc and copper, so take it with a zinc supplement that also includes copper.

VITAMIN B COMPLEX

Vitamin B complex is important because it is needed for GS to be properly processed in the body and to stop the buildup of homocysteine in tissues.

Low vitamin B_5 (pantothenic acid) levels have been found to cause a failure of healthy cartilage growth. For some people with OA, as little as 12.5 milligrams of B_5 daily have significantly reduced symptoms.[23] GS particularly needs B_6, B_{12}, and folic acid. Find a good B-complex that contains all of these.

Dosage
Take 1 to 2 tablets daily.

VITAMIN C

The vitamin C–dependent enzyme prolyl hydroxylase is the catalyst that enables collagen to form. Without vitamin C, prolyl hydroxylase cannot maintain activity, collagen cannot form fibers properly and bones, cartilage, and skin cannot heal efficiently. During collagen synthesis, vitamin C acts as an essential co-enzyme. For this reason collagen is usually high in vitamin C and deficiencies have been found to reduce cartilage repair and synthesis.

Dosage
Take 1,000 to 3,000 milligrams daily.

Cautions
Vitamin C at high doses will cause gas, flatulence, and, eventually, diarrhea. It is usually taken tbt or "to bowel tolerance" (sometimes tbd or "to bowel dose"). It is possible to build up tolerance to higher doses over time. It may also cause digestive disturbance; some physicians prefer giving it intravenously for this reason. While vitamin C can be useful in some kidney conditions, you should not use vitamin C if you are on hemodialysis, or suffer from recurrent kidney stones, severe kidney disease, or gout.

VITAMIN E

Because vitamin E potentiates both vitamin C and selenium in cartilage tissue, it is important to include.

Dosage
Take 400 to 800 international units daily.

WATER

We tend to dry out as we get older. While our wit benefits from this, cartilage does not. If you can imagine backbone cartilage as somewhat like tiny water balloons sitting in between the vertebrae, cushioning them from each other, you can get an idea of why water is important. Although the fluid is more of a gel, it needs water to retain its characteristics.

Dosage
Drink 4 to 6 glasses per day.

ARTHRITIS TEA

To make an arthritis tea, combine one pound dried, cut, and sifted (i.e., not whole or powdered) each of: nettles, horsetail, dandelion leaf, peppermint leaf, celery seed, turmeric, devil's claw, and meadowsweet and mix well. Add one cup of the mixed herbs to half a gallon of nearly boiling water and allow to steep covered overnight. Drink 3 to 4 cups daily.

Special Considerations for Rheumatoid Arthritis

Poor intestinal health has been found to be consistently present in people with RA and in some instances simply addressing the problem by helping the digestive system has produced significant improvement in symptoms. A significant number of people with RA have been found to have *small intestine bacterial overgrowth* (SIBO) and abnormal bowel permeability (leaky gut syndrome). A modified fasting program and a vegetarian/cold-water fish diet (e.g., mackerel, salmon, sardines, herring) have been found to alleviate both symptoms and the progression of RA. For more on this type of diet, see Chapter 11.

GOUT

The same uric acid that can form certain types of kidney stones can also concentrate in joints and cause gout. Although a number of joints can be affected, 90 percent of the time (no one knows why) it is in the big toe. The pain is as severe as kidney stones and as crippling. Even the weight of a bed sheet can be agony. Men suffer gout far more often than women.

As cells die and their DNA decomposes, purines (a part of DNA) are released and *they* decompose, in part, into uric acid. White blood cells, doing their normal scavenging to keep the body healthy, ingest them and release an enzyme that causes inflammation. This only becomes a problem if uric acid levels are very high. Normally, uric acid is excreted by the kidneys; however if levels are too high, the kidneys cannot excrete it fast enough, it builds up in the body, and an attack of gout (or uric acid kidney stones) can result.

Quite often a severe gout attack is initiated by a heavy night of drinking. You go to bed fine and wake up at three A.M. in acute agony. This is because high levels of alcohol significantly increase uric acid production through increasing purine breakdown. It also slows the effectiveness of the kidneys' ability to clear uric acid in the urine. This dynamic is often exacerbated in people who consume a high meat (or purine-rich) diet. The more meat you eat, the more uric acid the kidneys have to process. The primary treatment for gout is to reduce the intake of alcohol.

It usually takes a few agonizing days for a severe gout attack to subside. Other than pharmaceutical painkillers, the only immediate help for the pain is cold. Because it is so painful to put anything on the inflamed toe, the easiest approach is to soak the toe in ice-cold water. Large quantities of water and anti-uric acid herbs can help to decrease the duration of the episode. Long-term treatment is through diet alteration, enhancing kidney function, and the use of herbs that help eliminate uric acid from the body.

Natural Care for Gout

For One Week to Three Months
> Celery seed, 1 teaspoon tincture three times a day or 2 to 4 tablets daily
> Gravel root, ½ teaspoon tincture three times a day
> Devil's claw, 1 teaspoon tincture three times a day or 500 milligrams three times a day
> Nettle, 300 to 1,200 milligrams daily (or add to the diet)
> Java tea, 1 teaspoon steeped 15 minutes in 8 ounces of water, three times a day

Cherries (or equivalent), half a pound fresh or canned daily

Avoid alcohol

Avoid high purine foods (organ meats, red meat, shellfish, yeast, herring, mackerel, anchovies, mushrooms, peas, beans)

Avoid aspirin and niacin

Eat more fruits, vegetables, grains

Water, 48 ounces daily

CELERY SEED

Celery seed (*Apium graveolens*) is an antispasmodic, anti-inflammatory, and diuretic. It helps promote the excretion of uric acid from the body.

Dosage

Take 1 teaspoon of the tincture three times a day or 2 to 4 tablets daily.

GRAVEL ROOT

Gravel root (*Eupatorium purpureum*) has been used for at least three hundred years for the treatment of kidney stones and excess uric acid in the urine. It increases both urine flow and excretion of uric acid from the urine.

Dosage

Take ½ teaspoon of the tincture, three times daily.

DEVIL'S CLAW

Devil's claw (*Harpagophytum procumbens*) is a powerful herb for any inflammatory arthritic pain. It is powerfully anti-inflammatory and analgesic (comparable to the prescription drug phenylbutazone) and studies have found that it strongly promotes the excretion of uric acid from the body.

Dosage

Take 1 teaspoon of the tincture or 500 milligrams three times a day.

NETTLE

Nettles (*Urtica dioica*) have been found to lower uric acid levels and enhance kidney function in a number of studies.

Dosage
Take 300 to 1,200 milligrams daily or add to your diet.

Cautions
Mild side effects have occasionally been reported with the root, usually mild gastrointestinal upset. With the plant, only mild side effects are noted: skin afflictions such as rashes and mild swelling. *The Physicians' Desk Reference for Herbal Medicines* lists a contraindication for the plant in cases of fluid retention from reduced cardiac or renal action. No contraindications are noted for the root.

JAVA TEA

Numerous studies have found java tea (*Orthosiphon stamineus*) effective at enhancing kidney filtering and hormonal function, preventing uric acid buildup, and promoting uric acid excretion from the body. Java tea is best used as a tea.

Dosage
Steep one teaspoon of the dried herb for 15 to 20 minutes in 8 ounces hot water. Drink three cups per day.

CHERRIES

Cherries have been found to significantly lower uric acid levels and prevent recurrences of gout. Through a variety of mechanisms, the anthocyanidins in cherries help reduce inflammation and strengthen gout-prone areas of the body to better resist uric acid impacts. You can either eat a half pound of cherries daily (which quickly gets boring) or you can use a variety of other herbs or supplements instead. Hawthorn, bilberry, and blueberry are all effective and they possess tremendously beneficial actions for heart, brain, eyes, and ears as well. You can also use proanthocyanidin extracts made from pine bark or grape seed. These are all discussed in greater detail in other areas of the book; see the index for more information and dosages.

VEGETABLES, FRUITS, AND GRAINS

Adding vegetables, fruits, and grains to the diet (while reducing meats) will increase the alkalinity of the urine and reduce uric acid buildup.

WATER

The more water you drink, the more diluted the uric acid will be and the more easily it will be flushed from the body. Drink at least 48 ounces per day.

BURSITIS AND TENDINITIS

The bursae are viscous-fluid-filled sacs that help lubricate the joints in places where muscles and tendons meet bone. Bursitis occurs when these fluid-filled sacs become inflamed. The most affected areas are the shoulder (constant lifting), elbow (leaning on desks), knee (frequent kneeling), and hip. Tendinitis is an inflammation of a tendon, the strong elastic tissue that connects muscles to bones. The most commonly affected is the attachment of the biceps tendon at the shoulder. Both inflammations are painful and tend to limit movement.

The most immediate action you can take is to rest the injured joint or tendon, elevate it, and apply ice to reduce swelling. In the long run, finding ways to reduce impact on the joint or tendon, if at all possible, is essential.

Natural Care for Bursitis and Tendinitis

For One Week to Six Months
> Ginger, 100 to 300 milligrams three times a day
> Echinacea, 1 teaspoon tincture three times day
> Curcumin, 200 to 400 milligrams three times a day
> Bromelain, 250 to 750 milligrams three times a day
> Pine bark or grape seed extract (PCOs), 100 milligrams three times a day
> Pineapple, papaya, ginger, blueberry, turmeric juice, drink daily

GINGER

Ginger (*Zingiber officinale*) is a potent anti-inflammatory, analgesic, and blood circulatory stimulant. It has been found to be helpful for bursitis in a number of studies in Asia and contains many of the same powerful constituents (similar to bromelain) found in pineapple and papaya.[24] It can be used fresh or as tablets or capsules.

Dosage
Take 100 to 300 milligrams daily, up to 3 to 7 grams daily.

ECHINACEA

While echinacea (*Echinacea angustifolium, E. purpureum*) is most commonly known as an herb for colds, flu, and immune problems, it also has powerful actions on joints and connective tissue as well. Part of the way echinacea works is that it inhibits the action of a unique enzyme, *hyaluronidase*. Though this enzyme is normally present in the body, bacteria make it as well and use it to break through mucous membranes to the interior of the body. By inhibiting the enzyme, echinacea makes it harder for bacteria to gain access. This has particular use in cartilage and bursae problems. By inhibiting hyaluronidase, echinacea inhibits the breakdown of hyaluronic acid, the component in the joint cartilage and bursae that keeps them viscous. This helps promote healthy cartilage and bursae in degenerative or inflammatory joint conditions. Echinacea is also an anti-inflammatory, reducing swelling, which gives it a double impact for this type of problem.[25]

Dosage
Take 1 teaspoon of the tincture three times daily until pain and swelling are reduced.

Cautions
Large doses of echinacea are normally well tolerated. However, because of its actions on hyaluronidase, excessive echinacea doses may in very rare instances cause swelling in joint tissue. This normally occurs in people with *no* joint problems; they are taking echinacea for immune-stimulating purposes and notice their shoe size has increased. The large doses of echinacea

cause hyaluronic acid buildup in the joints by interfering with its breakdown. This condition subsides when the herb is discontinued. This action of the herb, however, makes it perfect for cartilage and bursae problems.

CURCUMIN

Curcumin is an extracted constituent of the turmeric plant that gives curry its yellow coloring. Curcumin has been found to be a highly effective anti-inflammatory in numerous studies. It has been found to be as effective, in fact, as cortisone and phenylbutazone but without their side effects.[26]

Dosage
Take 200 to 400 milligrams three times daily.

BROMELAIN

Bromelain is an isolated constituent of pineapple and has been found in a number of trials to be a powerful anti-inflammatory for conditions such as bursitis and tendinitis. Studies with athletes have consistently shown reduced swelling and faster healing times with the use of bromelain.[27]

Dosage
Take 250 to 750 milligrams three times daily.

PROANTHOCYANIDINS (OCPs)

Flavonoids such as proanthocyanidins, anthocyanidins, or citrus bioflavonoids have all been found to decrease the healing time of sports injuries to tendons and bursae. They are anti-inflammatory, protect collagen fibers from damage, and reinforce the cross-linking of collagen fibers to make them stronger.[28]

Dosage
Citrus bioflavonoids may be used (500 to 1,000 milligrams three times a day), anthocyanidins (standardized bilberry extract 80 to 150 milligrams three times a day), or proanthocyanidins from pine bark or grape seed extract (100 milligrams three times a day).

Anti-Bursitis/Tendinitis Fruit Drink

If you suffer recurrent bursitis or tendinitis, you may wish to add this drink to your diet daily as a preventative or even use it as a treatment during flare-ups. A number of people have found that the fresh pineapple or its juice (not just the extracted bromelain) can help alleviate these kinds of inflammations. Papaya contains the same kinds of constituents as pineapple, blueberry is high in anthocyanidins, and turmeric contains curcumin. Fresh ginger can be very intense in any quantity so start small to see if you like it. A piece about the size of your thumb from the top joint up is as big as you should begin with. And be warned, turmeric is *very* yellow and can stain anything.

Ingredients
>5 slices fresh pineapple
>¼ fresh papaya
>1 cup blueberries
>fresh ginger to taste
>2 teaspoons turmeric

Directions
Run the fruits and ginger through a juicer, add 2 teaspoons of turmeric, stir, and drink once daily.

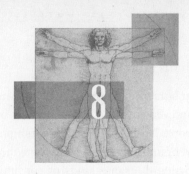

Energy: The Pancreas

The only conquests which are permanent, and leave no regrets, are our conquests over ourselves.

—NAPOLEON

The primary purpose of education is not to teach you to earn your bread, but to make every mouthful sweeter.

—JAMES ANGELL

I remember a friend from long ago who was tremendously kind, wise, and intelligent—one of the few people I have known who was really deserving of the term "saintly." He had had polio as a child and his hip did not work well. He took life slowly, was exceptionally attentive in all conversations, and was well loved by most everyone who knew him, which, in Boulder, Colorado, is saying something. Another friend, an expert in martial arts and a tremendously driven athlete, finally remarked in exasperation one day, "Look, he has to be nice, he can't run and he can't fight!"

I thought that was funny (I still do), but he had a point. Karate is for the young, aikido for the middle-aged, and tai chi for the old. All of them are effective, but in progression they are less dependent on power and more conscious of energy flow in producing the same results. I am not sure we are supposed to be calm, patient, and meditative when we are twenty. These are aspects of maturity and are supposed to come with time. Something causes that maturation process, it doesn't just happen out of thin air. We develop those skills when we are ready to do so, they come with the passing seasons and the changes attendant in the journey from youthfulness into middle age. For my friend, his illness had forced him to mature long before it is time for most of the rest us to do so.

In youth, energy supplies seem endless. We can go forever and never think about it. Tremendous exertion one day, a good sleep, and the next day, good as new. Somewhere between forty and fifty this begins to change; one day we step on the gas and the engine sputters. We stay up all night drinking and wake up the next morning incapacitated. We play a game of one-on-one and the next day are surprised to have trouble getting out of bed. We have to work to keep fit, when a few years earlier we could grow muscles lying on our parents' couches. Suddenly we find that even though we eat as we have always done, our waistline increases. Panicked, we diet, and it still increases. All this forces us to become conscious of things that we once took for granted. (Aging does seem to be a process of having to become aware of things we would generally prefer not to.)

One of the teachings of this movement into midlife is that energy is finite. It has to be husbanded (what a nice word for it)—that is, intentionally cultivated and used prudently. And this is crucial for our development as men; it forces us to consciously choose what we want to do with the energy we do have. In other words, if there is only a finite amount of energy, it forces us to ask the questions: "What do I want to use it for? What is really important to me?"

And so we start to slow down, begin to smell the flowers, and choose the path we walk. Our relationship with everything begins to change. We can no longer wolf a Big Mac, shake, and fries and not think about it. We can no longer take our energy levels for granted. Eventually, wheat grass juice enters our consciousness, jogging rears its ugly head, and bed at nine o'clock seems sensible. Our whole relationship with our energy begins to shift.

Many people I know who have gone through this transition say that while their energy levels are not the same as they were when they were twenty, their *stamina* is much greater. There is less wasted energy and they are more efficient in its use. From the experience of years of living, they have come to know themselves more deeply and now realize just how far they can push. They have learned how to go up to that edge and maintain it for hours. What they accomplish is much more potent, focused, and efficient than the accomplishments of their younger selves. And this consciousness has a benefit; life itself is more deeply savored, sweeter, and more poignant.

Like so many other things, this alteration of energy levels can become pathological. The most potent, and common, form of this is diabetes.

THE BODY'S ENERGY SYSTEM

It all comes down to sugar. All life on Earth fuels its energy by burning sugar, and all of that sugar comes from one source: plant transformation of the sun's energy through photosynthesis. The sap that plants use for food and as a circulatory transport mechanism is filled with many different types of sugars (and other chemistries), all made from sunlight. Many tree saps, like that of the maple, are so sweet that they have been used as foods for thousands of years. We get these sugars through the foods we eat: plant sugars, carbohydrates, and fats are all just different types of sugar. The most usable kind is called glucose. (Ordinary table sugar is a related, slightly more complex form of sugar called sucrose.)

When we eat, sugar is processed from our food and circulated through the blood (just as plants circulate sap) to wherever it is needed. All of our energy and bodily heat comes from this. Healthy levels of glucose or blood sugar are controlled by a complex assortment of endocrine glands and hormones. The pancreas and the pituitary, adrenal, and thyroid glands work together through the creation and release of hormones to maintain blood glucose homeostasis.

Not all the glucose entering the body is immediately used. If there is a surplus, it is converted into glycogen and stored short-term in both the liver and muscles. This commonly occurs after a meal when blood glucose goes very high. As blood sugar levels go down between meals, this temporary excess is converted back to glucose and used to keep blood sugar levels (and energy) where they need to be.

If there is a continual surplus, glucose is converted into fat and stored long-term. There is, unfortunately for Americans, little upper limit on how much fat the human body can store this way. The more glucose the body gets, the more it stores as fat and the more pants sizes we have in the closet.

However, if glucose levels are continually very high, the body's conversion process, even into fat, cannot keep up and excess glucose is excreted in the urine. This makes the urine sweet and gives rise to the origin of the term *diabetes mellitus*—honey fountain. . . . And yes, they actually used to taste urine to determine if someone had diabetes. ("Pee into this cup" had a whole different meaning a thousand years ago.)

Maintaining Blood Sugar

Four of the body's endocrine glands are intimately involved in maintaining and regulating blood sugar through their unique hormones. In the pancreas, the *islets of Langerhans* (IL) secrete two sugar-regulating hormones—*insulin* from the IL's beta cells and *glucagon* from their alpha cells. The beta cells also release another substance into the blood, *human islet amyloid polypeptide* or IAPP, about which little is known. (It plays an as yet unknown role in blood sugar metabolism.) The pancreas also creates and releases from other cellular structures three other important hormones: pancreatic polypeptide hormone (which increases the conversion of glycogen into glucose and regulates gastrointestinal activity), somatostatin (which inhibits glucagon and human growth hormone release), and finally, each day the pancreas releases about one and a half quarts of pancreatic fluid to the small intestine as a part of the digestive process.

Insulin decreases the amount of glucose in the blood by accelerating the movement of glucose through cell membranes (so that the cells can get sufficient sugar to fuel their metabolism). Insulin also increases the activity of an important enzyme, called *glucokinase*. Glucokinase helps the cells utilize glucose once it has been transported through the cell walls. This enzyme is also essential for the body to turn glucose into glycogen for short-term storage.

Glucagon from the IL's alpha cells increases the amount of glucose in the blood by increasing the activity of the enzyme *phosphorylase*. Phosphorylase accelerates the conversion of liver glycogen to glucose and its release into the bloodstream.

The pituitary gland gets involved by creating and releasing three hormones: human growth hormone (HGH), adrenocorticotropic hormone (ACTH), and thyroid-simulating hormone (*thyrotropin*).

HGH decreases the conversion of carbohydrates to sugar and increases the conversion of fats to sugar (thus increasing blood sugar levels). Less fat is stored in the body when HGH is active and more of the stored fats are used up (which is why people are interested in using it for weight control).

ACTH also increases blood sugar by stimulating the adrenal cortex to make and release more glucocorticoid hormones, essentially cortisol and corticosterone. These hormones accelerate the breakdown of protein (basically muscles) into amino acids, which are circulated to the liver via the blood, where they are converted into glucose. Too much cortisol on a regular basis will cause increased loss of muscle tissue from the body and steadily rising blood sugar levels. Glucocorticoids also heavily affect the distribution and use of fat cells by the body. With constant high cortisol levels, the body shifts to a fat-based (rather than a carbohydrate-based) metabolism, spends more time converting sugars to fats, and stores fats in such a way as to maximize their conversion back into glucose. In effect, this causes a shifting of fat storage to the face, shoulders, waist, and hips, and an increasing hunger for fat in the diet.

Thyrotropin from the pituitary gland increases the thyroid's production of thyroid hormone. This increases the body's metabolism, increasing energy levels and the body's use of sugar. Blood sugar levels go down when thyrotropin is active.

Epinephrine (aka adrenaline) is made in the adrenal glands and increases blood glucose levels. It is released by the body in response to stress or threat (the so-called fight-or-flight response). Epinephrine causes the liver and muscles to release stored glycogen and convert it quickly into glucose for immediate use. (The reason cola drinks are so biologically potent is that the sugar goes directly into the blood while the caffeine stimulates adrenaline production, thus increasing blood glucose levels even more. The end result is a tremendous burst of energy from two different mechanisms in a short period of time.)

Normally, through complex feedback loops, the body continually adjusts blood glucose levels to maintain health. The glands, in essence, compare notes and shift their hormone production depending on where the homeostasis of the body needs to go. The most commonly malfunctioning organ of the body's energy system is the pancreas (and its insulin). This malfunction is called diabetes.

Diabetes

There are two types of diabetes from (primarily) two different causes. Type I diabetes is caused when the pancreas's beta cells do not produce insulin or produce very little. This type of diabetes usually occurs in childhood or adolescence. Type II, the more common form, occurs later in life, often in middle age, and comes from cellular insensitivity to insulin. In Type II, or adult-onset diabetes, the pancreas generally makes plenty of insulin, the cells just don't respond to it as they used to. As a result, glucose doesn't get transported across cellular membranes, energy levels are low, blood sugar is high, and the urine can be filled with it.

No one really knows why Type I, or insulin-dependent diabetes mellitus (IDDM), occurs (though there are a lot of theories). People with this form of diabetes have to inject insulin daily for the rest of their lives. While natural protocols cannot reverse Type I diabetes of long standing, they can often slow the side effects of the disease and help keep the body healthy. Of the twelve million or so diabetics in the United States, about 90 percent are Type II, only a million or so are Type I.

Some of the more interesting new research on Type II diabetes has linked it with the same kind of deterioration that is found in the brain of Alzheimer's patients. The same kind of amyloid proteins that accumulate as a plaque during Alzheimer's disease have also been found in the pancreas. Rather than affecting the neural synapses, as they do in the brain, they build up in pockets and affect the pancreas's beta cells. This type of plaque is found almost exclusively in overweight people with Type II diabetes.

Researchers have found that as weight increases, the amount of IAPP, or amyloid proteins, that are produced in the beta cells increases substantially. The increased IAPP cannot be processed efficiently by the blood and it begins to accumulate in the pancreas as a plaque, destroying the beta cells. The proteins themselves, much like those in the brain and those that cause mad cow disease, once formed, cause other proteins to malfunction. The result in all three diseases is a spongy mass instead of healthy functional cells. Ninety percent of autopsied Type II diabetics have been found to have these plaques in their pancreas after death. Because this occurs with increasing body-fat levels, the finding lends weight to the belief that Type II diabetes is hormonal, diet, and body-fat-content related.

Type II diabetes, a relatively uncommon disease one hundred years ago, is now the seventh leading cause of death in the United States. It is increasing in frequency at about 6 percent per year, the number of diabetics doubling every fifteen years. While there naturally is a lowering of cellular sensitivity to insulin as we age, the increases in diabetes in men in the Western world are almost exclusively from the lowering of free testosterone levels, the increased androgen/estrogen imbalance, and our modern diet.

TESTOSTERONE AND DIABETES

As free testosterone levels fall in middle age and the androgen/estrogen balance begins to move toward the estrogenic side of the equation, men also begin to gain weight. Testosterone naturally increases the production of lean muscle tissue in the body and decreases fat production. (Which is why as teenagers most young men can and do eat anything and remain skinny.) Testosterone is in fact an anabolic steroid (though not a synthetic one). Anabolism means a constructive or building metabolism and testosterone builds muscle tissues. Catabolism, on the other hand, is a destructive or tearing-down metabolism. Men's bodies become more catabolic as their androgen balance moves more toward the estrogenic in middle age. Cortisol is intimately involved in this process; it tends to rise as testosterone levels fall. In part, this is because, at least in men, estrogens directly increase the body's production of cortisol. The estrogens bind to sites in the kidney and influence production of cortisol in the adrenal glands. What is important is not so much that cortisol is a "bad" hormone but more that the imbalance in androgens and estrogens allows more cortisol activity in the body. This has increasing impacts on diabetes as people age. For one thing, high cortisol and low testosterone levels naturally produce more fat in the body, usually distributed around the hips and waist.

As the number of fat cells in the body increases, the more likely people are to have diabetes and heart disease. In fact, most Type II or non-insulin dependent diabetes mellitus (NIDDM) occurs in middle-aged people who are overweight. One of the reasons is that many fat cells possess a unique enzyme, HSD-1, that initiates cortisol activity inside fat cells. The cortisol is cell-specific and never enters the bloodstream, much as significant quantities of cellular, DHEA-converted testosterone never enter the bloodstream. The more fat cells there are, the more active cortisol there is in the body.

Cortisol makes cells less sensitive to insulin and increases blood sugar levels, and can, by itself cause diabetes.

Both DHEA and cortisol are made in the same part of the adrenal gland. As estrogens rise, the adrenal spends more time making cortisol and less making DHEA. And, in fact, one of the potential markers to use to determine health levels is the body's DHEA/cortisol ratio. It is closely related to the androgen/estrogen ratio. Both help to give a picture of hormone activity in the male body.

Interestingly, one of the primary regulators of cortisol levels is the heart's ANF hormone. The happier people are, the more ANF their heart makes and the less catabolic their system becomes. A number of studies have confirmed the impact of ANF in diabetes. People who are unhappy and depressed are much more likely to contract Type II diabetes, and this is independent of weight gain and other factors.[1] Both ANF and natural androgens possess the ability to reduce the activity of the HSD-1 enzyme that activates cortisol within fat cells and to decrease cortisol production in the adrenal gland.

Another interesting aspect of testosterone's relationship to diabetes is that low levels of nitric oxide (NO) have been linked to impaired glucose utilization. Nitric oxide, necessary for vascular dilation and hence sufficient oxygen to tissues, also increases glucose transport in skeletal muscle cells. However, nitric oxide activity and production are both impaired in insulin-resistant individuals.[2] Because nitric oxide is essential for healthy heart function, blood circulation, vasodilation, and penile erection, this reveals another aspect of diabetic-related diseases: heart disease, arteriosclerosis, diabetic retinopathy, and erectile dysfunction. It also explains why, in part, testosterone and androgen supplementation can help diabetes. They both increase the amount and activity of NO in the body.

DIET AND DIABETES

It should come as no surprise that the easiest way to remedy Type II diabetes in men is to decrease the number of fat cells in the body, decrease cortisol levels, and improve androgen levels. To achieve all this, modification of diet is essential.

One of the surest indications of the relation of diabetes to Western diet is that the condition is extremely rare in indigenous societies who eat a wild food diet. People who leave traditional cultures and begin eating a Western diet tend to develop diabetes at the same rates we do in this country. Returning them to a traditional diet will, in most instances, reverse adult-onset diabetes. Part of the problem in Western diets is the ready availability of both fats and sugar. Neither of these substances are easily available in pure form in nature. Evolutionarily, the human body is not used to them in large quantities or in pure form.

The problem with sugar is that it is quickly absorbed into the bloodstream, which causes a rapid rise in blood sugar. The pancreas responds by releasing large quantities of insulin in order to normalize blood sugar levels. This causes the blood sugar to rapidly drop, which alerts the adrenal glands to release adrenaline to bring levels up again. This essentially overstimulates the system and years of cola drinks, candy bars, and sugar rushes cause the system to malfunction. The constant high insulin level from years of massive sugar intake have caused cells to become less insulin-sensitive, so the pancreas has to increase levels to maintain the same levels of blood glucose. The adrenal glands start to become exhausted and begin having more trouble producing adrenaline. At the same time, the diet has often been very high in fats. Fat is a problem because it is cortisol specific. The more the body gets used to constant high levels of fats as a glucose source the more the body uses cortisol to process it. This increases cortisol levels and moves the body to a fat-based metabolism dynamic that is very hard to stop. The increased cortisol activity also interferes with cellular insulin sensitivity and a vicious cycle develops.

As the cycle continues, the body has more and more difficulty dealing with glucose intake (whether as fats or sugars). The blood becomes saturated with sugars and the kidneys begin excreting glucose to try and bring levels back down. In order to keep the sugar dissolved so that it can be excreted, the kidneys have to make more urine. One of the more common first signs of diabetes is increased urination and constant thirst.

High levels of sugar in the blood bring their own problems as well. High blood sugar causes a narrowing of the small blood vessels throughout the body, producing poor circulation problems in the extremities. Especially hard hit are the feet, eyes, and, in men, the genitals. Over time, the kidneys begin to fail, wound healing becomes poor, cholesterol builds up, and cardiovascular disease becomes a serious problem. The higher the blood sugar level, the more the blood vessels constrict, the worse the circulation becomes. Long-term complications are erectile dysfunction or impotence in men, amputation of the feet, and blindness (diabetic retinopathy). Quite often wound healing is so poor that recovery from amputation is extremely difficult and many amputees die as a result. About half of all the amputations in the United States are caused by diabetes—a grim picture.

Because of such negative long-term side effects, being diagnosed with diabetes is often frightening. The good news is that natural approaches are exceptionally effective for Type II diabetes and the majority of its complications: atherosclerosis, cardiovascular disease, macular degeneration, and erectile dysfunction. *Simply losing weight, for many people, will reverse adult-onset Type II diabetes completely.* Even the side effects of Type I diabetes can be significantly helped. (For more on specific physical problems from diabetes see also: Chapter 3, "Erectile Dysfunction," Chapter 4, "Atherosclerosis" and "Cardiovascular Disease," and Chapter 9, "Diabetic Retinopathy.")

Cautions

Type I diabetics should discuss any natural health protocols with a health-care provider. Many of these herbs, supplements, and foods can alter insulin requirements, sometimes considerably. A number of trials have shown that certain herbs and supplements can actually reverse Type I diabetes of short duration (five years or less). Information on this can be found in Michael Murray and Joseph Pizzorno's *Encyclopedia of Natural Medicine* (Prima, 1998) or on the Internet. Protocols for this need to be tightly monitored and controlled and should be under a health-care provider's supervision.

Type II diabetics are of two types. Most (90 percent) are overweight, with elevated insulin levels in the blood. The second kind of Type II diabetic is usually thin and their pancreas has quit producing sufficient levels of insulin. There is more insulin than in Type I diabetes, but not enough to maintain blood sugar. Given that a large number of substances are specifically antagonistic to the body's beta cells, it is thought by a number of people that external chemical antagonists (and sometimes viral diseases) are responsible. One potential culprit is the nitrates in smoked meats, such as bacon, smoked salmon, ham, and so on. These N-nitroso compounds are very close in structure to streptozotocin, a synthetic compound that destroys beta cells. Type II thin diabetics with low insulin levels (in addition to general anti-diabetes supplements and diet modification) need to follow a protocol that enhances beta cell production, protects beta cells from further deterioration, and increases insulin levels, in essence, to concentrate on pancreatic tonic herbs and supplements. Some of the following herbs and supplements have been found to both protect the beta cells and increase their insulin production.

Natural Care for Diabetes

For Six Months to Two Years
   Vijaysaar, 250 milligrams, one to three times daily
   Gurmar, 200 to 400 milligrams once to twice daily
   Fenugreek, defatted powder, 50 milligrams a day
   Bitter gourd, 1 to 2 ounces fresh juice three times daily
   Androgen replacement or DHEA, minimum 50 to 100 milligrams
      daily
   Alpha lipoic acid, 600 milligrams daily
   Pine bark or grape seed extract (PCO), 150 to 300 milligrams daily
   Chromium, 100 micrograms daily
   Biotin, 8 to 16 milligrams daily
   Manganese, 30 milligrams daily
   Vitamin E, 800 international unit daily
   Zinc, 20 to 40 milligrams daily
   Diet alteration (essential)

VIJAYSAAR

Vijaysaar (*Pterocarpus marsupium*), or pterocarpus, is a Southeast Asian herb that has long been used in the Ayurvedic treatment of diabetes. It is from the bark of a large deciduous tree and contains a great many important flavonoids, among them epicatechin. Although epicatechin is considered to be the active constituent of pterocarpus, the whole herb has been found to be as effective as the isolated constituent in treating diabetes. At its most basic, pterocarpus lowers blood glucose levels and increases insulin sensitivity. More significantly, the plant is a potent tonic for the pancreas. Pterocarpus is specifically protective of the beta cells of the pancreas, similar to the way milk thistle is for the liver. Not only will it protect the beta cells from extremely powerful beta-antagonist chemicals such as alloxan and streptozotocin, but it also accelerates regeneration of beta cells in a compromised pancreas, again much like milk thistle does for the liver.

The herb has been tested extensively on animals and a limited number of clinical trials have also been conducted. Giving test animals pterocarpus before giving them glucose reduced their blood sugar by nearly 50 percent in one hour. The herb appears to suppress sugar absorption in the intestine. Clinical trials with diabetics have found that the herb reduces blood sugar, increases insulin sensitivity, reduces sugar in the urine, reduces urine output, reduces excessive thirst, and reduces excessive caloric intake.[3] While effective for all diabetics, this herb is especially useful for thin Type II diabetics with low insulin levels.

Both the herb and epicatechin are exceptionally well tolerated in the body. No side effects have been reported. A number of companies are now offering this herb alone or in combination with the most powerful of the pancreatic herbs for use in diabetes (e.g., GlucoCare, Pancreas Tonic, Gymnemosupium). All are widely available through health-food stores and the Internet. A standardized extract of pterocarpus, called Silbinol, is also available.

Dosage
Take 250 milligrams one to three times daily.

GURMAR

Gurmar (*Gymnema sylvestre*), aka gudmar and gymnema, grows throughout India, Southeast Asia, tropical Africa, and Australia and is a traditional Ayurvedic plant for the treatment of diabetes. Like pterocarpus, it has been found effective for both Type I and Type II diabetes. The herb is highly specific for a damaged pancreas, specifically targeting damaged beta cells; people without diabetes who take it show no effects at all on blood sugar or insulin. Significant evidence exists from animal (and some human) studies that the herb enhances beta cell production of insulin and actually regenerates beta cells in the pancreas. Clinical trials with Type I diabetics have shown that gymnema reduced their insulin requirements while some Type II diabetics were able to manage their diabetes with gymnema alone. Blood sugar levels have been found to decrease by half after ingestion of gymnema. Animal studies have found that in alloxan-treated rats (this destroys their beta cells), a month of gymnema treatment could restore most of their physiological values to normal. While in an alloxan-damaged pancreas, some beta cells will naturally regenerate, with streptozotocin they will not. Still, even with total beta cell destruction (from streptozotocin) in some sections of the pancreas, gymnema extracts have regenerated beta cells. The number of beta cells were found to increase as much as eighty-two times. Of further importance is that when non–beta cell damage has occurred in the pancreas, extracts were also found to initiate pancreatic regeneration and a renormalization of pancreatic function as measured by the other hormones released by the pancreas and by pancreatic fluid. Gymnemic acid, which is sometimes considered to be the active constituent of the plant, has been found irrelevant to regeneration in the pancreas.[4]

Interestingly, values normalized by the herb include chondroitin sulfates. These, important components in cartilage, typically decrease in people with osteoarthritis. Studies with rabbits and dogs have shown similar outcomes. While effective for all diabetics, this herb is especially effective for thin Type II diabetics with low insulin levels or Type I of short duration.

No side effects have been found from the use of gymnema. Again, a number of companies have produced combinations of this herb with many of the other most powerful pancreatic herbs (see pterocarpus). One company, PharmaTerra, is marketing a proprietary extract called ProBeta, upon which they have apparently done extensive studies.

Dosage
Take 200 to 400 milligrams once to twice daily.

FENUGREEK

Fenugreek (*Trigonella foenum-graecum*) contains a half-dozen compounds that help regulate blood sugar. Animal studies have consistently shown its ability to lower blood glucose levels and increase insulin sensitivity. One clinical trial with diabetics found that after using the herb for twenty-one days, all participants in the trial had achieved a more balanced glucose level and an enhanced insulin response. Others have consistently found that the herb can reduce urinary glucose excretion by half and improve glucose processing throughout the body.[5] This is true for both Type I and Type II diabetics. The herb acts much like a glucose-system adaptogen, that is, it normalizes the process. If sugar is too high, it lowers it. If sugar is too low, it brings it up.

Dosage

Take 15 grams of powdered fenugreek daily or 50 milligrams of defatted powder a day.

BITTER GOURD

Bitter gourd (*Momordica charantia*), aka bitter melon or balsam pear, is a Chinese herb often used in food and medicine. It is cultivated as a food throughout much of the world, especially in Africa, Asia, and South America. A significant number of clinical trials in Asia and India have shown consistently good results in the treatment of Type II diabetes. Seventy-three percent of those taking the fresh juice experienced improvement in blood sugar and other diabetic markers. The plant contains a large number of compounds that work synergistically in affecting diabetes. It enhances insulin activity through chemical mimicry and possesses a powerful glucose lowering constituent that is more powerful than tolbutamide, a synthetic hypoglycemic drug.[6]

Although the powdered herb can be used effectively for controlling blood sugar, the preferred method is the juice of the fresh fruit—a green, cucumber-shaped gourd. Simply juice 1 gourd to get 1 to 2 ounces of juice (take three times daily). Or juice enough for the whole day and consume it before meals as needed.

The effects of bitter gourd accumulate over time; the longer it is taken the more comprehensive the results. The fresh plant can be readily found in Asian grocery stores. It is *very* bitter, as its name suggests. Adding it to orange juice does help.

Dosage

Take 1 to 2 ounces of the fresh juice three times daily or 5 grams (2 teaspoons) of the powder daily. Take before meals.

ANDROGEN REPLACEMENT (DHEA AT MINIMUM)

A comprehensive androgen balancing protocol can help move the body back to an anabolic rather than a catabolic dynamic. This will help lower the fat content of the body, reduce cortisol activity, increase insulin sensitivity, and balance glucose metabolism. In a number of double-blind, placebo-controlled trials, DHEA has been shown to increase insulin sensitivity and decrease blood glucose levels. An even larger number of studies in rats have shown the consistent insulin lowering effects and blood glucose moderating effects of DHEA. Increasing levels of free testosterone have been found to decrease blood glucose levels and an imbalance in the testosterone/estrogen ratio toward the estrogen side has been shown to cause a mild form of diabetes in and of itself. Although direct research is lacking, overviews of testosterone replacement therapies indicate that diabetes in men receiving testosterone is exceptionally rare. Long-term clinical results from a number of physicians have shown that testosterone replacement is highly effective in decreasing vasoconstriction, arteriosclerosis, anginal pain, blood glucose levels, wound healing time, and even in curing diabetic gangrene.[7]

More powerful androgenic supplements such as testosterone, DHT, and 4-diol seem to provide more consistent results in the treatment of diabetes. While DHEA has, in some instances, provided significant results, it is important to note that many studies with DHEA have shown mixed results. No one is quite sure why this is so. While the rat research is consistent, when DHEA has been used in people the outcomes are not. In some studies DHEA has shown little or no impacts on blood glucose and insulin. DHEA seems to provide excellent help for some people (most often women) while other people have no response. However, what is clear is that DHEA and androgen replacement therapies do consistently show a reduction in most of the side effects associated with diabetes, especially heart disease, atherosclerosis, and erectile dysfunction. A number of studies have shown that diabetic men with erectile dysfunction are hypogonadic, with low testosterone levels. For that reason alone DHEA supplementation or an androgen replacement protocol is essential to consider.

Dosage

Androgen replacement therapy or 50 milligrams of DHEA once or twice a day.

ALPHA LIPOIC ACID (ALA)

A number of trials have shown that alpha lipoic acid normalizes blood sugar and significantly reduces or even reverses many of the symptoms of Type II diabetes. ALA is normally present in the liver throughout life though it begins decreasing as we age—about the same time as DHEA and other androgens. ALA facilitates glucose uptake by the cells of the body, thus lowering blood sugar. Additionally, ALA increases the body's levels of glutathione, a potent antioxidant, and has been shown to reduce such diabetes-associated problems as eye disease, diabetic nerve damage, cholesterol levels, memory and mental confusion, and erectile dysfunction.[8]

Dosage

Take 600 milligrams per day.

Cautions

Diabetics should use only after review with their physician. ALA strongly affects blood sugar levels and will affect medical protocols. N-acetyl cysteine (NAC) is an effective substitute for ALA at 1,200 milligrams daily.

PINE BARK OR GRAPE SEED EXTRACT (OPC)

Pine bark and grape seed extracts are high in proanthocyanidins, extremely powerful plant flavonoids that are some fifty times more powerful than vitamin C as antioxidants. Recent research has shown that flavonoids such as OPCs can promote insulin secretion by the pancreas and inhibit sorbitol accumulation within cells. Sorbitol, a byproduct of glucose metabolism, can build up in the cells of diabetics and cause severe eye, nerve, and pancreatic problems. OPCs inhibit sorbitol increase and promote capillary strength throughout the body, especially within the eye.

One of the more important reasons to use OPCs in diabetes is the recent understanding that amyloid plaques are significant contributors to beta cell malfunction and pancreatic disease. The proteins that make up the amyloid plaques that form in the pancreas can be reduced in number through the use of exceptionally strong antioxidants like OPCs. (See "Alzheimer's Disease.")

Dosage
Take 150 to 300 milligrams daily.

Cautions
Standardized Extracts: Pine bark extracts may be synergistic with "blood-thinning" medications such as warfarin, heparin, clopidogrel, pentoxifylline, and aspirin and should, therefore, be used with caution or under the supervision of a health-care practitioner if you are using these drugs. Side effects are rare: mild allergic reactions and digestive upset have been reported.

Herbal Extracts: Some people are sensitive to pine products—seeds, pollen, bark, resin, and so on. Negative reactions can run from mild allergies to anaphylactic shock. **If you have a history of allergies to pollen or severe reactions to bee stings, you should proceed with caution to make sure that your reactions do not extend to pine products.**

CHROMIUM

Diabetics are usually low in chromium and a number of clinical studies have shown that chromium alone can significantly help normalize glucose levels in the blood. Chromium has been found to increase glucose utilization, decrease insulin resistance (chromium resensitizes the cells to insulin), lower insulin levels, and normalize blood cholesterol levels. Chromium has also been linked to reversing the body's move to a catabolic rather than an anabolic metabolism. Chromium supplements alone have been found in clinical trials to increase the body's lean muscle mass and decrease fat accumulation, thus helping reverse the trend toward a more diabetic body type.[9]

Most natural chromium supplements are from brewer's yeast in the form of chromium polynicotinate. This form is some 300 percent more bioavailable than chromium picolinate and 600 percent more bioavailable than chromium chloride.

240

Dosage

Most trials used 100 to 500 micrograms daily. Suggested dosage is 100 to 200 micrograms daily.

BIOTIN

Biotin is made in the intestines from the bacteria that normally live there. It is essential to health, especially in diabetes. Keeping the digestive system healthy is important to make sure that enough of this substance is available in the body. (Though you can also take biotin as a supplement.)

Several clinical trials have shown that biotin can help increase insulin sensitivity, normalize blood glucose, and improve glucose control by the body. Biotin works in part by increasing the activity of glucokinase, one of the important enzymes that controls the glucose/glycogen conversion process. Diabetics normally have little functional glucokinase in their bodies. Biotin increases biotin levels and also its effectiveness.[10]

Dosage

Take 8 to 16 milligrams daily.

MANGANESE

Diabetics have commonly been found to be deficient in manganese, often having only half the normal levels. Manganese is crucial to the enzymes that regulate blood sugar, thyroid function, and energy metabolism in the body. Decreasing manganese intake in guinea pigs will cause them to become diabetic and lead to their offspring being born without a pancreas.[11] Manganese is a pancreas-specific mineral and necessary for healthy pancreatic functioning.

Dosage

Take 30 milligrams daily.

VITAMIN E

Vitamin E has been found to be a key vitamin in helping regulate blood sugar. A number of clinical studies have shown that vitamin E alone improves glucose utilization and insulin sensitivity in diabetics. This kind of supplementation has also been shown to lower an individual's propensity to develop Type II diabetes later in life.[12]

Dosage
Take 800 to 1,200 international units per day.

ZINC

Zinc is essential in maintaining a healthy immune system, regulating blood sugar, and facilitating wound healing. Zinc, in fact, is intimately involved in nearly all aspects of insulin activity in the body, including protection of the beta cells of the pancreas. Diabetics tend to lose much of their zinc through excess excretion in the urine. Both Type I and Type II diabetics have shown improvements in their insulin dynamics when given zinc as a supplement.[13]

Dosage
Take 20 to 40 milligrams per day. It is generally recommended to not exceed 40 milligrams of zinc per day.

Cautions
Over time, zinc intake can cause copper depletion in the body. To counteract this, most zinc supplements come with copper added. At very high doses, zinc can cause nausea and upset stomach, skin rashes, depression, folate deficiency, and lower tolerance to alcohol.

DIET MODIFICATION

Because weight loss (lowering fat-cell density in the body) alone has been shown to reverse Type II diabetes in a majority of cases, it should be one of the first things considered by anyone who is diabetic and overweight. A complete diet modification program is included in Chapter 12. And since diabetes is so closely linked with the foods commonly eaten in Western industrialized diets, it is crucial to modify the intake of foods known to be associated with the onset of diabetes. Even if you do not lose weight, eating different foods can help diabetes and its symptoms significantly.

In general, it is exceptionally important to eat a low-fat diet filled with foods that are known to reverse Type II diabetes, that are effective in preventing or reversing atherosclerosis, that increase peripheral circulation, and that moderate glucose balance in the blood.

About Diabetic Neuropathy

Some diabetics have problems with diabetic neuropathy, basically a diabetes-caused nerve disease often accompanied by a tingling, then burning, sensation in the feet, which often progresses to severe pain in the digestive tract and other parts of the body. Vitamin B supplements, especially B_6 and B_{12}, have been found highly effective in helping this problem. Both of these B vitamins, when deficient, cause the same symptoms that accompany diabetes with such neuropathies. Diabetics are consistently deficient in both B_6 and B_{12} and in many instances supplementing with these vitamins will reverse the problems. Alpha lipoic acid supplementation has also been found to reverse diabetic neuropathy within as little as three weeks.[14]

Foods for Diabetes

Onions and garlic
Beans
Burdock root, dandelion root, jerusalem artichoke
Prickly pear cactus
Oats, psyllium, and soy
Foods high in potassium
Cold-water fish (omega-3 and -6 fatty acids)

ONIONS AND GARLIC

Garlic and onions will help clear blood vessels and improve blood flow. They also help regulate blood sugar. Garlic and onions have a long history of folk usage in Asia, Europe, and the Middle East in the treatment of diabetes. A number of clinical trials have been carried out both with whole garlic and several isolated garlic constituents, and blood sugar levels have consistently lowered. Sulfur-containing compounds in onions (allyl propyl disulfide [APDS] compounds) have been found to have a specific effect on both blood sugar and insulin levels in people. Garlic and onions can be eaten either raw or cooked and still produce the same benefit. And of course, the powerful ability of these herbs to prevent or ameliorate atherosclerosis makes them essential in the diet for anyone with diabetes. (In addition, onions contain large amounts of quercetin, which has been shown to help eye problems such as diabetic retinopathy.)[15]

Dosage

The more the merrier: ¼ to ½ onion per day (1 to 7 ounces); 1 to 3 garlic cloves per day. Studies have shown that the more that is consumed, the better blood sugar and insulin levels, and health of blood vessels, become.

BEANS

Beans (and other high-fiber foods) have been found in numerous studies to help reduce blood sugar in people with diabetes. Essentially, they help reduce the high glucose spike that occurs just after eating a meal. Part of the reason that high-fiber diets help is that they contain mucilages and gums, two plant substances that, among other things, reduce the availability of sugar to foraging bacteria in order to protect damaged plant tissues from infection. This reduced-sugar-availability activity of the two substances is of considerable benefit whenever lots of fiber is added to the diet. The absorption of sugars across the intestinal wall is impeded, keeping blood sugar lower than with other foods.

If you are also suffering from erectile dysfunction, you should add fava or ox-eye beans as they contain L-dopa and can help as erection stimulants (see Chapter 3).[16]

Dosage

Add 4 to 5 servings weekly in the diet.

BURDOCK ROOT, DANDELION ROOT, JERUSALEM ARTICHOKE

All these roots have been found (in clinical trials) to help lower the blood glucose levels that occur after a meal, in part because they contain inulin, a blood sugar–lowering compound. All are exceptionally good tonics, especially dandelion and burdock roots. Burdock can be found fresh in Asian (and some natural food) grocery stores and fresh dandelion root in most health-food stores of any size. Dandelion and burdock are primarily liver tonics, while burdock also exerts beneficial effects on immune function. Prior to World War II, they were common foods for most Americans and Europeans.[17]

Dosage

Enjoy regularly in the diet. Normally they are steamed. Burdock root tastes much like a firm asparagus, dandelion root like a parsnip with flavor.

PRICKLY PEAR CACTUS

Prickly pear cactus has been a traditional indigenous food in the Americas for thousands of years. Both the fruit (something like a tiny spine-covered papaya, though quite different in taste) and the pads of the cactus are eaten. Researchers, noting that indigenous peoples eating a traditional diet did not have diabetes, connected food use to the traditional use of prickly pear in Mexican folk medicine for the treatment of diabetes. Supplementation with the plant, either as food or a powder, does in fact lower both blood sugar and insulin as an increasing number of human trials have shown. Trials found that glucose lowered 17 percent and insulin 50 percent.[18]

Dosage

Add 100 to 500 grams (3 to 15 ounces) of the powdered plant per day or fresh as a regular part of the diet. The 100-gram dose was, in general, as effective as higher doses. But the plant seems better if used as a food additive rather than a supplement. Effects are cumulative.

Cautions

Not for thin Type II or Type I diabetics. The plant can most easily be found in Mexican or South American grocery stores, often fresh. They will tell you how to prepare it. Needless to say, the spines have to be removed. It is worth it, as prickly pear is very tasty and there are a number of wonderful traditional dishes that use the plant.

OATS, PSYLLIUM, AND SOY

Oatmeal has been found to be an excellent food for diabetics in a number of trials, increasing the body's glucose utilization and decreasing insulin levels. Psyllium, both seed and husk, has been found in a number of clinical trials to reduce insulin levels (17 percent) and reduce blood glucose. Glucose transport and utilization was improved in all those using it. And soy, as a grain or tofu, has been found effective as well in lowering blood sugar and decreasing insulin levels.[19] All of these foods work in part because of their high fiber content.

Dosage

Take 50 grams of oats per day as oatmeal. Various dosages of psyllium were used in the clinical trials—5, 10, and 15 grams daily. All were found effective. Take 15 grams of soy daily.

FOODS HIGH IN MAGNESIUM

Magnesium deficiency is high in diabetics and that contributes to a number of problems, such as diabetic retinopathy. The best way to get magnesium is from the diet: beans, tofu, seeds, nuts, whole grains, green leafy vegetables such as kale, spinach, beet greens, dandelion greens, nettle, and so on.

Magnesium is better assimilated with at least 50 milligrams daily of vitamin B_6 in the diet.

Dosage

Eat at least one serving of a high-magnesium food daily. The more, the merrier.

COLD-WATER FISH

Eating fish high in omega-3 fatty oils has been shown to increase glucose utilization and decrease glucose intolerance in a number of men with diabetes. This kind of meat also helps control blood fat levels and reduce or prevent atherosclerosis.[20] Mackerel, sardines, albacore tuna, and salmon are all good examples of high omega-3 fish.

Dosage

Eat seven ounces per week. It is better if consumed in two separate meals during the week.

Other Foods

Other foods that have been found helpful in diabetes include macadamia nuts, olive oil, black and green tea, carrots, apples, beets, figs, turmeric, and okra.

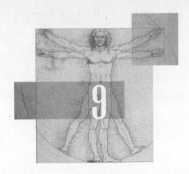

Seeing and Hearing

Sight is a faculty; seeing is an art.

—George Marsh

"Are you listening to me?"
"Uh-huh."   —Anonymous

The continual focusing of our eyes on the external world, over time, literally wears them out. This is especially true if our focus is on tiny exteriors, such as words in books, organisms in microscopes, or the jewels seen through a jeweler's loupe. We spend our youth focusing on the outer world and, after a time, the eye tires, the outer world becomes blurry, and somewhere in our mid to late forties, we start to hold things farther away from ourselves in order to see them clearly. The aging of our eyes forces us into a detachment from the external world and begins directing our gaze inward. We turn to our interior worlds and an examination of the landscapes we have built within us—there is a reason that the personal revelation of deep meaning in a thing is called *insight*. It comes from looking within things (including ourselves), instead of focusing on their outer form. This cultivation of insight accompanies maturing; it rarely belongs to the very young. It comes as our eyes begin to lose their ability to focus clearly and we are forced to develop our latent capacity to see with faculties other than the merely physical. This particular kind of depth perception allows us to see much that lies hidden to the young—patterns of life, patterns of living—in ourselves and in each other.

It is interesting then, in this light, to note that the more our technology has urged us to focus outward, the more our eyesight dims, forcing us inward. Cultures without books become nearsighted at nowhere near the levels that afflict the technologically developed. Of course, in response, a new industry arises, supplying eyeglasses by the millions. Instead of focusing inward, the determination to focus outward becomes all the more insistent.

At the same time that our sight alters, the acuity of our hearing also starts to decrease, forcing us inward through another mechanism. Perhaps it is so we can begin to hear the call of those things most important to us, those things that are crucial to living a fulfilled life. Perhaps it also allows us to begin finding that small, still, quiet place that is within each of us.

Natural Care for Eyes and Ears

Although it seems right that as we age we begin to look, and hear, inward, sometimes the process is exacerbated by outside factors. Sometimes it goes farther, perhaps, than it should, forcing us not merely inward but into darkness, not merely into internal listening but into permanent silence. Here, again, there are many herbs and supplements that can be of help.

The most common problems that afflict eyes as they age are macular degeneration, diabetic retinopathy, glaucoma, and cataracts. For ears it is tinnitus, presbycusis, and vertigo. I find it highly interesting that, with slight variations, the same herbs, foods, and supplements can be successfully used for all of them.

MACULAR DEGENERATION (MD)

MD refers to the deterioration of the *macula*, the central region of the retina at the back of the eye. The macula is the most sensitive portion of the nerve-rich retina, where all finely focused images are formed. From age fifty to sixty, this portion of the eye sometimes begins to break down or degenerate. About one-fourth of people over age sixty-five experience MD. The form it takes can range anywhere from mild symptoms to legal blindness. Usually it is a progressively degenerative disease. Not surprisingly, it is closely connected to the quality of the blood flow in the body. Tiny blood vessels like those in the eye are the first to experience difficulty in such diseases as atherosclerosis. As the blood supply diminishes, oxygen flow to the nerves decreases, and they begin to degenerate. Free radicals that cause oxidation in different portions of the eye have also been implicated in the degeneration of the macula (see "About Free Radicals" on page 251).

There are two types of macular degeneration. The most common type is "dry," which affects between 80 and 95 percent of people with MD, and "wet," which affects the remainder. In dry MD, the central area of the retina gradually accumulates sacs of cellular debris known as *lipofuscin*. This distorts the macula, causing people to lose vision in the central part of the eye. They still possess good peripheral vision; they just cannot see what is right in front of them. In contrast, wet MD is caused by the growth of abnormal blood vessels. Wet MD can often be effectively, and easily, treated early in its progression by laser surgery. There is no effective medical treatment for the more common dry form of MD.

Natural Care for Macular Degeneration

For One to Twelve Months
Bilberry, 40 to 80 milligrams three times daily (standardized extract)
Ginkgo, 40 to 80 milligrams three times daily (standardized extract)
Vincamine, 20 milligrams three times daily
Pine bark or grape seed extract, 150 to 300 milligrams daily
Vitamin C, 1,000 milligrams three times daily (effervescent salts)
Vitamin E, 800 international units per day
Beta-carotene, 50,000 international units daily (mixed carotenoids)
Zinc, 40 milligrams daily

BILBERRY

Also called European blueberry, bilberry (*Vaccinium myrtilis*) is closely related to cranberries, blueberries, and huckleberries. Like most of the berry bushes in this family, it is a short, shrubby plant (in this instance usually a foot or so tall) fond of growing in thickets and covering large areas. While there is a closely related plant (the bog bilberry) that prefers bogs (like cranberries do in the United States), the bilberry prefers the high ground. Europeans have collected the fruit for centuries.

According to anecdotal stories, modern research on bilberry began when Royal Air Force pilots reported that their night vision improved after eating bilberries. Studies have shown that constituents in bilberry, espe-

ABOUT FREE RADICALS

Free radical is a funny, 1960s sort of term much bandied about as a primary cause of pretty much everything. Free radicals are short-lived, highly reactive molecular fragments that contain one or more unpaired electrons. While they can form from a number of molecules, the ones that are generating the most concern are those that form from oxygen molecules.

Contrary to common sense, oxygen is a highly toxic substance. Five hundred million years ago or so the oxygen content of the atmosphere was only about 1 percent. For plant life to colonize the land masses a higher oxygen content was necessary. Fires require oxygen—rapid fires, like that of wood burning—and slow fires—such as those that occur during oxidation. Oxidation is the rusting of iron and what happens in our muscles when we run. Large muscle tissue can only work when atmospheric oxygen is above 10 percent; fires only begin to burn when it rises above 15 percent. However, at 25 percent, fires will rage uncontrolled. (Normally, a highly volatile atmosphere such as the one we have would "run down" to a more stable state. It was this long-term constancy of an unstable atmosphere that stimulated James Lovelock to perceive the Earth as a living organism, Gaia, not just a collection of parts.) So, oxygen enables much more vigorous processes to occur—land life, larger plants, and animals can develop—but at a price. Oxygen is toxic. It is mutagenic (causes genetic mutations), carcinogenic (causes uncontrolled cellular growth or cancer), and oxidative (causes cellular damage from oxidation).

Oxygen is used for an incredible variety of chemistries in living organisms. When plants take in carbon dioxide (CO_2) they break the molecules apart into oxygen and carbon, and they use these molecules (along with nitrogen and hydrogen) to make all the chemicals they need. These new molecules make up their sap, chlorophyll, and all the thousands of secondary chemistries in their bodies, many of which make them powerful medicines for human beings. But when living organisms use such plant compounds to produce and maintain life, oxygen is continually broken off from more complexly formed chemicals. These free oxygen atoms, or free radicals, can do serious damage to living tissues (oxidation) unless they are reused. So, all living organisms have what are called free-radical scavengers whose primary job it is to find and capture oxygen atoms and re-process them. Plants, because they are so much older than we are and have been at it a lot longer, have scores of different free-radical scavengers within them. We have evolutionarily developed to get many of the free-radical scavengers we need from our food, most of which historically have come from an incredibly rich plant diet made up of at least several hundred different plant foods and herbs eaten throughout the year. Without substantial numbers of free-radical scavengers in our diet, the levels of free radicals in our bodies can build up and, as levels rise, more and more cellular damage occurs. Our skin and other sensitive tissues, especially the nerves and the eyes, are particularly vulnerable to free-radical damage.

cially the *flavonoids* and the *anthocyanosides* (a special type of flavonoid), increase intracellular vitamin C levels, strengthen capillaries (reducing breakdown and hemorrhages), stimulate circulation to peripheral blood vessels (especially cerebral blood vessels), and are potent antioxidants.

Other constituents of bilberry seem to have a particular affinity for the macular area of the retina, and numerous studies have found the herb effective in treating such things as diabetic retinopathy, macular degeneration, cataracts, retinitis pigmentosa, and night blindness. Among the many studies showing its effectiveness in treating eye diseases is one revealing that the daily use of 400 milligrams of bilberry (combined with 20 milligrams of beta-carotene) improves night vision and enlarges visual fields.[1]

Dosage
Take a standardized extract 80 to 160 milligrams daily.

Note
Bilberry is generally used medicinally as a standardized extract. The anthocyanoside content is considered the most important factor by many clinicians and is generally standardized to 25 percent. The usual dose is 80 to 160 milligrams of the standardized extract three times per day. However, the use of antioxidants like pine bark, which contains *proanthocyanidins*, substances much more powerful than those in bilberry, shows that while highly useful, they have no *specific* affinity for the eye. Bilberry itself, and

not the anthocyanosides, possesses some natural affinity for eye tissue that has not yet been identified, making the use of the herb itself, standardized or not, important. It is not merely the anthocyanosides that are doing the work.

The fruit can also be used, consumed in any quantity desired throughout the day. Blueberry and huckleberry (and their juices) have the same effects. Blueberries, a close relative of bilberries, have been shown in clinical studies with aging rats to improve balance, coordination, and short-term memory. The rats in the studies consumed the human equivalent of a half cup of blueberries daily for eight weeks. Their coordination, balance, and memory improved to nearly youthful levels.[2]

GINKGO

Both researchers and clinicians have found ginkgo (*Ginkgo biloba*—GBE) specific for cerebral and peripheral vascular disorders, specifically those that affect the brain (see Chapter 10), penis (see Chapter 3), eyes, and ears. There are numerous clinical trials using ginkgo for treating diseases of the eye and ear. Macular degeneration, cataracts, tinnitus, cochlear deafness, and vertigo have all been found to respond to the herb.

In one instance, twenty-four people were tested in a randomized, double-blind study. After the use of 160 milligrams of ginkgo per day for four weeks, a significant increase in the sensitivity of the damaged areas of the retina was seen. *Only* the damaged areas of the retina were affected by the GBE.

In another case, after six months of GBE use, ten people in a placebo-controlled trial experienced a significant improvement in long-distance visual acuity.[3]

Dosage
Normal dosage in these conditions runs from 40 milligrams three times per day to 40 milligrams four times per day of an extract standardized to 24 percent ginkgoflavonglycosides.

Cautions
Some people have shown sensitivity to ginkgo preparations. Caution should be used if you are taking antithrombotic (anti-blood-clotting) med-

ications. Uncommonly, side effects are mild gastrointestinal upset or head-ache and, very rarely, allergic skin reactions. In very large doses, ginkgo can cause diarrhea, irritability, and restlessness. Because ginkgo is a PAF in-hibitor, it should be avoided before surgery.

PINE BARK (OR GRAPE SEED) EXTRACT (OPCS)

Pine bark has been found to possess a number of important actions as a medicinal agent. It is a potent antioxidant, a free-radical scavenger, a lipid peroxidation inhibitor, an anti-inflammatory, and a strong collagen and elastin stabilizer. Pine bark extract has, in fact, been found to be one of the most potent antioxidants known.

Pine trees contain a family of chemicals known as oligomeric proan-thocyanidin complexes (OPCs), or sometimes procyanidolic oligomers (PCOs), or sometimes simply (so to speak) proanthocyanidins, which are closely related to the anthocyanosides in bilberry and the procyanidins in hawthorn, but have a much higher degree of antioxidant activity. Pine bark extracts are a combination of some forty different OPCs isolated and con-centrated from the inner bark of different kinds of pine trees. Usually the French maritime pine is used. Their modern discovery and use came out of the research of Jacques Masquelier of the University of Bordeaux in France in 1951. He went on to discover and also popularize the use of grape seeds, again for their OPC content and antioxidant actions. Grape seed extract can be used interchangeably with pine bark extract.

While vitamin E as an antioxidant scavenges fat-soluble free radicals, and vitamin C scavenges water-soluble ones, pine bark or OPCs do both. OPCs are synergistic with vitamin C, extending its life span and potentiat-ing its activity in the body. OPCs have been found to be twenty to fifty times more powerful in their actions than either vitamin C or vitamin E.

OPCs are specifically effective for venous insufficiency, especially in the lower extremities, in treating such diseases as intermittent claudica-tion, phlebitis, and varicose veins. There have been a significant number of clinical trials for these conditions showing the compounds' effectiveness. OPCs also strengthen and preserve connective tissue and the elasticity of the skin. They have been found to increase blood circulation to the eye and to increase the strength of capillaries. There have been a scattering of trials conducted on OPC use in treating eye disease. One six-week study showed that of one hundred healthy volunteers who received 200 milligrams of OPCs daily, most experienced significant improvement in night vision. Other studies have shown their effectiveness in diabetic retinopathy and macular degeneration.[4]

The OPCs from pine bark and those from grape seed are generally considered interchangeable. The OPCs from grape seed are available to some extent in red wine, explaining in part the powerful health attributes of red wine in relation to the heart and the cardiovascular system.

Dosage
Take a standardized extract of 150 to 300 milligrams daily.

Note
Most of the pine bark extracts that have been used in clinical studies are essentially some form of standardized extract sold under trade names like Pycnogenol (the gold standard) or Enzogenol. Pine bark extracts made from the raw pine bark itself are not the same thing, though they will, to a lesser extent, possess the same actions. Comparable dosages have not been established between the two forms of extract.

Standardized Extracts: A therapeutic dose is twenty milligrams twice a day for every 20 pounds of body weight to (usually) 300 milligrams per day (typically 150 to 300 milligrams per day). A tonic dose is 50 milligrams per day.

Herbal Extracts: Although a number of herbalists have begun using pine bark from various species as a dietary supplement, most research has been on the combined complex of chemical extracts from the bark. That the bark will also be effective can be seen from its historical use as both a food and a medicine. The inner bark of many pines can be removed in long, pastalike strips and cooked much the same way. The taste and texture differ depending on the species, but some of them are very much like a piney-tasting noodle. The inner bark was also regularly collected, dried, powdered, and used to make exceptionally tasty cakes and breads in cultures throughout the world. Pine shoots were also traditional pot herbs though a bit tougher than those of other evergreen species. Pine and other evergreen needles were regularly used to make tea, one of the primary sources of vitamin C in nonindustrial cultures. The proanthocyanidins in the bark are synergistic with the vitamin C in the needles, enhancing its physiological effects considerably. Native peoples rarely *ever* suffered from scurvy or other collagen-related diseases.

Generally, dosage with the herb is 500 to 1,500 milligrams up to three times a day.

Cautions

Standardized Extracts: Pine bark extracts may be synergistic with "blood-thinning" medications such as warfarin, heparin, clopidogrel, pentoxifylline, and aspirin and should, therefore, be used with caution or under the supervision of a health-care practitioner if you are using these drugs. Side effects are rare: mild allergic reactions and digestive upset have been reported.

Herbal Extracts: Some people are sensitive to pine products—seeds, pollen, bark, resin, and so on. Negative reactions can run from mild allergies to anaphylactic shock. **If you have a history of allergies to pollen or severe reactions to bee stings, you should proceed with caution to make sure that your reactions do not extend to pine products.**

VINCAMINE

Vincamine is a constituent isolated from the lesser periwinkle (aka *Vinca minor*) in the 1950s. Hundreds of papers have been written on its effects, and numerous double-blind trials and lengthy clinical use in Germany have regularly shown it to be effective in treating vertigo and dizziness, Meniere's disease, tinnitus, presbycusis, and impaired blood flow to the retina of the eye. Like ginkgo and bilberry, vincamine appears to be specific for cerebral vascular disorders. It increases blood flow to the brain and smaller blood vessels in the ears and retina, and acts as a general vascular tonic for those areas.[5] The isolated constituent is considered more reliable than the herb itself, and it is upon vincamine that all studies have been done. (For more on vincamine, see Chapter 10.)

Dosage

The normal dose is 20 milligrams three times per day. Vincamine as a supplement is readily available on the Internet and at many health-food stores (see the Resources section).

Cautions

Generally, the acceptable safe dose is considered to be 40 milligrams daily. Normally zinc should not be taken in doses exceeding that amount unless under health-care supervision. Over time, zinc intake can cause copper depletion in the body. To counteract this, most zinc supplements come with copper added. At very high doses, zinc can cause nausea and upset stomach, skin rashes, depression, folate deficiency, and lower tolerance to alcohol.

DIABETIC RETINOPATHY

Diabetic retinopathy is a type of eye deterioration that occurs in the eyes of some diabetics, usually after ten years or so of the disease. As with MD, there are two types: nonproliferative (NPDR) and proliferative (PDR). In many ways they are very similar to the two forms of MD. With NPDR, the capillaries begin to weaken and eventually the eyes suffer continual hemorrhages of blood into the retina. It is a sort of hemorrhoid in the back of the eye: the blood vessels weaken, engorge, and sooner or later begin leaking fluid and blood. The macula is affected, central vision goes, and sometimes blindness occurs. In the second form, there is abnormal blood vessel growth and scarring in the retina. Like wet MD, this latter form can be remedied with laser surgery. There is little medical help for NPDR. In general, diabetic protocols can help the eyes heal and stay healthy (see Chapter 8). More specifically, a diabetic retinopathy protocol is sometimes called for.

Natural Care for Diabetic Retinopathy

For Six Months to Two Years
    Diabetic protocol daily
    Bilberry, 40 to 80 milligrams three times daily (standardized extract)
    Ginkgo, 40 to 80 milligrams three times daily (standardized extract)
    Vincamine, 20 milligrams three times daily
    Pine bark or grape seed extract, 150 to 300 milligrams daily
    Vitamin C, 1,000 milligrams three times daily (effervescent salts)
    Vitamin E, 800 international units day

Beta-carotene, 50,000 international units daily (mixed carotenoids)

Zinc, 40 milligrams a day

BILBERRY

Bilberry leaf (*Vaccinium myrtilis*) tea has been used in Europe for nearly a thousand years as a treatment for diabetes and eye problems. In fact, research has shown that the tea does decrease blood sugar levels, even when glucose is injected intravenously at the same time. Normally, Europeans consumed the leaf tea and berries as a regular part of their diet, using the herb over time to control the symptoms of diabetes. It is exceedingly interesting that the herb is also specific for one of the primary problems associated with diabetes—diabetic retinopathy. At the same time bilberry controls blood sugar, it is also healing, protecting, and strengthening the eye.

The constituents of bilberry seem to have a particular affinity for the macular area of the retina, and numerous studies have found the herb effective in treating such conditions as diabetic retinopathy, macular degeneration, cataracts, retinitis pigmentosa, and night blindness. The use of bilberry for diabetic retinopathy has been standard medical practice in France since 1945, and French physicians continually report good results from use of the herb.[9]

Dosage

Take a standardized extract of 80 to 160 milligrams daily.

Note

See "Macular Degeneration," above.

GINKGO

Ginkgo (*Ginkgo biloba*—GBE), not surprisingly, has been shown to be effective in treating eye conditions similar to diabetic retinopathy. Forty-six people with either glaucoma or severe degenerative vascular retinal disease were given 160 milligrams of GBE for four weeks, followed by 120 milligrams thereafter. Mild improvements were seen in visual acuity, visual field, and intraocular pressure.[10]

Dosage

Normal dosage in these conditions runs from 40 milligrams three times per day to 40 milligrams four times per day of an extract standardized to 24 percent ginkgoflavonglycosides.

Cautions

Some people have shown sensitivity to ginkgo preparations. Caution should be used if you are taking antithrombotic medications. Uncommonly, side effects are mild gastrointestinal upset or headache and, very rarely, allergic skin reactions. In very large doses, ginkgo can cause diarrhea, irritability, and restlessness. Because ginkgo is a PAF inhibitor, it should be avoided before surgery.

PINE BARK (OR GRAPE SEED) EXTRACT (OPCS)

Several studies have shown the effectiveness of OPCs in the treatment of diabetic retinopathy.[11] (Also see "Macular Degeneration," above.)

Dosage

Take a standardized extract of 150 to 300 milligrams daily.

Cautions

Standardized Extracts: Pine bark extracts may be synergistic with "blood-thinning" medications such as warfarin, heparin, clopidogrel, pentoxifylline, and aspirin and should, therefore, be used with caution or under the supervision of a health-care practitioner if you are using these drugs. Side effects are rare: mild allergic reactions and digestive upset have been reported.

Herbal Extracts: Some people are sensitive to pine products—seeds, pollen, bark, resin, and so on. Negative reactions can run from mild allergies to anaphylactic shock. **If you have a history of allergies to pollen or severe reactions to bee stings, you should proceed with caution to make sure that your reactions do not extend to pine products.**

VINCAMINE

In numerous studies vincamine has been shown to be effective for impaired blood flow to the retina of the eye. It is specific for numerous cerebral vascular disorders, increases blood flow to the brain and smaller blood vessels in the ears and retina, and acts as a general vascular tonic for those areas.[12] The isolated constituent is considered more reliable than the herb itself, and it is upon vincamine that all studies have been done. (For more on vincamine see Chapter 10 and "Macular Degeneration," above.)

Dosage

The normal dose is 20 milligrams three times per day. Vincamine as a supplement is readily available on the Internet and at many health-food stores (see the Resources section).

Cautions

Extreme overdoses can cause serious drops in blood pressure. Vincamine is contraindicated in brain tumors and in cases of intracranial pressure. Use the supplement under the care of a health practitioner if you currently have low blood pressure. Vincamine may occasionally cause nausea. If it does, lower the dosage or discontinue use.

BETA-CAROTENE (MIXED CAROTENOIDS)

Beta-carotene is specifically indicated in these kinds of eye diseases. See "Macular Degeneration," above.

Dosage

Take 200,000 international units daily.

VITAMIN C

Vitamin C is indicated in the treatment of diabetic retinopathy because of its strong antioxidant activity. Trials have shown its effectiveness for other similar eye disorders such as glaucoma, cataracts, and macular degeneration.

Vitamin C is best taken as effervescent salts. Much like Alka-Seltzer in nature, this form tastes good and can be taken in the high dosages necessary.

Dosage
Take 1 gram three times daily.

Cautions
Vitamin C at high doses will cause gas, flatulence, and, eventually, diarrhea. It is usually taken tbt or "to bowel tolerance." It is possible to build up tolerance to higher doses over time. It may cause digestive disturbance; some physicians prefer giving it intravenously for this reason. While vitamin C can be useful in some kidney conditions, you should not use vitamin C if you are on hemodialysis, or suffer from recurrent kidney stones, severe kidney disease, or gout.

VITAMIN E

Vitamin E is a synergistic antioxidant. Vitamin C, selenium, glutathione, and beta-carotene all work better when taken with vitamin E. For this reason its use is indicated in these kinds of eye diseases. Vitamin E reduces blood clotting (blood "thinner") and is a powerful antioxidant for fat-soluble free radicals. Often, it is difficult to get enough vitamin E from dietary sources. It is highest in certain oil-rich seeds and nuts like Brazil nuts and plants such as fresh purslane and turmeric.

Dosage
Take 400 to 800 international units daily.

ZINC

Because zinc is such an essential mineral and has been found to play essential roles in such cerebral vascular disorders as macular degeneration and tinnitus, its use is indicated in similar conditions such as diabetic retinopathy.

Dosage
Take 20 to 40 milligrams daily.

Cautions

The usual acceptable daily dose for zinc is 40 milligrams. Generally zinc should not be taken in doses exceeding that amount unless under health-care supervision. Over time, zinc intake can cause copper depletion in the body. To counteract this, most zinc supplements come with copper added. At very high doses, zinc can cause nausea and upset stomach, skin rashes, depression, folate deficiency, and lower tolerance to alcohol.

GLAUCOMA

Glaucoma is an increase in the amount of the internal fluid of the eye, which creates an abnormal pressure inside the eyeball. Collagen deterioration is strongly implicated in the development of this condition. In essence, the collagen in the eye breaks down and is not processed properly, so it builds up in the fluid of the eye. This blocks the drainage of intraocular fluid out of the eye, creating increased interior pressure. As pressure increases, the optic nerve can be damaged. This causes blurred vision, loss of peripheral vision, halo effects around lights, blind spots, eye pain, and redness. Emerging research indicates that glutamate, an important neurotransmitter in the eye, can rise to two to six times the normal levels in people who have glaucoma. These high levels of glutamate can damage the optic cells of the eye, causing cellular death. Free-radical damage and vasoconstriction have both been connected to these higher levels of glutamate. (In some instances glaucoma can be caused by a low-functioning thyroid, and simply normalizing the thyroid has corrected the problem.) Marijuana is one of the most reliable herbs for lowering intraocular pressure. It is widely used for this purpose in some countries overseas (e.g., Holland). Unfortunately, it is illegal in this country.

Natural Care for Glaucoma

For One to Twelve Months
Bilberry, 40 to 80 milligrams three times daily (standardized extract)
Ginkgo, 40 to 80 milligrams three times daily (standardized extract)
Pine bark or grape seed extract, 150 to 300 milligrams daily
Vitamin C, 1,000 milligrams three times daily (effervescent salts)

Vitamin E, 800 international units a day

Beta-carotene, 50,000 international units daily (mixed carotenoids)

Magnesium, 200 to 600 milligrams a day

Chromium, 200 to 400 micrograms a day

BILBERRY

The constituents of bilberry (*Vaccinium myrtilis*) seem to have a particular affinity for the macular area of the retina, and numerous studies have found the herb to be effective in treating such conditions as diabetic retinopathy, macular degeneration, cataracts, retinitis pigmentosa, and night blindness. Bilberry has been found to be useful in helping reverse glaucoma: its constituents interact with vitamin C to stabilize collagen synthesis in the eye.[13]

Dosage
Take 80 to 160 milligrams of a standardized extract daily.

Note
See "Macular Degeneration," above.

GINKGO

Ginkgo (*Ginkgo biloba*—GBE) has been found to be effective in treating a number of similar eye conditions. At least one trial has focused on its use in treating glaucoma. Forty-six people with either glaucoma or severe degenerative vascular retinal disease were given 160 milligrams of GBE for four weeks, followed by 120 milligrams thereafter. Mild improvements were seen in visual acuity, visual field, and intraocular pressure.[14]

Dosage
Normal dosage in these conditions runs from 40 milligrams three times per day to 40 milligrams four times per day of an extract standardized to 24 percent ginkgoflavonglycosides.

Cautions
Some people have shown sensitivity to ginkgo preparations. Caution should be used if you are taking antithrombotic medications. Uncom-

monly, side effects are mild gastrointestinal upset or headache and, very rarely, allergic skin reactions. In very large doses ginkgo can cause diarrhea, irritability, and restlessness. Because ginkgo is a PAF inhibitor, it should be avoided before surgery.

PINE BARK (OR GRAPE SEED) EXTRACT (OPCS)

OPCs strengthen and preserve connective tissue and the elasticity of the skin. They increase blood circulation to the eye and strengthen capillaries. Numerous studies have found that OPCs stabilize collagen, which gives them a role in the treatment of glaucoma. See also "Macular Degeneration," above.

Dosage
Take a standardized extract of 150 to 300 milligrams daily.

Cautions
Standardized Extracts: Pine bark extracts may be synergistic with "blood-thinning" medications such as warfarin, heparin, clopidogrel, pentoxifylline, and aspirin and should, therefore, be used with caution or under the supervision of a health-care practitioner if you are using these drugs. Side effects are rare: mild allergic reactions and digestive upset have been reported.

Herbal Extracts: Some people are sensitive to pine products—seeds, pollen, bark, resin, and so on. Negative reactions can run from mild allergies to anaphylactic shock. **If you have a history of allergies to pollen or severe reactions to bee stings, you should proceed with caution to make sure that your reactions do not extend to pine products.**

BETA-CAROTENE (MIXED CAROTENOIDS)

Beta-carotenes are essential in protecting the retina of the eye from oxidative damage. Mixed carotenoids from palm oil contain the highest amounts of the carotenoids needed to support the eye. Check the source of the beta-carotenes on the product label when purchasing.

Dosage

Take 200,000 international units daily.

VITAMIN C

Vitamin C has been shown to lower intraocular pressure in glaucoma. Clinical studies have consistently shown reductions in intraocular pressure as long as doses were high enough, generally ranging from 2 to 35 grams per day.[15]

Vitamin C is best taken as effervescent salts. Much like Alka-Seltzer in nature, this form tastes good and can be taken in the high dosages necessary.

Dosage

Take 1 gram three times daily. While vitamin C can be useful in some kidney conditions, you should not use vitamin C if you are on hemodialysis, or suffer from recurrent kidney stones, severe kidney disease, or gout.

Cautions

Vitamin C at high doses will cause gas, flatulence, and, eventually, diarrhea. It is usually taken tbt or "to bowel tolerance." It is possible to build up tolerance to higher doses over time. It may cause digestive disturbance; some physicians prefer giving it intravenously for this reason.

VITAMIN E

Vitamin E is a synergistic antioxidant. Vitamin C, selenium, glutathione, and beta-carotene all work better when taken with vitamin E. For this reason it is indicated for use in eye conditions such as glaucoma, especially so since glaucoma has been linked to oxidative damage.

Dosage

Take 400 to 800 international units daily.

MAGNESIUM AND CHROMIUM

Magnesium has been found to be essential in the maintenance of intraocular pressure and acts as a sort of natural calcium channel blocker, relaxing constricted blood vessels in the eye. One study with ten people suffering from glaucoma found that a dose of 120 milligrams of magnesium twice daily for four weeks significantly improved visual field and blood supply to the eye. In studies with up to 400 people, chromium deficiency has been linked to higher incidences of glaucoma. Decreases of chromium levels in the body have been found to directly cause increases in intraocular pressure.[16]

Dosages
Magnesium: Take 120 milligrams twice daily; chromium: take 200 to 400 *micro*grams per day.

Cautions
Magnesium is normally well tolerated. However, people with certain conditions, such as high-grade atrioventricular block, should only use magnesium under the supervision of a health-care provider.

CATARACTS

Cataracts occur when the clear protein structure of the lens of the eye becomes cloudy. The clear lens begins to go opaque (often whitish), causing impaired vision and sometimes blindness. Over time, most people experience some clouding of the lens of the eye. For the majority, it never becomes serious. In others, the lens-clouding process continues until sight is severely impaired or lost. The primary reason appears to be that the lens of the eye is highly susceptible to the actions of free radicals or oxidative damage. The lens begins to cloud, much like clear plastic that is exposed to sunlight for long periods of time. People who consume higher quantities of antioxidant-containing foods and supplements have been found to be less susceptible to cataracts.

The standard treatment for cataracts is surgery. The cloudy lens is removed and an artificial one inserted in its place. About half a million such operations are performed each year at a cost of more than $3.5 billion. The best approach is, of course, to never get them in the first place. The regular use of antioxidants is a good way to help prevent them from developing.

Natural Care for Cataracts

For One to Twelve Months
> Bilberry, 40 to 80 milligrams three times daily (standardized extract)
> Hachimijiogan formula, 150 milligrams three times daily
> Pine bark or grape seed extract, 150 to 300 milligrams daily
> Vitamin C, 1,000 to 3,000 milligrams three times daily (effervescent salts)
> Vitamin E, 800 international units day
> Beta-carotene, 200,000 international units daily (mixed carotenoids)
> Alpha lipoic acid, 150 to 300 milligrams twice a day
> (or N-acetyl cysteine, 500 to 600 milligrams twice a day)
> Selenium, 400 micrograms a day

HACHIMIJIOGAN

One particularly effective herbal formula for cataracts is called *Hachimijiogan*. This is a combination herbal formula that has been used for millennia in China for treating cataracts. It seems to be especially effective in the early stages of cataract formation. In one clinical trial, 60 percent of those treated experienced significant improvement while 20 percent had no worsening of their cataracts. Only 20 percent of the participants experienced any cataract progression. At least five other long-term trials have been conducted, the largest with 380 people, almost all of whom had both eyes affected. All studies reported similar outcomes.[17] The formula normally contains the following herbs: *Rehmania glutinosa, Poria cocos sclerotium, Dioscorea opposita, Cormus officinalis, Epimedium grandiflorum, Alisma plantago, Astragalus membranaceus, Cinnamomum cassia.* See the Resources section for sources.

Dosage
Take 150 milligrams three times daily.

BILBERRY

Studies have shown that constituents in bilberry (*Vaccinium myrtilis*), especially the *flavonoids* and the *anthocyanosides* (a special type of flavonoid), increase intracellular vitamin C levels, strengthen capillaries (reducing breakdown and hemorrhages), stimulate circulation to peripheral blood vessels (especially cerebral blood vessels), and are potent antioxidants. The constituents of bilberry seem to have a particular affinity for the macular area of the retina, and numerous studies have found the herb to be effective in treating such conditions as diabetic retinopathy, macular degeneration, cataracts, retinitis pigmentosa, and night blindness. In one study, bilberry (in combination with vitamin E) stopped the progression of cataracts in forty-eight of fifty people using it.[18]

Dosage
Take 80 to 160 milligrams of a standardized extract daily.

Note
Also see "Macular Degeneration," above.

PINE BARK (OR GRAPE SEED) EXTRACT (OPCS)

Because OPCs from plants such as pine bark are such potent antioxidants, free-radical scavengers, lipid peroxidation inhibitors, and strong collagen and elastin stabilizers, they are especially indicated in the treatment of cataracts. Pine bark extract is one of the most potent antioxidants known. OPCs have been found to be effective in treating a number of eye conditions such as diabetic retinopathy and macular degeneration (see "Macular Degeneration" above).

Dosage
Take 150 to 300 milligrams of a standardized extract daily.

Cautions
Standardized Extracts: Pine bark extracts may be synergistic with "blood-thinning" medications such as warfarin, heparin, clopidogrel, pentoxi-

fylline, and aspirin and should, therefore, be used with caution or under the supervision of a health-care practitioner if you are using these drugs. Side effects are rare: mild allergic reactions and digestive upset have been reported.

Herbal Extracts: Some people are sensitive to pine products—seeds, pollen, bark, resin, and so on. Negative reactions can run from mild allergies to anaphylactic shock. **If you have a history of allergies to pollen or severe reactions to bee stings, you should proceed with caution to make sure that your reactions do not extend to pine products.**

SELENIUM AND ALPHA LIPOIC ACID (ALA)

Two of the best antioxidants for cataracts are selenium and alpha lipoic acid (ALA). Recent research has found selenium, one of the most important minerals in the human body, to be an essential antiviral. Perhaps this antiviral activity explains why a great many viruses, from hepatitis C to HIV to the flu, have specific mechanisms for deactivating it in the human body. Selenium is also a potent antioxidant and free-radical scavenger. Selenium levels in the eyes of people with cataracts have been found to be substantially lower than those in people with healthy eyes.[19] Of further interest, studies have shown that the level of hydrogen peroxide in cataract-afflicted eyes is up to twenty-five times the normal. Excess hydrogen peroxide is linked to increased free-radical activity and damage to the eye's lens. Glutathione peroxidase, which depends on selenium, is responsible for the breakdown of hydrogen peroxide. Alpha lipoic acid is important in that it is an essential precursor to the formation in the body of glutathione. (N-acetyl cysteine, or NAC, can also be used for the same purpose.) A number of studies have found that cataracts can be prevented through the regular use of ALA.[20] Glutathione, one of the most powerful of the body's antioxidants, is a small protein. It is so small, in fact, that it can act inside cells instead of merely outside them (like vitamin C). Like selenium, glutathione is also a powerful antiviral. Because the body cannot usually assimilate glutathione supplements, it is important to take glutathione precursors, such as ALA or NAC, and let the body make its own. Glutathione normally exists in high levels in the lens of the eye and is significantly diminished in the eyes of most cataract sufferers.

Dosage
Selenium: Take 50 to 200 *micro*grams per day; alpha lipoic acid: take 600 milligrams per day. (N-acetyl cysteine: Take 1,200 milligrams daily.)

Cautions
Selenium can be highly toxic. Although dosages can range as high as 400 micrograms per day, this may become toxic over the long run. The dosage range for safety should be between 50 and 200 micrograms daily. Signs of toxicity are nausea and vomiting and emotional instability. The metabolism of N-acetyl cysteine can deplete the body's zinc and copper, so take it with a zinc supplement that also includes copper.

BETA-CAROTENE (MIXED CAROTENOIDS)

Beta-carotenes are essential in protecting the retina of the eye from oxidative damage and as such is especially indicated in the treatment of cataracts. Studies have shown that regular supplementation with carotenoids can reduce the risk of cataracts. Mixed carotenoids from palm oil contain the highest amounts of the carotenoids needed to support the eye. Check the source on the product label when purchasing.

Dosage
Take 200,000 international units daily.

VITAMIN C

A number of studies have shown that vitamin C can halt the progression of and sometimes reduce cataracts. One study with 450 patients found that most of those using 1 gram daily of vitamin C over the four years of the study showed a significant reduction in cataract development. This study has been repeated at least once with the same outcome.[21]

Vitamin C is best taken as effervescent salts. Much like Alka-Seltzer in nature, this form tastes good and can be taken in the high dosages necessary.

Dosage
Take 1 gram three times daily.

Cautions

Vitamin C at high doses will cause gas, flatulence, and, eventually, diarrhea. It is usually taken tbt or "to bowel tolerance." It is possible to build up tolerance to higher doses over time. It may cause digestive disturbance; some physicians prefer giving it intravenously for this reason. While vitamin C can be useful in some kidney conditions, you should not use vitamin C if you are on hemodialysis, or suffer from recurrent kidney stones, severe kidney disease, or gout.

VITAMIN E

Lack of sufficient vitamin E has been implicated in the formation of cataracts in a number of studies.[22] Vitamin E is a synergistic antioxidant. Vitamin C, selenium, glutathione, and beta-carotene all work better when taken with vitamin E, and for this reason should be considered in treating cataracts. Vitamin E reduces blood clotting (blood "thinner") and is a powerful antioxidant for fat-soluble free radicals. Often, it is difficult to get enough vitamin E from dietary sources. It is highest in certain oil-rich seeds and nuts like Brazil nuts and plants such as fresh purslane and turmeric.

Dosage

Take 400 to 800 international units daily.

TINNITUS AND PRESBYCUSIS

Tinnitus is a chronic ringing, whining, roaring, or whooshing in the ears. Like the eyes, the ears contain highly sophisticated nervous structures: some thirty thousand nerves are involved in the process of hearing. Fluid in one organ in the ear, the cochlea, a snail-shaped tube, vibrates in response to sound and moves thousands of tiny hairs in the ear's organ of Corti. These hairs connect to the numerous nerves that send impulses to the hearing centers of the brain. Tinnitus occurs when these nerves experience stimulation without an external sound source. Often this is caused by lesions or tears at the base of the hairs in the organ of Corti, which stimulates the nearby nerves.

Presbycusis is a sensorineural hearing loss that gradually increases with age. Initially, high-frequency sounds become difficult to hear (this can begin as young as age twenty), and gradually this expands into the lower ranges by fifty-five to sixty. Stiffening of the ear membranes and deterioration of hair cells, nerve structures, and cochlear nuclei seem to be the primary causes. Men seem to experience this more often than women, perhaps from more exposure to loud noises in their work.

The four primary causes of tinnitus and presbycusis appear to be: (1) pharmaceutical drugs, (2) loud noises—short- or long-term (airplanes, firearms, firecrackers, machinery, loud music, and so on)—which cause tearing and lesions in the ear, (3) decreased blood flow to peripheral systems (such as the nerves in the ear), and (4) ear inflammation with a subsequent fluid buildup in the inner ear.

Drugs that can cause tinnitus include interferon, aspirin, calcium channel blockers, lidocaine, benzodiazepines, glutamate, and atropine. Drugs causing presbycusis include aminoglycoside antibiotics, aspirin and other salicylates, quinine and synthetic malarial drugs, ethacrynic acid, and furosemide. Many of these drugs are particularly toxic to the organ of Corti.

Insufficient blood supply to the vessels supplying the nerves in the ear is an important causative factor as well, and restoring blood supply can often help. High blood pressure itself, basically vasoconstriction of the blood vessels, can cause tinnitus. This will stop once the blood vessels relax.

Natural Care for Tinnitus and Presbycusis

For One to Six Months
   Ginkgo, 40 to 80 milligrams three times daily (standardized extract)
   Vincamine, 20 milligrams three times daily
   Magnesium, 200 to 400 milligrams per day
   (For tinnitus) Vitamin B_{12}, 2,000 micrograms twice daily for 30 days, 1,000 micrograms per day thereafter
   (For presbycusis) Vitamin B_{12}, 300 to 1,000 micrograms daily
   Zinc, 40 milligrams per day

GINKGO (GBE)

In a double-blind study, 103 people with recent-onset tinnitus were given either placebo or ginko (*Ginkgo biloba*—GBE). A majority of those using

GBE experienced a decrease of the progression of tinnitus, decreased impairment, or complete remission. In another study over a nine-week trial period, of thirty-three people who took GBE, twelve experienced remission and five a reduction in symptoms.

In a trial treating acute cochlear deafness, one double-blind study found significant improvement in those taking GBE.[23]

Dosage

Normal dosage in these conditions runs from 40 milligrams three times per day to 40 milligrams four times per day of an extract standardized to 24 percent ginkgoflavonglycosides.

Cautions

Some people have shown sensitivity to ginkgo preparations. Caution should be used if you are taking antithrombotic medications. Uncommonly, side effects are mild gastrointestinal upset or headache and, very rarely, allergic skin reactions. In very large doses, ginkgo can cause diarrhea, irritability, and restlessness. Because ginkgo is a PAF inhibitor, it should be avoided before surgery.

VINCAMINE

Vincamine is a constituent isolated from the lesser periwinkle (aka *Vinca minor*) in the 1950s. Hundreds of papers have been written on its effects, and numerous double-blind trials and lengthy clinical use in Germany have regularly shown it to be effective in treating vertigo and dizziness, Ménière's disease, tinnitus, presbycusis, and impaired blood flow to the retina of the eye. Like ginkgo and bilberry, vincamine appears to be specific for cerebral vascular disorders. It increases blood flow to the brain and smaller blood vessels in the ears and retina, and acts as a general vascular tonic for those areas.[24] The isolated constituent is considered more reliable than the herb itself, and it is upon vincamine that all studies have been done. (For more on vincamine see Chapter 10.)

Dosage

The normal dose is 20 milligrams three times per day. Vincamine as a supplement is readily available on the Internet and at many health-food stores (see the Resources section).

Cautions

Extreme overdoses can cause serious drops in blood pressure. Vincamine is contraindicated in brain tumors and in cases of intracranial pressure; use it under the care of a health practitioner if you currently have low blood pressure. It may occasionally cause nausea. If it does, lower the dosage or discontinue use.

ZINC

Taking 60 to 120 milligrams of zinc per day has been found to be effective in helping tinnitus in several studies. Zinc deficiency is sometimes associated with tinnitus and certain types of hearing loss.[25]

Dosage

Take 20 to 40 milligrams daily.

Cautions

Generally zinc should not be taken in doses exceeding 40 milligrams per day unless under health-care supervision. Forty milligrams is considered to be the normal self-dosage level. Over time, zinc intake can cause copper depletion in the body. To counteract this, most zinc supplements come with copper added. At very high doses, zinc can cause nausea and upset stomach, skin rashes, depression, folate deficiency, and lower tolerance to alcohol.

VITAMIN B_{12} AND MAGNESIUM

About half the people with tinnitus have been found to be deficient in vitamin B_{12}, a vitamin essential to the health maintenance of the organs in the ear.[26] Sometimes, simply increasing the dietary intake of B_{12} can clear up the problem. (Two signs of B_{12} deficiency are weak and brittle nails and chronic digestive disturbances.) Magnesium has also been found to be vital in protecting hearing. One double-blind, placebo-controlled study with three hundred young, healthy military recruits found that hearing loss from exposure to noise was reduced in those given 167 milligrams of magnesium per day. Magnesium depletion is common in animals and people who suffer noise-induced hearing loss (NIHL). Through a variety of mechanisms, reduced magnesium causes reduced blood flow to the inner ear and increases intracellular calcium, both of which can cause damage to the hair cells.[27] Tinnitus may, in fact, be an early warning sign of reduced levels of magnesium. Simply increasing magnesium has been found to prevent and correct hearing impairment in a number of instances.

Dosages

Vitamin B_{12} for tinnitus: 2,000 *micrograms* twice daily for thirty days, 1,000 micrograms per day thereafter; vitamin B_{12} for presbycusis: 300 to 1,000 micrograms daily; magnesium (for both conditions): 200 to 400 milligrams daily.

Cautions

Magnesium is normally well tolerated. However, people with certain conditions, such as high-grade atrioventricular block, should only use magnesium under the supervision of a health-care provider.

VERTIGO

Vertigo, or dizziness, is a loss of balance that is often caused by problems in the inner ear. Seasickness, a well-known type of vertigo, is caused by the rolling of a ship on water. This sloshes the inner ear fluid about, upsets stomachs, and, to the dismay of sufferers, sometimes entertains those not so afflicted. *Vertigo* comes from the latin *vertere*, meaning "to turn," which, in essence, describes how one feels. A particularly intense form of vertigo, Ménière's disease, can be quite debilitating.

Vertigo often occurs from the deterioration of the hairlike cells that line the inner membranes of the ear. Normally, as the head or body moves, ear structures called *otoliths* shift and press on the hairlike cells, which then transmit position-shift information to the brain. Over time, cellular damage occurs in these hairlike cells, much like the damage that occurs in tinnitus. False signals are sent to the brain, and people feel dizzy or have vertigo. Restoration of healthy blood circulation to the ear can, in many instances, help restore the sense of balance.

Natural Care for Vertigo

For One to Six Months
    Ginkgo, 40 to 80 milligrams three times daily (standardized extract)
    Vincamine, 20 milligrams three times daily
    Ginger, 1 gram daily
    Vitamin B_{12}, 300 to 1,000 micrograms daily
    Zinc, 40 milligrams per day

GINKGO

Forty-seven percent of people using ginkgo (*Ginkgo biloba*—GBE) in a double-blind trial for vertigo became symptom-free after three months. In another study, GBE was found to be better than placebo in a double-blind trial of people experiencing vertigo or dizziness.[28]

Dosage
Normal dosage in these conditions runs from 40 milligrams three times per day to 40 milligrams four times per day of an extract standardized to 24 percent ginkgoflavonglycosides.

Cautions
Some people have shown sensitivity to ginkgo preparations. Caution should be used if you are taking antithrombotic medications. Uncommonly, side effects are mild gastrointestinal upset or headache and, very rarely, allergic skin reactions. In very large doses, ginkgo can cause diarrhea, irritability, and restlessness. Because ginkgo is a PAF inhibitor, it should be avoided before surgery.

VINCAMINE

Vincamine is a constituent isolated from the lesser periwinkle (aka *Vinca minor*) in the 1950s. Hundreds of papers have been written on its effects, and numerous double-blind trials and lengthy clinical use in Germany have regularly shown it to be effective in treating vertigo and dizziness, Ménière's disease, tinnitus, presbycusis, and impaired blood flow to the retina of the eye. Like ginkgo and bilberry, vincamine appears to be specific for cerebral vascular disorders. It increases blood flow to the brain and smaller blood vessels in the ears and retina, and acts as a general vascular tonic for those areas.[29] The isolated constituent is considered more reliable than the herb itself, and it is upon vincamine that all studies have been done. (For more on vincamine see Chapter 10.)

Dosage

The normal dose is 20 milligrams three times per day. Vincamine as a supplement is readily available on the Internet and at many health-food stores (see the Resources section).

Cautions

Extreme overdoses can cause serious drops in blood pressure. Vincamine is contraindicated in brain tumors and in cases of intracranial pressure; use under the care of a health practitioner if you currently have low blood pressure. It may occasionally cause nausea. If it does, lower the dosage or discontinue use.

GINGER

Ginger has been found in numerous clinical studies to relieve vertigo.[30] Although the majority of these trials were with motion- or seasickness, ginger can help alleviate some, or all, of the problems associated with vertigo. In part this comes from ginger's ability to stimulate circulation to the tiny capillaries throughout the extremities of the body.

Dosage

Take 1 gram powdered, encapsulated gingerroot, one to three times daily.

VITAMIN B_{12} AND MAGNESIUM

Because B_{12} and magnesium are so essential to the maintenance of the healthy physiology of the ears, their use should be considered in vertigo.

Dosage

Vitamin B$_{12}$: 300 to 1,000 micrograms daily; magnesium: 200 milligrams daily.

Cautions

Magnesium is normally well tolerated. However, people with certain conditions, such as high-grade atrioventricular block, should only use magnesium under the supervision of a health-care provider.

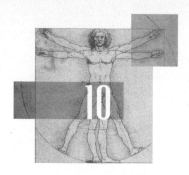

The Mind

I think therefore I am.   —RENÉ DESCARTES

What was I saying?   —ANONYMOUS

One of the primary horrors of aging, for many people, is the altering of the mind, the undependability of memory, the change in mental functioning that seems inevitable. Part of the reason that mental changes are so feared is that they are only compared to what is considered normal in younger life. The alterations age brings to the mind are rarely examined in and of themselves or in light of what memory should actually be like for us as we age. So, the changes often seem abnormal; to the young they *appear* pathological. But there may, in fact, be important, non-pathological reasons why our memories alter with middle age and even more so in old age.

It is an odd sensation, to be sure, when I can clearly see an actor's face in my mind but cannot recall his name. Coffee cups, eyeglasses, pens, papers, books, all disappear into the general clutter of life even though I had them just a minute ago. *Things* have taken on much less importance and hence are not worth remembering. What has come alive now are the deeper meanings in life, the experiences shared with others or myself. The maturing of self has caused a *change of mind*. And the brain literally does change. James Hillman quotes researchers who note that:

> For every decade after age fifty, the brain loses 2 percent of its weight. . . . The motor area of the frontal cortex loses between 20

and 50 percent of its neurons; the visual area in the back loses about 50 percent; the physical sensory part on the sides also loses about 50 percent.

However, at the same time:

The higher intellectual areas of the cerebral cortex have a significantly lower degree of cell disappearance. . . . It may even be that the fewer neurons increase their activity. . . . Recent research suggests that certain cortical neurons seem actually to become more abundant after maturity . . . the filamentous branchings (dendrites) of many neurons continue to grow in healthy old people. . . . Neuroscientists may actually have discovered the source of the wisdom which we like to think we can accumulate with advancing age.[1]

In fact, it may actually be important to embrace this change of mind as a necessary component of maturing. What will we find if we let go and allow ourselves to delve into this altered way of remembering? Will we worry less about things that in the long run really do not matter? Will we concentrate more on the things that are truly important? Might not this alteration in the brain's memory and thinking patterns be occurring so that the memories stored in the heart can come into our consciousness? Might it not be so that these older stored memories can be more deeply worked, processed, and assimilated into our characters?

Perhaps this is why the brain begins to shut down in certain ways, so that the brain of the heart can offer up its memories to the less busy mind. It could be that much of this process is not pathological at all, that it is simply a shift in the type of thinking we are supposed to do as we age. It could be that it is something intended for the maturation of the soul.

A number of factors, however, are interfering with this natural process. Two of the most prevalent forms of the pathologizing of memory and mental function are Alzheimer's disease and cerebrovascular disease, or stroke.

ALZHEIMER'S DISEASE

Alzheimer's disease, named after Bavarian psychiatrist Alois Alzheimer, who first described it in 1907, is accompanied by significant cognitive failure, loss of memory, and disorientation. There is usually cortical atrophy and a reduction in the metabolism of the posterior cortex and temporal lobe of the brain. Alois Alzheimer commented that his patients' brains (he liked to cut them open after, you see) contained scattered deposits of what he called a "peculiar" substance. What Alzheimer was describing was amyloid beta-protein, a 40-amino-acid-long protein fragment that, during the progression of Alzheimer's, concentrates in the brain as an *amyloid plaque.* The primary speculation is that it builds up in pockets and causes abnormalities and degeneration in the neural structures of the brain. Nerve filaments around the hippocampus, the brain's memory center, begin to deform as the plaque thickens. The discovery that the heart produces BNF, or brain natriuretic factor, has lent weight to a newer perspective that the plaque may be secondary to nerve damage.

BNF stimulates the production of a unique protein, beta-amyloid precursor protein, the function of which is to protect neurons from stressor damage, especially in the hippocampus. It may be, in fact, that the amyloid beta-protein that accumulates in the brain does so in attempting to protect brain neurons from high levels of stressors. In any event, as neurons begin to deform, they tangle, interfering with information retrieval and formation. At the same time, there is also a disruption of neurotransmitter actions in the brain.

Acetylcholine, an essential neurotransmitter closely connected to both memory and learning, facilitates the transmission of impulses from one nerve fiber to another in the brain. It is formed by an enzyme, *choline acetyl transferase,* from precursors (basically, acetyl and choline) in the brain. As acetylcholine forms, it binds to receptor sites, activating them, essentially completing the message sent from nerve to tissue. Once used, the acetylcholine is broken apart—back into its precursors—by another enzyme called *acetylcholine esterase.* In Alzheimer's disease, choline acetyl transferase progressively becomes less active, resulting in smaller quantities of acetylcholine in the brain. Alzheimer's patients usually have 60 to 90 percent less acetylcholine in their brains.

During Alzheimer's disease, both the neurons and the neurotransmitter chemistries necessary to neuron functioning break down. To counter this, one of the primary medical approaches is the use of what are called *cholinesterase* inhibitors, which block the breakdown of acetylcholine. This keeps acetylcholine levels higher, more neurotransmitter action occurs, and more memory retrieval and learning takes place. This doesn't stop the progression of Alzheimer's but does help deal with the memory and learning problems associated with it. Other treatment approaches include: preventing the formation of the amyloid plaque, increasing the amounts of acetylcholine in the brain from outside sources such as supplements and food, and supplying nutrients known to protect brain integrity.

Amyloid proteins are essential to the body's health. They occur, for instance, not only in neuronal tissues but also in the walls of peripheral blood vessels, the pancreas, and virtually every other cell in the body. As tissues deteriorate, these proteins can enter the bloodstream and be carried to the brain where they congregate. Maintaining the integrity of cellular tissue, blood vessels, and capillaries reduces the amount of amyloid proteins entering the blood. Additionally, maintaining the integrity of the brain's neuronal structures prevents the overproduction of beta-amyloid precursor protein by the heart's BNF hormone and the subsequent accumulation of plaque.

Diet and external pollutants have also been found to play an essential role in the development of Alzheimer's; low levels of zinc and vitamin B_{12} are common in people with Alzheimer's, as are high brain levels of aluminum and mercury. There is also significantly less DHEA and (because there are fewer androgens to metabolize) fewer estrogens in the brains of men and women with Alzheimer's.

Estrogens and Alzheimer's

Converted in the brain from the steroidal precursors DHEA, androstenedione, and testosterone, estrogens such as estrone and estradiol are necessary for healthy brain function. They are crucial for the development and continual maintenance of the density of the brain's axons, dendrites, and neuronal filaments. When estrogen levels decline, neuronal filaments retract and thin, memory begins to fail, and learning is impeded. Additionally, estrogens are an important catalyst to the production of choline acetyl transferase in the brain. Low brain estrogens directly translate into lower levels of acetylcholine. Men who have low androgen levels are at much greater risk for Alzheimer's disease and other cognitive disorders because there are fewer androgens to be converted to estrogens in the brain. In fact, researchers have found that men with the greatest cognitive problems have significantly lower DHEA levels than men without cognitive problems. DHEA levels in Alzheimer's patients are generally half or less than those of people the same age without the disease.[2] Even more interesting is that in men over eighty-five the level of the potent estrogen estradiol in their brains is a direct indicator of mental functioning and well-being.[3] The higher the estradiol, the better their mental functioning. The importance of estrogens in mental functioning was first noticed by physicians working with estrogen replacement therapy (ERT) for women. They found that significantly fewer women on ERT developed Alzheimer's disease.[4]

To a large extent, Alzheimer's appears to be a physiological response to three factors: (1) lower levels of androgens in the brain, (2) our contemporary lack of plant foods that have historically supported healthy chemistry in the brain, and (3) environmental pollutants. An essential part of any Alzheimer's program is to make sure that no aluminum is entering the body. This may sound odd but aluminum is an ingredient in a great many more common substances than is commonly known (see "Foods for Alzheimer's").

Natural Care for Alzheimer's Disease

For One to Three Years
  Huperzine A, 50 to 100 micrograms twice a day
  Ginkgo, 120 milligrams a day
  Hawthorn, 600 to 900 milligrams a day
  Bilberry, 400 milligrams a day
  (Possibly) periwinkle (vincamine), 20 milligrams three times a day
    (see "Stroke")
  L-acetylcarnitine, 500 milligrams three times a day
  DHEA, 50 to 100 milligrams a day
  Zinc, 50 milligrams a day
  Sage, rosemary, nettles, and garlic, daily in diet

HUPERZINE A

Huperzine A, a constituent of the common club moss *Huperzia serratum*, has a number of potent impacts on the functioning of the brain, which makes it highly useful for conditions like stroke and Alzheimer's disease.

It is a neuroprotector, a neural tonic, a cholinesterase inhibitor, a butyro-cholinesterase inhibitor, an antiamnesic, antiglaucomic, antimyasthenic, memorigenic, anti-inflammatory, a febrifuge, an antihemorrhoidal, and a capillary tonic.

The club moss from which huperzine A comes is traditionally used in Chinese medicine, where it is called either *qian ceng ta*, meaning "thousand layered pagoda," or *jin bu huan*, meaning "more valuable than gold." It has been commonly used for fevers, inflammatory disorders (arthritis and rheumatism), and general vascular weakness that causes bruising, bleeding from the lungs, or hemorrhoids. A similar species, *Lycopodium clavatum*, has been used for thousands of years in Ayurvedic medicine in much the same way but also for dizziness, epilepsy, irritable bladder, and nighttime urination problems. The American Eclectic botanical physicians, during the late nineteenth and early twentieth century, also used it for urinary gravel and kidney stones. American Indians, for several thousand years, used the various lycopodiums for exactly the same things. It is exceedingly interesting that this type of plant has been commonly used for such problems as vascular insufficiency, central nervous system problems such as epilepsy, arthritis, and problems with nighttime urination. All these problems are related to aging to some extent, especially if you expand "epilepsy" to include such nervous disorders as dementia, Parkinson's, and multiple sclerosis. The fact that vascular weakness has been implicated as a contributing factor in Alzheimer's because of the transfer of amyloid proteins to the brain is interesting as well.

Chinese physicians isolated huperzine A from this species, then known as *Lycopodium serratum*, in 1980 and isolated huperzine-B five years later. *Huperzia serrata* contains other interesting chemistries such as the alkaloid fordine, which has been found *in vivo* to possess similar actions to the huperzines, speeding up learning, reversing impaired learning, and protecting against hippocampal and cortical damage of the brain.

Chinese researchers found that the two alkaloidal constituents of huperzia, huperzine A and huperzine B, exert potent effects on brain function, huperzine A being some ten times stronger than huperzine B (which is why it is usually used). Of specific interest is the huperzines' ability to prevent the breakdown of acetylcholine, to prevent the destruction or deformity of neuronal networks in the hippocampus and cerebellum, and to promote the dendrite outgrowth of neuronal cultures.

Interestingly, huperzine A has been found to be *brain specific*. Acetylcholine is active not only in the brain but in other parts of the body where it is also broken down much as it is in the brain. Huperzine A works on acetylcholine *only* in the brain, while at the same time protecting the breakdown of neuronal networks and promoting dendrite density and complexity. This brain-specific activity of huperzine A causes fewer side effects than those associated with the pharmaceutical cholinesterase inhibitors that are often used for Alzheimer's and that affect acetylcholine indiscriminately throughout the body. Toxicology studies have shown that huperzine A is nontoxic even when given at fifty to one hundred times the human therapeutic dose. The extract also continues to be active in the brain far longer than pharmaceuticals, up to six hours at a dose (*in vivo*) of 2 micrograms per kilogram (2.2 pounds) of body weight. This has been averaged to 150 micrograms twice a day in clinical trials.

The research and clinical trials are impressive. One placebo-controlled, double-blind trial with 160 people suffering from Alzheimer's found huperzine A to be significantly superior to placebo, the pharmaceutical tacrine, and another cholinesterase inhibitor, physostigmine. They found huperzine A to be active for three hours versus two for tacrine and thirty minutes for physostigmine. Patients and caregivers reported significant improvement in clearheadedness, memory, and language over both placebo and other medications. In another instance, a double-blind, placebo-controlled trial was conducted with 103 people with Alzheimer's disease. Half the people were given huperzine A (100 micrograms twice daily), half placebo, for eight weeks. All participants were evaluated with the following scales: Wechsler memory, Hasegawa dementia, mini–mental state examination, activity of daily living, treatment of emergency symptoms. Significant changes were seen in 58 percent of the people taking huperzine A in memory, cognitive, and behavioral functions. Clinical studies have also taken place with fifty-six people with stroke (multi-infarct dementia) and one hundred with senile memory disorders. Both studies showed significant improvement in those taking huperzine A. Another study gave huperzine A to thirty-four pairs of middle school students who had complained of memory problems. One group was given huperzine A (two 50-microgram capsules twice daily), the other a placebo for four weeks. Learning and test scores were significantly enhanced in the huperzine group.[5]

Dosage

Most commonly what is used is the purified extract *huperzine A,* normally in 50-microgram capsules. Typical dosage is 50 to 100 micrograms twice daily. (Huperzine is often found combined with other memory herbs such as ginkgo. Normally, each tablet or capsule will contain a minimum of 50 micrograms of huperzine A.)

The whole herb itself has traditionally been used as a tincture, a whole powder, or a tea. No one has, to my knowledge, tried the herb by itself in the treatment of memory disorders, nor have I been able to find exactly how much huperzine A is present in sample quantities of the plant.

Cautions

This herb, sometimes called *jin bu huan* in Chinese medicine, should not be confused with the patent remedy containing tetrahydropalmatine, which is also confusingly called Jin Bu Huan.

GINKGO (GBE)

Ginkgo (*Ginkgo biloba*) has been found to be truly impressive for treatment of what is generally called dementia. This includes Alzheimer's disease and multi-infarct dementia (more commonly known as stroke). At least sixty trials have been carried out throughout the world, many of them placebo-controlled, double-blind, randomized, crossover studies. The studies have looked at anywhere from twenty-five patients to as many as thirteen thousand. Irrespective of the cause, ginkgo has been found effective. Some highlights:

- Fifty patients aged fifty to seventy-six years of age who received 150 milligrams per day showed significant improvement in five separate tests of mental, social, and behavioral functioning after three weeks. Indicators continued to improve the longer the herb was taken.

- An in-depth analysis of four randomized, placebo-controlled, double-blind trials with Alzheimer's patients showed that ginkgo provided significant improvement in symptoms.

- An examination of the practices of 1,357 physicians who had treated 13,556 people (42 percent stroke, 26 percent Alzheimer's, 32 percent mixed-type dementia) found that ginkgo improved symptoms with less than 2 percent of patients reporting any side effects.

- A fifty-two-week placebo-controlled, double-blind, fixed-dose, parallel-group, multicenter study with Alzheimer's and stroke patients with mild to severe impairment found that ginkgo improved symptoms. Symptoms for those in the placebo group significantly worsened during the same period. Ginkgo even helped those patients who were severely impaired. While such improvement was slight there was no worsening of their symptoms, as there was in the placebo group.

- Ginkgo was tested in a clinical study against the cholinesterase inhibitors tacrine, donepezil, rivastigmine, and metrifonate. Tacrine was found to possess significant side effects when compared to ginkgo and the other pharmaceuticals. Researchers concluded that ginkgo was *equally* effective in the treatment of Alzheimer's as the commercial pharmaceuticals and possessed fewer side effects.

- Ginkgo has been found to normalize the activity of acetylcholine receptors in the hippocampus and increase acetylcholine transmission.[6]

Ginkgo has been found to be effective in a number of areas for both Alzheimer's and stroke patients. Here are some of the overall research findings:

- Both caregivers and patients agree it improves symptoms.

- It improves both cognitive function and social behavior.

- Attention, concentration, short-term memory, visual memory, absent-mindedness, confusion, and fatigue problems all improve.

- Ability to cope increases and depression decreases.

- While most studies have been with mildly to moderately impaired people, ginkgo was still found to help severely impaired patients. More important, it significantly slows the worsening of symptoms.

- Researchers consistently note that "Ginkgo delays the progression of dementia."

- Ginkgo increases alpha brain wave activity when tested by EEG.

- While improvements could be seen in as little as three weeks, improvement became obvious at six weeks and improvement continues the longer the herb is taken.

Dosage

Ginkgo is (usually) standardized to 24 percent ginkgo flavonglycosides. These compounds are not normally present in unstandardized formulations in sufficient amounts to be effective. Five pounds of ginkgo are processed to yield one pound of standardized herb. Essentially, standardized ginkgo preparations are highly concentrated. All clinical studies have been with standardized preparations.

The normal dose is 120 milligrams per day, though trials have used from 40 to 240 milligrams. It is important to note that most improvements were seen after at least twelve weeks of use.

Cautions

Some people are sensitive to ginkgo preparations. Caution should be used if you are taking antithrombotic medications. Uncommonly, side effects are mild gastrointestinal upset or headache, and very rarely, allergic skin reactions. In very large doses, ginkgo can cause diarrhea, irritability, and restlessness. Because ginkgo is a PAF inhibitor, it should be avoided before surgery.

HAWTHORN AND BILBERRY

Hawthorn (see Chapter 4) is a well-known heart-normalizing herb with strong effects on the circulatory system. Bilberry, a relative of huckleberry and blueberry, is best known for its effects in preventing or reversing macular degeneration in the eye (see Chapter 9). However, both these herbs can play a role in helping alleviate or slow Alzheimer's disease. Bilberry is exceptionally good for increasing circulation and this is why it is so effective for eye disease. Bilberry also contains compounds known as anthocyani-dins. Numerous studies show that these compounds break down the plaque deposits that sometimes line the arteries and help prevent blood clots. Hawthorn is a circulatory stimulant and tonic to the entire blood and circulatory system. Beyond this, however, they are both extremely good at strengthening fragile capillaries. Basically, they improve the integrity of the walls of blood vessels. This can help to reduce the amount of amyloid pro-teins moving into the bloodstream from degeneration of blood vessel walls.

Dosages
Take 600 to 900 milligrams of hawthorn per day and 400 milligrams of bil-berry a day.

L-ACETYLCARNITINE (LAC)

L-acetylcarnitine (LAC) is naturally found in the human brain and re-searchers have found that it mimics the actions of acetylcholine. To some extent, LAC acts like an acetylcholine supplement. In at least six placebo-controlled trials with Alzheimer's patients, LAC was found to consistently improve function in all the areas studied, including memory, cognition, and behavior. Other studies with age-related mental impairment found the same kinds of improvement. Dosage range in most of the studies was 1,500 to 2,000 milligrams per day.[7]

Dosage
Take 500 milligrams three times a day.

DHEA

Both DHEA and androstenedione are converted in the brain to estrogens, upon which the brain depends for healthy functioning. This especially af-fects memory, cognition, mental clarity, alertness, and the density and health of the neural networks in the brain. A significant number of studies and clinical trials have found that DHEA levels are low in men and women with dementia, increasing DHEA levels enhances mental alertness and physical control over their bodies, and sufficient DHEA (and subsequently estrogen) levels in the brain are essential for healthy brain and mental functioning. *The importance of increasing androgen levels in the brain cannot be overstated.*

One study with male nursing home residents between the ages of 57 and 104, for instance, found that DHEA levels were inversely related to both the level of assistance the men needed and their levels of dementia. Eighty percent of those needing total care had abnormally low levels of DHEA. Other studies have found that DHEA replacement helps reverse many of the problems of dementia in aging people. And still other studies show that DHEA actually prevents neuronal damage and deterioration in brain tissue.[8]

Because androgen replacement therapy raises both androgen and testosterone levels and balances the androgen/estrogen ratios, the entire range of androgen replacement supplements are applicable. The brain contains ample supplies of the aromatase enzyme that converts testosterone to estrogens. In essence, the higher the levels of androgens (testosterone and its precursors like DHEA and androstenediol) the more estrogen the brain is able to make when it needs it. Physicians working with testosterone replacement therapy have consistently noted that when testosterone levels fall in aging men, brain function begins to fail rapidly.[9] Testosterone replacement therapies, as a result, usually have immediate effects on mental clarity.

Some newer research is showing that testosterone supplementation directly affects the neurofibrillary tangles that often form in the brain of people with Alzheimer's disease. A key enzyme that stimulates the formation of the tangles (glycogen synthase kinase-3-beta or GSK-3-beta) is inhibited by testosterone from becoming overactivated in the brain. Rats given testosterone supplementation were protected from the formation of neurofibrillary tangles in their brains.

Dosage
Take 50 to 100 milligrams a day.

Cautions
Some clinicians think DHEA can exacerbate the mania stage of manic depression, others believe it is contraindicated for men whose PSA (prostate-specific antigen—an indicator for prostate disease level) is high. The only literature-noted side effect is masculinization (facial hair, etc.) in some

women and the case of one woman who developed jaundice and liver problems after one week of use. It is not known if the latter side effect was related to the use of DHEA. Women seem most at risk of side effects.

ZINC

A number of studies have found that zinc levels are chronically low in
aging populations. Zinc levels in Alzheimer's patients are often extremely
low. There has been some preliminary evidence that the neurofibrillary tangles in the brains of Alzheimer's patients are exacerbated by zinc deficiencies. One controlled study with ten Alzheimer's patients found that eight
improved significantly with 27 milligrams of zinc supplementation, one
seventy-nine-year-old man miraculously so.[10]

Dosage
Take 40 milligrams a day. It is generally recommended to not exceed 40 milligrams of zinc per day.

Cautions
Over time, zinc intake can cause copper depletion in the body. To counteract this, most zinc supplements come with copper added. At very high
doses, zinc can cause nausea and upset stomach, skin rashes, depression,
folate deficiency, and lower tolerance to alcohol.

OTHER SUPPLEMENTS

Emerging research is showing a connection between Alzheimer's disease
and long-term high levels of homocysteine in the blood. Surveys of people
with high homocysteine levels have shown that, over time, they have nearly
two times the risk of developing Alzheimer's disease. Experimental studies
with rats have also shown a consistent relationship between homocysteine
levels and Alzheimer's-like deterioration in the brain. Increasing folic acid as
well as vitamin B_{12} and B_6 intake has been found to reduce the effects of homocysteine on brain cells. Homocysteine is thought to accelerate damage to
the neural cells of the brain. Folic acid seems especially important in that it
acts to protect the neural cells from damage and also deactivates the homocysteine molecule. Vitamins B_{12} and B_6 also help deactivate homocysteine.

A good-quality B-vitamin complex daily is suggested as is the regular consumption of green leafy vegetables, which tend to be high in folic acid. Other foods that contain folic acid are citrus fruits, tomatoes, and pinto, navy, and kidney beans. The recommended daily amount of folic acid is 400 micrograms.

SAGE AND ROSEMARY

Sage, rosemary, nettles, and garlic have all been found to possess attributes that are strongly supportive of healthy brain function or are specifically antagonistic to dementia.

Rosemary's colloquial name is "the herb of remembrance" and it has been used to improve memory for at least two thousand years. It does contain at least six compounds that have been found to help prevent the breakdown of acetylcholine in the brain. Many of these compounds can be absorbed through the skin. For this reason, Jim Duke, in his *Green Pharmacy*, suggests using rosemary shampoos, rosemary in the bathwater, and lots of rosemary tea. It is, as well, very good in food.

This is also true of sage. British researchers have found that sage possesses a number of strong compounds that also possess anticholinesterase action. John Gerarde, in 1597, was the first to remark on this. In his famous herbal he noted sage's efficacy for memory disorders, recommending it to "helpeth a weak braine or memory." Both sage and rosemary were plants commonly used in diets until recently. Sage ale was one of the most plentiful ales consumed in the middle ages. Rosemary ale, while not one of the top five, was also exceptionally common in both tavern and cottage life.

Suggested Use
Try a combination sage and rosemary bath extravaganza: shampoo, soap, and bath oil. Also use liberally in food.

Foods for Alzheimer's

There are a number of foods that contain acetylcholine and can be helpful in keeping levels in the body high: kale, bell pepper, carrot, cherries, potatoes, and spinach. Add them liberally to the diet. Nettles are also high in acetylcholine and were once a very common pot herb, cooked much like spinach. They were historically one of the most heavily consumed herbs of early spring; nettle beer was also a staple and was consumed in huge quantities until early summer. Beyond their use as food, nettles can be taken as a supplement. In this case, use the *freeze-dried* plant, not the root. Dosage range is 300 to 1,200 milligrams per day.

Because garlic is so good for circulatory health and preventing or healing atherosclerosis and blood pressure problems, it only makes sense to liberally include it in the diet for Alzheimer's relief. (For more, see Chapter 4.)

Avoid the Following

It is very important to avoid bodily intake of aluminum if you have or are at risk for Alzheimer's. Aluminum can be found in a number of forms in the following substances (read *all* product labels):

- Many antacids

- Many antidiarrheal preparations (e.g., Pepto-Bismol)

- Many antiperspirants

- Baking and cooking items: baking powder, self-rising flour, cake mixes, frozen doughs, sliced processed cheese; each of these can contain from 5 to 70 milligrams of sodium aluminum phosphate

- Nondairy creamers

- Some table salt; aluminum is included to prevent clumping

- Aluminum cans; aluminum can leach into anything inside an aluminum can (e.g., beer and soft drinks); buy glass instead

- Juice boxes; these aluminum-coated waxed containers also leach aluminum; buy glass instead

- Shampoos; many antidandruff shampoos contain either magnesium aluminum silicate or aluminum lauryl sulfate

- Buffered aspirin

- Aluminum cookware; to be avoided always

STROKE

Some 500,000 people have strokes each year in the United States. Most of them are from blood clots in the brain (ischemic stroke), about 20 percent are hemorrhagic strokes that are caused by a bursting blood vessel. Much of the information in Chapter 4 about heart disease applies here as well since stroke is specifically a cardiovascular problem. However, the treatment for stroke is essentially identical to that of Alzheimer's. The same herbs and supplements, especially ginkgo, have been found to both help prevent and to heal brain damage and the side effects from stroke. For stroke, however, the use of herbs that support capillary strength and healthy blood are also essential. Three important additions are vincamine, garlic, and vitamin E. LAC, while it can be of benefit, is not as essential.

Vitamin E, in a number of long-term studies, has shown benefit in helping patients recover from stroke, in preventing stroke, and in supporting a healthy cardiovascular system.[11] Garlic has shown many of the same properties and is an essential herb in the treatment of cardiovascular disease (see Chapter 4). Androgen supplementation is also essential as low levels of testosterone have been closely tied to cardiovascular disease (see Chapters 3 and 4). Basically, lower testosterone levels and an imbalance in the androgen/estrogen ratio have been tied to: (1) higher stroke levels in men, (2) increased fibrinogen levels (the basis of most blood clots), (3) decreased plasminogen (a natural anticlotting factor in the blood), (4) decreased arterial dilation, and (5) increased arterial plaque.

Natural Care for Stroke

For Six to Twenty-Four Months

Huperzine A, 50 to 100 micrograms twice a day

Ginkgo, 120 milligrams a day

Periwinkle (vincamine), 20 milligrams three times a day

Bilberry, 400 milligrams a day

Hawthorn, 600 to 900 milligrams a day

Garlic, 600 to 900 milligrams a day

DHEA, 50 to 100 milligrams a day

Zinc, 50 milligrams day

Vitamin E, 400 to 800 international units daily

PERIWINKLE (VINCAMINE)

The periwinkles (vincamine) (*Vinca minor, V. major*) have been used for thousands of years as herbs for stopping bleeding, diarrhea and dysentery, nervous disorders, headaches, vertigo, and memory difficulties. A relative, the Madagascar periwinkle (*Vinca rosea*), a historical diabetic tonic, is better known today as the source of the cancer drugs vinblastine and vincristine.

Vincamine was isolated from the lesser periwinkle, *Vinca minor,* in the early 1950s and some three hundred papers have been written on it since. Vincamine has specific effects on cerebral blood flow—it increases flow, increases oxygen consumption by the brain, and enhances brain-blood glucose utilization. Vincamine exerts a tonic effect on the cerebral arterioles and revitalizes cerebral metabolism. Double-blind trials and ECG readings have consistently shown that vincamine improves electrical activity in the brain, memory, concentration, behavior and speech disorders, irritability, vertigo, headaches, concentration, tinnitus, and blood flow in the retina of the eye. Researchers comment that the supplement is of special use in cases of stroke and arteriosclerosis. Improvement normally begins to be seen after three to six weeks of use.

As only one example: A twelve-week, double-blind trial of vincamine (30 milligrams twice daily) was conducted with 142 men and women between the ages of fifty and eighty-five who had been diagnosed with either Alzheimer's or multi-infarct dementia. All the participants were in either psychogeriatric centers or nursing homes. By the end of the study, vincamine was found to be significantly superior to placebo in the treatment of both types of dementia. All the patients were found to have improved by six different scales of measurement, including need for help by nursing staff.[12]

Dosage

Take 20 milligrams vincamine three times a day (or 30 milligrams twice a day). Vincamine is the form used for clinical trials and is widely available on the Internet and through health-food stores.

Take 1 teaspoon of the dried plant per cup of boiling water, steeped fifteen minutes, up to three times a day.

Take 1 to 2 milliliters (¼ to ½ teaspoon) of the tincture three times a day.

Cautions

Extreme overdoses of vincamine can cause serious drops in blood pressure. Contraindicated in brain tumors and intracranial pressure, use under a health practitioner's care if you currently have low blood pressure. It may occasionally cause nausea; if it does, lower the dosage or discontinue use.

As the herb can lower blood pressure and is a powerful treatment for diarrhea, avoid it if you have low blood pressure or chronic constipation. Some people have reported stomach upset. The German Commission E Monographs suggest that the use of vincamine is of more benefit and more reliable than the herb itself.[13]

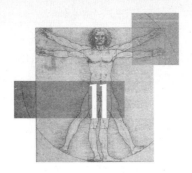

Inspiration: The Respiratory System

Inspiration (in'spa ra'shen) n. 1. The arousal within the mind of some idea, feeling, or impulse, especially one that leads to creative action. 2. Divine influence exerted upon the mind or spirit. 3. The act of drawing in the breath; inhalation. [OF inspirer < L inspirare to breathe into]

From Wakan Tanka, *the Great Spirit, there came a great unifying force that flowed in and through all things—the flowers of the plains, blowing wind, rocks, trees, birds, animals—and was the same force that had been breathed into the first man. Thus all things were kindred, and were brought together by the same Great Mystery.* —LUTHER STANDING BEAR

For human beings, breath has always had a connection to deeper transcendent truths. In all times and places, breathing—inspiration—has not only implied the simple act of breathing but a substance breathed into human beings at the beginning of their emergence on this planet, an original animating force, and transcendent states of mind. Even our own medical term for breathing—inspire—is connected to older, transcendent meanings. And, of course, to expire means not only to exhale but the end of breathing altogether, the departure of whatever it is that animated our bodies in the beginning.

One of the greatest pleasures of being a young man is the initial inspirations of a mature imagination. There is a time, somewhere between seventeen and twenty-three, that great winds begin to blow through the soul, something is breathing the imagination of the world into the newly mature self. Connections are seen everywhere, new ideas, images, spectacular thoughts, a deep-flowing river of *inspiration* has taken hold of the imagination. This early impact of the imagination of the world lays the foundation for the journey to middle age. The development of our characters is intimately bound up in those inspirations; the things that inspire us indicate a great deal about who we are and what motivates us. Our inspirations move us this way and that, setting a course for our life and the development of our characters that lies far outside our conscious thought.

But in middle age, there is an ending to that initial surge of inspiration and a letting go of the realities that gave it birth. It is not uncommon for men in middle age to feel devoid of *juice,* a loss of inspiration, or empty of imagination. For those who struggle through this *leaving,* there is on the other side a new kind of inspiration, a new kind of breathing. It is an inspiration that comes more out of a sense of historical time than newness of experience.

An emerging consciousness informs us that the breath we take is the exhale of the world (our exhale, its inhale). We no longer breathe an air untouched by other lungs, but air breathed by Shakespeare and whales, a street vendor in Beijing, dinosaurs, and our grandfathers. Our respiration connects us to all that has been and all that will be. And the inspirations, insights, and imaginations that begin to come to us, if we open to them and allow them entrance, are designed, like those of our younger selves, to shape the kind of men we are becoming. They give direction to us in our middle years, setting the course that sees us into old age.

The great truths that inspire us are not personal possessions. They exist outside the self. Like the wind, they flow into us, through us, and out again, just as they have done with our ancient ancestors and they will do with our descendants in times, long years from now, that none of us can know. This is perhaps one of the greatest teachings of the midlife passage.

But, we have polluted the world. It is no wonder that its air does more now than inspire us. It has also begun to make us ill. Chronic bronchitis, chronic sinusitis, and asthma are three of the fastest growing diseases of the industrialized world.

RESPIRATION AND THE LUNGS

The air we breathe comes in through the nose, circulates through the sinuses, travels down the pharynx (the throat), through the larynx (voice box), then the trachea (windpipe), and finally into the passages of the lungs. After the large primary bronchi enter the lungs, the air passages soon split into smaller secondary bronchi, split again into thousands of bronchioles, which all ultimately terminate in the countless alveolar ducts that are nestled in the lung tissue. Into and through this system we take ten to fifteen breaths a minute, twenty-five thousand breaths a day, 720 million breaths a lifetime to provide the oxygen and other gaseous chemistries we need to sustain our lives.

The world's forests provide much of the oxygen we need, just as we provide much of the carbon dioxide *they* need. Fascinatingly, our bronchial system looks much like a tree. Without the lung tissue that covers the bronchial passages, our airways from the trachea on down look like an inverted, leafless tree. The thousands of branches on the bronchial tree terminate in two sophisticated, yet delicate, membranes—the lungs. The lung membranes cover the outside of the bronchial tree much like leaves cover the terminal branches of trees in a deciduous forest. Each tiny branch of a tree terminates in leaves. Each tiny bronchial branch ends in a membrane of lung tissue. Leaves and lungs do the same thing; they provide a large surface area for gas exchange.

The Bronchial Passageway

The nose and sinuses warm and moisten the air, filter it for impurities, and chemically examine it for anything that might be irritating to the lungs. The sinuses also act as echo chambers, facilitating our ability to make sounds. Additionally, the nose serves as the location for olfactory (smell) sensors and the vomeronasal organ (VNO). The VNO takes molecules from the complex blend of gases we breathe and hooks them onto its special organ receptors. Information about the molecules' structures is sent to the brain for analysis. A single molecule, sometimes present at only one part per billion, is enough to cause the brain to entirely shift the physiology of the body in response. Substances present at only one part per million, for instance, have been found to shift the frequency, severity, length, and timing of women's menstrual cycles. Some people actually become sensitive to VNO activity and consciously learn to interpret the information it receives. (Some researchers are referring to this as a possible source of what has been called a sixth sense in human beings.)[1] The brain can also tell from VNO receptors whether something is harmful to the body or lungs and can alter lung functioning in response.

The pharynx is a muscular passageway for both air and food and it plays an important role in language. Certain vowel sounds can only be made by flexing the muscles of the pharynx, thus changing its shape. The larynx, in contrast, is made of both muscle *and* cartilage. Most of the rest of the bronchial tree, except the smaller bronchioles, is made of cartilaginous circles embedded in muscle tissue.

The largest cartilage formation in the larynx is the thyroid cartilage, so-named because the thyroid grows around the outside of its lower edge. (More commonly, it's called the Adam's apple.) Like all the airway passages of the body, the larynx is lined with mucous membranes. At one point in the larynx, the membranes fold and there is a narrow slit. Here, at the narrowest part of the larynx, are the vocal cords. Air flowing through the slit, like the air escaping through a balloon's stretched opening, causes a vibration. By altering the size and shape of the opening, language and other interesting sounds are made.

The trachea extends from the bottom of the larynx nearly to the lungs. It divides at the lower end into the two large bronchial tubes that enter the lungs. These primary bronchi, along with the large pulmonary blood vessels, enter through a slit in the side of each lung called the *hilum*. Shortly after they enter the lungs, the branches of the bronchi begin dividing into smaller secondary bronchi, which subdivide again into the thousands of bronchioles. This division process continues, each branching passageway getting smaller, until they are literally microscopic. At the terminal ends of these tiny branchioles are the alveolar ducts, which, like capillaries, consist of only a single layer of epithelial tissue. At the end of each duct is a cluster of grapelike sacs—the alveoli. Again, each microscopic alveolus is only a thin layer of simple epithelial tissue. Still, there are some 300 million of them in each lung. If they were opened up flat, they could cover nearly 240 square feet of space (a 10- by 24-foot room), some forty times the surface area of the body. There are scores of tiny gaps, infinitesimally small holes, in the thin walls separating alveoli that, when a breath is taken, allow the air pressure to equalize. Thus, all the alveoli receive the same volume of air simultaneously.

The pulmonary arteries that entered the lungs through the hilum have been branching too, so that every tiny alveolus is enveloped by a network of microscopic capillaries. Through a microscope, the alveoli look something like a cluster of grapes supported in a fine, netlike, expandable nylon bag. So many capillaries surround the alveoli, in fact, that the body's entire blood supply takes only a minute to flow through them.

The blood capillaries are fused to the alveoli through electrical polarity (magnetic attraction). The bond is so strong, the connection so tight, that the space between the two is fifty times thinner than the page on which these words are printed. This allows gases to move across the membranes very easily, facilitating the uptake of oxygen (and other chemistries in air that we need to remain healthy) and the discharge of excess carbon dioxide.

The Specialized Cells of the Lungs

The lungs, like the GI tract and skin, are a unique point of interface between the human being and the outside world, perhaps the most sensitive of them all. The exterior atmosphere is drawn inside us, where it comes into contact with a tremendously large surface area composed of extremely thin membranes. This membranous surface is designed to be easily penetrated by oxygen and complex carbon-chain molecules so that gas exchange can occur. *Anything* in the air we breathe can potentially penetrate it. This encompasses an incredible number of substances: oxygen, nitrogen, carbon dioxide, hydrogen, helium, dust, floating bacteria and viruses, the volatile oils given off by plants, pheromones, and synthetic pollutants—just to name a few.

In order to process the complex molecules that are entering the body, and to protect the lungs (and body) from damage, the entire surface area of the lungs and the respiratory tract contains billions of highly distinct, extremely specialized cells—over forty different kinds. Through sophisticated chemical actions and reactions they maintain the health of the lungs, protect the interior of the body from pathogens and contaminants, and promote the most effective gas exchange possible. The entire interior surface of the lungs is designed to sense anything and everything that comes into contact with it and then *do something* in response.

Among the cells that cover the interior surface of the respiratory tract are cilia (aka ciliated columnar cells), mucous (or goblet) cells, serous cells, myoepithelial cells, epithelial cells, neuroepithelial bodies, Kulchitsky cells, Clara cells, smooth muscle cells, membranous pneumocytes, granular pneumocytes, alveolar macrophages, fibroblasts, lymph cells, and mast cells (just to name some of the better known). All of these cells are highly sensitive, and reactive, to chemical communications from the outside world, whether that comes from bacterial organisms, synthetic petrochemicals, or the volatile terpenes released from evergreen trees.

This complex cellular community, the interior surface of the lungs, is covered by a special soaplike liquid (airway surface fluid—ASF), which is usually pH neutral, and a thin layer of mucus. Each lung is also sheathed in a slippery sac, then the whole encased inside another, similar sac, both of which are called pleura (which when inflamed cause the disease called pleuritis, or pleurisy). The spaces between the two pleurae are lubricated with a soaplike liquid, very similar to ASF, which allows the lungs to easily slide up and down as we breathe.

Maintaining the Mucosal Lining of the Lungs

Mucous, or goblet, cells make and release mucus to maintain the mucous blanket that lines the airways. The mucous blanket keeps the respiratory passageways and air we breathe moist and acts to contain lung-damaging agents (microbes, dust, pollutants) that come in with the air. In response to any kind of injury to or invasion of the respiratory tract, goblet cells can multiply rapidly, tremendously increasing their production of mucus. This traps and contains invading organisms, dust, or other particulate matter while, at the same time, coating and soothing the lung tissue.

Ciliated cells, under magnification, look somewhat hairlike. They cover most of the inside of the respiratory tract and move in a constant rhythmic pattern, about 1,000 to 1,500 cycles per minute. (In the lower airways, the cilia move slower, about 0.5 to 1 millimeter per minute, in the upper airways faster, about 5 to 20 millimeters per minute.) As goblet cells make mucus, the cilia that lie just under the mucosal surface slowly move it along. Most of it is moved up the throat and then down into the digestive system, some we cough out, some is processed through a special lymph drainage system in the lungs. The entire mucous blanket that covers the interior of the lungs is completely recycled in this way every twenty-four hours. Everything that accumulates in the lungs, including anything trapped in the mucus, is removed daily through this cephalad movement of the mucociliary escalator.

There are also a number of unique types of salivary glands, bronchial submucosal glands, located throughout the bronchi. They contain highly specialized mucous cells (which are somewhat different than goblet cells) and serous cells surrounded by a special myoepithelial tissue. The glands release mucus, mucins, lysozyme, and immunoglobulin A (IgA) into the airways, where the compounds are mixed with the mucus produced by the goblet cells to form the unique mucous coating that lines the lungs.

Lysozyme is a small enzyme that breaks the carbohydrate chains in bacterial cell walls, destroying their cellular integrity, causing the bacteria to burst open. It is part of the primary immune response in the lungs. Mucins are glycoproteins that combine with mucus to give it its particularly viscous and elastic qualities. IgA, made only in the respiratory and GI tract, is an immune (or secretory) antibody that is active against both bacteria and viruses. It is, as well, an important part of the lungs' immune response. IgA is extremely protective of the mucosal lining. These gland secretions are essential in protecting the lungs from the entry of pathogens into lung tissue. Thus, the healthier the submucosal glands, the healthier the lungs.

Submucosal gland secretion and release is controlled by the endocrine system through hormones and by Clara cell activity. The myoepithelial cells that surround the glands are composed of myofilaments and modified smooth-muscle cells. When they contract, in response to system communications, they expel secretions from the glands.

Clara cells are unique cells mostly located in the terminal, or smaller, bronchioles. They produce a watery, protein-filled secretion whose function is still mostly unknown. The secretion intermixes with the airway surfactant fluid, keeping it from becoming too thick. Some of the Clara cell–produced compounds act to control bronchial gland secretions, sometimes inhibiting, sometimes enhancing, their production. Clara cells are extremely sensitive to synthetic, petrochemically derived chemicals such as the dry-cleaning compound trichlorethylene. Such compounds can destroy or disable Clara cells when they are inhaled in tiny parts per million quantities, intermixed with the air we breathe.

The Alveoli

Alveoli are made up of at least four different types of cells: membranous pneumocytes, granular pneumocytes, macrophages, and fibroblasts.

A bit less than half of the cells in the alveoli are membranous pneumocytes (MPs) but they cover 92 percent of the alveolar surface area. MPs are extremely thin cells with very large surface areas. These are the cells across whose membranes the oxygen (and other gases) in the air diffuse into our blood. Some nutrients and fluids can also diffuse through these membranes, both into the blood and into the very thin layer of lymph fluid that flows between capillaries and alveoli. MPs cannot regenerate if they are damaged; they have to be replaced by new cells.

Granular pneumocytes (GPs), on the other hand, make up a bit more than half of alveolar cells. Much smaller in size, they only cover about 7 percent of the surface area. They manufacture and store the airway surface fluid that coats the inside of the lungs. ASF is crucial to lung function. Premature babies, often born before these cells are mature enough to make ASF, will die unless the cells can be matured quickly or a synthetic fluid inserted temporarily into the lungs. ASF reduces lung surface tension, helps equalize air pressures, and stabilizes and maintains the alveoli. GPs can regenerate themselves and they are the cells that are used to make more membranous pneumocytes when needed. Like Clara cells, GPs are extremely sensitive to organic solvents.

A tiny percentage, only about 1 percent, of the alveolar cells are special macrophages and fibroblasts. Alveolar fibroblasts produce a low molecular weight protein that stimulates the production of ASF by the GPs; they also help regulate blood flow through the capillaries. The alveolar macrophages are the main immune defense of the alveoli. They are special white blood cells that envelop and deactivate pathogenic organisms.

Once alveolar macrophages have enveloped a pathogenic organism they can either move up the mucociliary escalator (where they are processed through the digestive system or coughed out) or they can cross into the fluid between the capillaries and alveoli. If they move into this fluid, they are routed into the body's lymph system, often congregating in the lymph nodes during processing (and producing the familiar swelling). During any infection, the macrophages also release chemical signals that either call or activate neutrophils, eosinophils, and T lymphocytes in the lung tissue in order to promote immune response.

Because they are the main point of oxygen exchange, any infection or fluid buildup in the alveoli can cause difficulty in breathing. During pneumonia, for example, the alveoli become inflamed in response to pathogenic organisms, macrophages, and other immune cells multiplying by the millions, engulfing bacterial or viral organisms, and clogging the alveoli and the openings between them. The alveoli and alveolar ducts can, in fact, completely fill with thick, infectious mucus. The more alveoli that are affected, the less gas exchange that occurs. Unless the lungs can rapidly deactivate the organisms, liquefy the material clogging the alveoli, and then move it quickly into the lymph system for disposal, suffocation can occur. Similar blockages in the bronchial passageways during acute asthma attacks can also cause suffocation.

The lungs contain specialized lymph cells and channels in order to facilitate pulmonary drainage. To keep the lungs clear, excess mucus, cellular debris, used immune cells, and dead bacteria and viruses move through these channels and into the lymph system of the body for disposal.

Mast Cells

The lungs also contain other immune cells, called *mast* cells. Actually a specialized type of white blood cell, mast cells contain tiny packets or granules of inflammatory compounds. Some of these are preformed—histamines, heparin, tryptase, platelet-activating factor (PAF), and kininogenase—others are derived from arachidonic acid—leukotrienes, thromboxanes, and prostaglandins—and form only in response to chemical triggers. Mast cells also release other important inflammatory compounds—cytokines, GM-CSF, and TNFa. These compounds recruit and activate a number of inflammatory cells, causing them to cluster and bind tightly to sites of inflammation.

All these compounds have specific impacts on lung function. PAF, for example (which is also released from many other cells: neutrophils, basophils, eosinophils, macrophages, endothelial, and epithelial cells), stimulates an increased concentration and hyperactivity of immune cells in lung tissue. It decreases heart rate, constricts the bronchi, increases vascular permeability, increases water content (bloat) in lung tissues (pulmonary edema), and increases arachidonic acid release and eicosanoid production. PAF is some 100 to 10,000 times more potent than histamine in its inflammatory effects.

Histamine itself is extremely bioactive, causing lung inflammation when present at only 7 parts per million. The amount of PAF, or even leukotrienes, which are similarly potent, needed to induce inflammation is infinitesimally tiny.

Mast cells release their contents (and create other inflammatory compounds) in response to a flood of calcium ions into the mast cell. Though anything that causes intracellular calcium levels to rise will stimulate release, one major stimulant is immunoglobulin E (IgE). IgE is an amino acid antibody unique to the respiratory and GI tract. When it detects compounds that it feels are a danger to the respiratory system, it binds to mast cells and floods them with calcium ions, stimulating the mast cells to respond.

Lung Hormones

Although research on lung hormones is somewhat scanty, the lungs do, like most other organ systems in the body, make a number of unique hormones to control functioning. The Kulchitsky cells in the lungs are unique pulmonary hormone glands. They belong to a diffuse, poorly understood neuroendocrine system called the APUD (Amine Precursor Uptake and Decarboxylation) system. Kulchitsky cells occur in a number of locations in the lungs and bronchial passageways (and sometimes in other parts of the body) and contain dense neurosecretory granules that produce highly bioactive hormones, not all of which have been identified. This includes serotonin, calcitonin, and bombesin. These three hormones possess powerful impacts on lung functioning and play important roles in chronic lung diseases.

Calcitonin (which is also made in the thyroid gland) acts to control calcium concentrations, especially in the blood. Besides its impacts on intracellular levels of calcium in lung tissue, calcitonin affects the amount of calcium laid down in the intracellular matrix during bone formation.

Bombesin, widely distributed in the GI tract and brain, modulates smooth-muscle contractions, exocrine and endocrine gland actions, metabolism, and behavior. It stimulates gastric acid secretion, gallbladder contraction, pancreatic secretion, and proper functioning of the duodenum. (The duodenum is where most of the minerals—calcium, magnesium, potassium, and so on—are extracted from food.) Bombesin deficiency can cause impaired nutrient intake and glucose metabolism, reduced metabolic rate, mild obesity, and vasoconstriction. The lungs can, when there are insufficient minerals to maintain electrolytic balance, increase bombesin secretion to stimulate the duodenum's uptake of minerals from food.

Serotonin in the lungs, unlike that in the brain, causes contractions in smooth-muscle tissues. It is made from tryptophan by an enzyme, tryptophan hydroxylase. High serotonin levels in the body (not brain) cause increased muscle contractions.

Other pulmonary hormones are produced in the lungs' neuroepithelial bodies. The neuroepithelial bodies are clusters of neuroendocrine cells that are scattered throughout the alveoli and some of the bronchioles. Very little is known about them.

Besides making their own hormones, the lungs are also highly sensitive to steroid hormones, both androgens and estrogens. Just how important they are can be seen by their crucial impacts on the lung development of the fetus. (Premature infants often suffer life-threatening problems because of immature lung development.)

As the fetus moves toward birth, cellular chloride secretory pathways in the lungs diminish and sodium absorptive pathways increase. These chloride channels are more commonly called the cystic fibrosis transmembrane conductance regulators (CFTR) because they were discovered through cystic fibrosis (CF) research. People with CF have very poorly functioning CFTR channels, which causes their lungs to have a very thick mucus infused with high concentrations of salt. The CFTR is, however, involved in many other cellular functions besides merely regulating chloride channels. It is also an important conductance regulator. It helps move glutathione, an important antioxidant in lung tissues, into cells that have encountered oxidants, and it has also been found to affect a number of other ion channels in the cellular membrane. CFTR has in fact been found to play a significant role in regulating the influx of calcium ions into cells. The functional activity of CFTR channels is increased by androgens and decreased by estrogens. The more estrogens the lungs encounter, the more

CFTR action is inhibited. This can have a number of negative side effects if the pre-birth infant (or even a grown person) encounters too many estrogens. High estrogen levels have been found to consistently interfere with healthy ion transport in cellular tissues, being especially compromising to the CFTR system.[2] This may also explain why women, with their higher estrogen levels, tend to have more cystic fibrosis and chronic asthma, sinusitis, and bronchitis than men.[3] The lungs also convert DHEA to more highly active androgens like testosterone when they need them to maintain lung health. The maintenance of this androgen balance is crucial to the lungs' cellular homeostasis.

The Importance of Electrolytes

Healthy lung function and optimum gas exchange depends on a highly sophisticated balance of the intracellular salts (or electrolytes) that the kidney routinely monitors and routs within the body: calcium, chloride, magnesium, potassium, manganese, and copper.

Manganese and copper are used by the lungs in the formation of two superoxide dismutases (SODs), one copper-based and the other manganese-based, that it uses as antioxidants. Because the lungs are designed to transfer large quantities of oxygen from the air into our blood, and because free oxygen radicals are so toxic, the lungs have developed mechanisms for protecting themselves from oxidative damage. SODs are part of this protective mechanism, along with a sophisticated array of other antioxidants that include such things as antioxidant enzymes, catalase, and glutathione. The lungs encounter many different kinds of oxidants in the air, all of which cause different kinds of damage and so a different cascade of antioxidant defenses occurs, alone, in combination, or in sequence, depending on what the lungs breathe in.[4]

The other four salts—calcium, chloride, magnesium, and potassium—are used to control cell functioning and lung homeostasis. By opening and shutting different pathways or gates into and out of the cells, the intracellular levels of the various salts change, and lung function alters, sometimes dramatically in response. Which cellular gates are open and which are shut, control the flow of anions and cations—negative and positive electrolyte ions—across cellular membranes. If a cell receives a flood of calcium anions into itself, thus building up intracellular calcium levels, it acts completely differently than it does if positive potassium ions are accumulating within the cell.

Of extreme importance in diseases like asthma are the electrolytic balances in cells that control bronchial muscle relaxation and constriction. High intracellular calcium levels are a major component of asthma and other bronchopulmonary diseases because calcium anion influx causes muscle cells to contract. Potassium influx, on the other hand, causes them to relax. (High calcium additionally initiates the rapid cellular production of the potent inflammatory compound PAF.) Magnesium is an essential element in healthy lung function because of its regulatory impacts on calcium. When magnesium is deficient the actions of calcium are enhanced. High magnesium levels are antagonistic to the influence of calcium on cellular functioning. The body, in fact, cannot manage intracellular calcium levels without sufficient magnesium.

Cyclic adenosine monophosphate, or cAMP, also affects ion gating in lung tissue. Cyclic AMP is created through the action of an enzyme in the lungs, adenylate cyclase (AC). AC is activated by a number of different types of compounds, among which is the adrenal hormone epinephrine (aka adrenaline). When activated, cAMP relaxes the muscles that surround the bronchial passages, allowing more air to be inspired. Cyclic AMP also inhibits the degranulation of mast cells (thus stopping the release of inflammatory histamines and leukotrienes), increases heart muscle contractions, increases insulin secretion, and increases thyroid metabolism. Cyclic AMP is especially important because it regulates the levels of intracellular calcium in lung muscles and tissues.

CHRONIC RESPIRATORY DISEASES

Asthma, chronic bronchitis, and chronic sinusitis are all caused by an increased sensitivity and hyperreactivity of the tissues of the respiratory tract. People develop different patterns of tissue sensitivity in airways depending on their genetics, personal history, level of exposure to environmental pollutants, diet, and so on. Some people with asthma only respond to specific allergens they breathe in—so-called extrinsic asthma. Others are constantly sensitive and a large number of factors, even stress, can set off an acute episode—so-called intrinsic asthma. In chronic sinusitis, the sensitivity is usually limited to the sinus passages—in chronic bronchitis, the bronchi.

Again, in some people, certain allergens can set off sinusitis or bronchitis attacks; in others, the passages are constantly sensitive. Some people suffer all three conditions simultaneously. All of the conditions are increasing in incidence each year.

Between 1980 and 1994, asthma increased 102 percent. Between 1994 and 2002 it increased another 50 percent. In the industrialized world, asthma is increasing between 6 and 7 percent per year. In Switzerland, 8 percent of the population has asthma; twenty-five years ago it was only 2 percent. The less industrialized a nation is, the less chance someone will suffer the disease. In India, only about 2 percent of the people are sufferers. Somewhere between fifteen and twenty million people in the United States have asthma, 150 million worldwide.

Chronic bronchitis is considered to be a chronic inflammation of the lining of the bronchial tubes that lasts longer than one year. More women have it than men, about nine million people in the United States.

Chronic sinusitis is an inflammation of the lining of the sinuses that lasts longer than three months. It is the most common chronic condition in the United States, affecting an estimated thirty-seven million people.

All three respiratory diseases are marked by elevated IgE levels and cellular alterations in the mucosal lining of the respiratory tract. The mucosa thickens and becomes hypersensitive and hyperreactive to a variety of airborne pollutants and allergens. The primary cause of these changes in the respiratory tract is believed to be airborne pollutants.

Airborne Pollutants

The human lung evolved over an estimated million years immersed in a very specific atmosphere. Besides oxygen, human beings were surrounded by the highly bioactive and volatile carbon-based essential oils given off by thousands of different wild plants. The evergreen forests of the Earth, as only one example, give off two trillion pounds of volatile oils each year. These gaseous volatiles, along with trillions of tons more from other plants, float in the air and fall to the ground as a rain of highly bioactive complex terpenes. They are also breathed in by everything that inhales. Plant aromatics have a number of important functions, among which are disinfecting the air, enhancing respiration, and increasing organism growth. Many evergreen terpenes have distinct enhancement impacts on alveoli and transmit easily across alveolar membranes into the blood. The human lung is designed to breathe in these kinds of chemistries and to incorporate them into the body in a variety of ways. Scores of other gaseous compounds besides oxygen and carbon dioxide have crossed the human lung membranes throughout evolutionary time. They can all significantly affect lung function and bodily health in incredibly tiny quantities—parts per million or even parts per billion.

To understand the powerful impact of synthetic pollutants in the air, you need only to realize that most synthetic chemicals are carbon-based molecular structures. They are all made from petroleum, which is itself derived from long-buried plant matter. Such chemicals, for example, as the fumes from gasoline and diesel fuel, are close enough to evolutionary, complex-carbon, gaseous compounds that the lungs readily take them in. But these are new substances, evolutionarily speaking; our bodies are not used to processing them. The cellular population of the lungs have no evolutionary mechanism for dealing with them.

Because every cell in our lungs has been designed to be so sensitive to gases and small particulate matter, these synthetic pollutants have tremendous physiological impacts because of their chemical mimicry. Over time, the entire physiology of the respiratory passages changes and becomes highly sensitive, especially to bioactive synthetic chemicals.

Respiratory Inflammation

The constant influx of synthetic chemicals into the respiratory tract initiates inflammation either by activating IgE response or directly increasing intracellular calcium levels.

Most people with chronic respiratory diseases have significantly elevated levels of IgE in their airway mucosa. IgE can become sensitive to a wide range of substances. Activated, IgE binds to mast cells, where it can remain for months, ready to respond to any new influx of the substances (allergens) to which it is sensitive. Any allergen influx activates IgE response, which causes the release of inflammatory compounds from mast cells by increasing their intracellular calcium levels.

Importantly, mast cells can also be set off by anything else that increases intracellular calcium. Low body magnesium, certain drugs, including some used for asthma, a malfunctioning or depressed cystic fibrosis transmembrane regulator (CFTR), oxidative damage to the mucosal lining of the respiratory tract, and many synthetic chemicals can all increase intracellular calcium. Different substances increase calcium ions in different cells in lung tissue, all of which can release PAF when so stimulated. Calcium influx into cells, in fact, initiates a cascading series of inflammatory responses, of which PAF release is only one factor.

As intracellular calcium levels rise, mast cells degranulate, releasing their preformed contents. The cellular enzyme *cystolic phospholipase A2* is activated, causing cell membrane phospholipids to break apart. This releases lyso-PAF and arachidonic acid (AA). Lyso-PAF is then enzymatically converted to PAF, while arachidonic acid metabolism gives rise to leukotrienes, thromboxanes, and prostaglandins—all highly potent inflammatory agents.

The preformed contents in mast cells cause an initial, early-phase inflammatory response within fifteen or twenty minutes of release. PAF activation is also fairly rapid, leading to a clustering and hyperactivity of immunoactive cells. The arachidonic acid derivatives take several hours to synthesize and their effects occur most strongly some five to six hours later. All of these inflammatory actors, plus cytokines and a battery of tissue-damaging enzymes and reactive oxygen molecules, work in concert, exacerbating airway tissue inflammation.

Because of the pervasiveness of airborne pollutants in industrialized nations and a general tendency to low body magnesium, these inflammatory reactions continually occur at a low level in many people for years. (Part-per-million quantities of sulfur dioxide, nitrogen oxides, diesel exhaust, and fly ash are all particularly powerful in their impacts on the respiratory passages. Diesel exhaust itself is a potent stimulant of IgE production.) Normally, the body is able, through its delicately balanced control over cellular function in the lungs, to decrease inflammation after contact with an irritant or infectious agent. Unfortunately, the continual presence of synthetic chemicals in the atmosphere never allows the lungs to escape exposure long enough to completely recover. The continuing inflammatory stimulation of tissues by synthetic pollutants eventually results in actual cellular alterations of the respiratory passageways. The mucosal lining thickens and, over time, becomes hypersensitive and hyperreactive. There is more mucus production, greater vascular permeability, eosinophil penetration of the mucosa, and the cellular functions of the airways become abnormal. Electrolyte imbalances are common, enzyme production is skewed, lung antioxidant production is chronically depressed, and hormone production is upset. The pH of the lungs becomes more acidic (altering lung enzyme activity even more) and the lungs begin producing excess nitric oxide. For people who develop asthma, the hyperreactive bronchial passageways become more susceptible to acute attacks with each passing year.

In an acute asthmatic attack, the mucosal lining of the airways becomes highly inflamed, which narrows the respiratory opening. The muscles in which bronchial cartilage is embedded become tightly constricted, narrowing the airway openings. And the bronchial passages produce tremendous amounts of a very thick mucus that blocks the airways. In very acute episodes it is sometimes impossible to get air into or out of the lungs.

The common medical intervention for asthma is beta2-adrenergic receptor agonists. These are very similar to epinephrine and cause the bronchial tubes to expand. Recent studies have shown that long-term use of these compounds may cause asthma to worsen, in part because they cause more calcium ion concentration in lung tissue. Anticholinergic pharmaceuticals are also often prescribed to relax the muscles that surround the bronchial passages. Sometimes these may also be used for chronic sinusitis and bronchitis. Both these approaches do nothing to treat the underlying abnormal condition of the respiratory system.

Natural Care for Chronic Asthma, Bronchitis, and Sinusitis

To reverse chronic asthma, sinusitis, and bronchitis it is crucial to strengthen the underlying structure of the lungs, reestablish electrolyte balance, and reverse the hyperreactivity and hypersensitivity of the respiratory passages. There are a number of highly effective herbs and supplements that will help in this process. One of the most interesting is coleus.

Note: This protocol is for helping correct chronic conditions only. Acute episodes of asthma can be life-threatening. Interventive pharmaceuticals are, in many instances, necessary and can be lifesaving.

> Coleus, standardized extract, 50 milligrams two to three times daily (or forskolin 10 milligrams twice daily)
> Tylospora, 200 milligrams daily

Desmodium adscendens, tea daily

Khella, 250 to 300 milligrams daily

Ginkgo, 80 milligrams three times daily

Reishi, three 1-gram tablets three times daily

Pine bark or grape seed extract, 100 milligrams three times daily

DHEA, 25 to 50 milligrams daily

Magnesium, 200 to 400 milligrams three times daily

N-acetyl cysteine, 1,200 milligrams daily

Vitamin B_6, 50 to 100 milligrams twice daily

Vitamin C, 1 to 2 grams daily

Selenium, 200 micrograms daily

Sinupret (sinusitis), as directed

Bromelain (sinusitis and bronchitis), 250 to 750 milligrams three times daily

Diet alteration

Onions, lots daily

Yoga, massage, meditation

COLEUS

Coleus (*Coleus forskohlii*), an attractive, aromatic, perennial member of the mint family, is a traditional Ayurvedic medicinal plant from India. Historically, the root of the plant has been used for a number of conditions: asthma, respiratory disorders, heart disease, intestinal spasms, kidney stones, insomnia, painful urination, and convulsions. One specific compound in coleus, forskolin, has been found especially effective in the treatment of asthma.

Forskolin activates the important cellular enzyme adenylate cyclase (AC), which, when activated, increases the amount of cyclic adenosine monophosphate (cAMP) in cells. Forskolin increases cAMP some six- to four hundredfold, depending on the cell in which AC is activated. The cAMP activation stimulates the muscles of the bronchial passageways and the pulmonary blood vessels to relax, inhibits histamine release by preventing mast cell degranulation, inhibits PAF immune cell activation, and enhances the thyroid regulatory mechanisms that have direct impacts on lung function. It specifically increases thyroid hormone production and release, which increases body metabolism and enhances the regulation of calcium by the thyroid's production and release of calcitonin. Forskolin has also been found to inhibit platelet activating factor (PAF) formation in lung tissue. This inhibits the congregation of immune cells in the lungs, decreases neutrophil formation, decreases vascular permeability, and also helps reduce bronchial constriction by reducing inflammation. Because it is a specific PAF antagonist, forskolin is strongly antiallergenic, reducing the impacts of allergens on bronchial tissues. Forskolin has also been found to have direct impacts on a number of other lung enzymes, membrane transport proteins, and the potassium and calcium ion channels that affect cellular functioning. It affects which ions are transported across membranes, altering intracellular ionic electrolytes. It especially affects the cystic fibrosis transmembrane regulator (CFTR), enhancing its activity. Forskolin stimulates an uptake of nitric oxide by muscle cells (potentiating their relaxation) and moves lung tissue and airway surface liquid from an acidic to a more normal pH.

One of the more intriguing things about forskolin is that it increases androgenic hormone levels. Forskolin increases the production of DHEA in the adrenals and enhances 3-beta-hydroxysteroid (3BHSD) activity, which increases the conversion of androstenediol into testosterone. Forskolin increases the activity of 3BHSD sevenfold and increases the production of androstenedione fivefold. Forskolin has also been found to increase sperm motility and to help erectile dysfunction, showing that it has broad impacts on the male reproductive system.

Because low DHEA and testosterone are common in men with chronic obstructive pulmonary diseases (COPDs) such as asthma and bronchitis, forskolin is supportive not only through relaxing tissues, lowering sensitivity to allergens, and increasing the health of the bronchial tissues, but also through elevating androgen levels.

At the same time, forskolin helps chronic pulmonary diseases by reducing fat levels in the body. It increases lipolysis (the breakdown of fat for fuel), thus reducing the body's fat levels (shifting the body from an estrogenic/cortisol to a more androgenic/DHEA metabolism). It also increases nutrient absorption in the small intestine. A number of early studies are showing that forskolin is extremely efficient in lowering the fat content of the body. This could be exceptionally helpful in the long-term treatment of asthma, as several studies have shown a positive correlation between asthma and excess body fat.

There is speculation that some of forskolin's effects come from stimulating more efficient functioning of the lungs' Kulchitsky cells—enhancing bombesin and calcitonin secretion and decreasing serotonin.

Depression in asthma is fairly common. Low adenyl cyclase activity (the enzyme that initiates cAMP formation) has been linked to depression (especially in men) and forskolin has been found to help lower depression levels in people because it increases enzyme activity and cAMP levels.

Over five thousand research studies have been carried out on forskolin's impacts on cellular metabolism, especially on cAMP formation. A number of clinical trials have also been conducted with forskolin in the treatment of bronchial asthma.

In one randomized, placebo-controlled, double-blind, crossover trial, sixteen people with asthma used either forskolin capsules or the pharmaceutical fenoterol as inhaled gas or encapsulated powder. Within 120 minutes of ingestion, all the compounds caused bronchodilation and increased airway conductance. While the forskolin was not quite as strong in its effects as the fenoterol, it possessed markedly fewer side effects and caused less finger tremor with no decrease in blood potassium levels.

Another study with twelve healthy volunteers found that forskolin and fenoterol had equal bronchodilating effects after five minutes of inhalation. And though fenoterol's impacts lasted longer, the protective effects of forskolin against inhaled acetylcholine was as good as those of fenoterol after three to five minutes of inhalation.

While most clinical and lab studies have used the concentrated extract, the standardized whole herb has actually been found to be more inhibitive of PAF than forskolin.

Forskolin has also been found to reduce lung tumor colonization by 70 percent and to reduce intraocular pressure in glaucoma (when applied as drops to the eyes).[5]

Dosage

Normally, the forskolin content in coleus is increased through concentrated standardization to about 18 percent. Normal dosage is 50 milligrams two to three times daily of a standardized extract (which will give a forskolin dose of 9 milligrams two to three times daily). Purified forskolin is also available in 10-milligram tablets. Normal dosage is one tablet two to three times daily.

Cautions

No side effects have been noted; however, it is not suggested for those with gastric ulceration or low blood pressure. Because forskolin also affects heart function through a number of mechanisms, it should not be taken concurrently with pharmaceutical heart medications unless under the supervision of a health-care provider.

TYLOSPORA

Tylosporas (*Tylospora asthmatica, T. indica*) are perennial climbing plants common throughout India. The leaves of two species have long been used as traditional Ayurvedic medicine for hay fever, sinusitis, bronchitis, and asthma (as the Latin name for one of them indicates).

Tylospora relaxes bronchial smooth muscles, prevents mast cell degranulation—especially inhibiting the release of histamines—inhibits the chemoattraction of immune cells to the mucosal walls of the respiratory tract, and is specifically anti-anaphylactic—desensitizing tissues to allergens. The herb is specifically anti-inflammatory to the respiratory system, stabilizes mast cells, inhibits the release of inflammatory agents, acts to correct the thickening of the respiratory mucosa, and desensitizes the respiratory system to allergens.

A number of *in vitro, in vivo,* and human studies have been carried out and have verified the traditional use of the herb for respiratory disorders.

In a double-blind, placebo-controlled, crossover study of 103 people with asthma, after six days of 40 milligrams daily of tylospora, participants showed marked improvement over placebo. While the improvements diminished with time, the beneficial impacts of only six days of use were still measurable three months after the study.

Another study of 135 people with asthma who took 200 milligrams twice daily of tylospora for six days, showed marked improvements in symptoms and respiratory function over placebo. Improvements were still measurable two weeks after treatment ceased.

Double-blind, crossover trials that compared tylospora with pharmaceutical anti-asthmatics have found it comparable in effect. One found that tylospora was more effective than the bronchodilator isoprenaline.

Trials have also found the herb effective for other respiratory conditions such as bronchitis, sinusitis, and allergic rhinitis.[6]

Because the herb possesses long-term corrective effects and seems to stabilize mast cells, normalize mucosal membranes, prevent attachment of immune cells to the mucosa, and desensitize the respiratory passages to allergens, it seems indicated, if it can be tolerated (see below), as a regular part of an anti-asthmatic regimen.

Dosage
Take 200 to 400 milligrams daily of the dried herb (200 milligrams twice daily).

Cautions
About 10 percent of people using tylospora experience side effects such as vomiting, nausea, mouth soreness, and loss of taste for salt. Side effects are more common in people using the fresh leaf (up to 50 percent) or an alcoholic extract than in those using capsules or tablets.

DESMODIUM

A number of herbs that are specific for kidney stones are, not surprising, also specific for asthma and bronchitis. This is because the herbs, like coleus (which is also used for kidney stones), are calcium antagonists. They balance the body's cellular metabolism of electrolytes, shifting it away from calcium ion influx. Additionally, some of the herbs, like desmodium, have powerfully inhibitory impacts on inflammatory processes in airway tissues.

Desmodium adscendens, a close relative of the beggar's-lice used for kidney stones, is an herb that has been used both in Ghana and South America for a wide range of complaints. Desmodium, called *amor seco* in South America, is a multibranched, weedy perennial herb, about eighteen inches high, that is harvested and dried for use, usually as a tea. Indigenous to many tropical regions, it has been used very successfully by folk herbalists in Ghana for hundreds of years in the treatment of asthma and other bronchopulmonary conditions.

The plant has been found in a number of studies to contain the most potent potassium channel opener known. Other studies have shown that the herb inhibits allergic smooth-muscle contraction at multiple sites, it inhibits antigen-induced bronchopulmonary contractions, and it inhibits the activity of inflammatory leukotrienes in airways. It is also anti-anaphylactic, inhibitory of histamine-induced contractions, and reduces the amount of smooth-muscle-stimulating substances released from lung tissue during allergic responses. Other studies have discovered that the plant inhibits the synthesis of prostaglandins and leukotrienes from arachidonic acid precursors. One major mode of action seems to be the inhibition of the arachidonic acid (AA) cascade. Stopping AA conversion reduces inflammatory substances in the lungs and reduces the incidence of asthma attack and daily compromise in lung tissue.

One 1977 clinical trial found that 3 grams of the dried and powdered herb given in three divided doses daily resulted in remission or significantly alleviated symptoms in all the patients in the study.[7]

Desmodium can be added to other lung-specific herbs as a respiratory tea if desired. Goldenrod, couch grass, nettles, plantain, Iceland moss, lungwort, and peppermint are all specific for bronchopulmonary conditions and make a good blend.

Goldenrod, also a kidney herb, has profound effects as an anticatarrhal in bronchial conditions and has long been used for bronchopulmonary conditions. Couch grass is considered specific for asthma as a calcium antagonist. Nettles are a potent antihistamine and studies have found them to powerfully inhibit inflammatory responses in the lungs. Plantain, Iceland moss, and lungwort are all specifics for bronchitis, commonly used in European medicine. Peppermint is a powerful antispasmodic and adds an excellent taste to the tea.

Dosage

As a tea add 1 teaspoon dried herb to 6 ounces of hot water, steep for 15 minutes, and drink three times daily. As a tincture take ¾ to 1 teaspoon twice daily. As capsules or tablets take one to five grams twice daily.

To make a tea, combine sixteen ounces of desmodium and eight ounces each of goldenrod, couch grass, nettles, plantain, Iceland moss, lungwort, and peppermint and mix well. Add one cup of the mix to one quart of hot water and let it steep overnight. Strain and drink throughout the day as often as desired (at least three times daily). One quart daily.

Cautions

No side effects have been noted with use of the herb. However, in acutely sensitive individuals, especially those with pollen or grass allergies, the dust from the herbs may provoke an allergic response. Have someone else prepare the tea.

KHELLA

While khella (*Ammi visnaga*) is better known for its effects on the heart, it is also highly effective for asthma. The herb is a member of the carrot family (which it looks very much like) and stands about three feet tall; the dried berries (seeds) are used. Khella is common throughout the Mediterranean region and it was a primary medicinal used by the ancient Egyptians, listed in the very ancient Ebers papyrus. Its primary historical use, like many herbs for asthma and the heart, was the treatment of kidney stones. Like so many of those other herbs, it has a strong regulatory effect on the body's metabolism of calcium while at the same time being strongly antispasmodic. This has the effect in respiratory diseases of lowering intracellular calcium levels, acting somewhat as a calcium channel blocker (thus reducing muscle contractions) and expanding the respiratory passages. Khella is especially active on the smaller bronchi and bronchioles, the relaxation effects lasting about six hours. The effects of khella on bronchial tissue accumulates over time; the more it is used, the better and longer its impact. The herb is especially useful at night. Taken before bed, it helps maintain an uninterrupted sleep. (It has been found very helpful at nighttime for those with emphysema as well.) Khella's activity is enhanced when used with other herbs or supplements that affect the bronchial passages either through different modes of action or in different locations (i.e., higher passageways). A combinations of plants and supplements, including khella, produce a highly effective, synergistic impact on lung diseases.

There have been a considerable number of studies on the herb and its various constituents, mostly in Germany, and the clinical results (from physician practice) are impressive. While there are many clinical studies on the use of khella for angina, there is only one trial (as opposed to the clinical practice experience of German physicians) I have been able to locate using it for chronic asthma. The study was with twelve people with asthma and emphysema. Half improved, some significantly, after the use of khella.[8]

Dosage

Take 250 to 300 milligrams daily or ¼ teaspoon of the tincture twice daily, morning and evening, just before bed. The herb is most often standardized for 18 percent khellin content. The tincture is often preferred because it is absorbed rapidly through the mucous membranes of the mouth, where it then produces almost immediate effects on lung function.

Cautions

Photosensitization can sometimes occur—extremely light-skinned people should be cautious in their sunlight exposure when taking the herb. At high doses, liver inflammation and jaundice, in very rare instances, can occur. These conditions clear upon discontinuing the herb.

GINKGO

Ginkgo (*Ginkgo biloba*) has been widely, and very successfully, used in China for the treatment of asthma. Gingko contains unique compounds known as *ginkgolides,* which are strongly antagonistic of platelet activating factor (PAF). One particular ginkgolide—BN 52021—because it is so strongly inhibitive of PAF, is a standard compound in laboratory studies of platelet-activating factor. In numerous studies, BN 52021 has improved antioxidant defenses in damaged lungs, reduced neutrophil adherence to and penetration of endothelial cells, reduced pulmonary arterial pressure and capillary permeability, and inhibited the synthesis of arachidonic metabolites. Besides BN 52021, ginkgo contains at least four other potent ginkgolides, each one a powerful PAF antagonist.

Ginkgo's ginkgolides have been shown to be highly effective in a number of double-blind studies of people with asthma. PAF activity was inhibited, respiratory function improved, and—best of all—bronchial hyperreactivity was reduced. The trials were conducted with pure ginkgolides, which are, unfortunately, commercially unavailable. (Ginkgo is normally standardized for 24 percent flavonglycosides and 6 percent terpenoid ginkgolides.) However, at least one placebo-controlled clinical trial has been carried out in Japan using a standardized, concentrated ginkgo extract. It significantly reduced airway hyperreactivity and improved clinical symptoms and pulmonary function.[9]

Dosage
Take 80 milligrams three times daily.

Cautions
Some people are sensitive to ginkgo preparations. Caution should be used if you are taking antithrombotic medications. Uncommonly, side effects are mild gastrointestinal upset or headache, and very rarely, allergic skin reactions. In very large doses, ginkgo can cause diarrhea, irritability, and restlessness. Because ginkgo is a PAF inhibitor, it should be avoided before surgery.

REISHI

Reishi (*Ganoderma lucidum*), a largish reddish, woody mushroom, has a very long history of use in Asia for many complaints, especially liver and lung diseases. In clinical studies, reishi has shown consistent inhibition of allergic responses in bronchopulmonary tissues. Reishi inhibits histamine release from mast cells, desensitizes bronchial tissues (thus lowering hyperreactivity), and relaxes smooth muscles in the respiratory tract. It has been found to inhibit both histamine inducers and IgE-mediated allergic reactions. Through a number of mechanisms, reishi exerts strong anti-inflammatory activity. It also increases the amount of superoxide dismutases in the lung tissues. Reishi has, in consequence, consistently shown potent antioxidant activity, lowering free radicals in tissues up to 50 percent.

There have been a number of trials using reishi for the treatment of bronchopulmonary diseases. While a number of them have shown that it helps alleviate asthma, the larger studies have explored its use in the treatment of chronic bronchitis. One extremely large clinical study in China examined the use of reishi by over two thousand people with chronic bronchitis. Within two weeks, 60 to 90 percent of the participants showed significant improvements in their condition, including a number who also suffered from bronchial asthma.[10]

Dosage

Take three 1-gram tablets three times daily.

PINE BARK OR GRAPE SEED EXTRACT (OPCS)

Flavonoids, most notably quercetin, can be highly effective in the treatment of asthma. These kinds of flavonoids, even more prevalent in grape seed and pine bark extracts, are powerful inhibitors of histamine release from mast cells. They also interfere with the production of leukotrienes and other inflammatory mediators in the lungs. The proanthocyanidins (OPCs) in grape seed and pine bark have been found to specifically inhibit mast cell degranulation, the release of histamine, and AA synthesis of leuko-trienes.[11] OPCs also inhibit the action of the enzyme histidine decarbox-ylase, which enables the production of histamine.

Dosage

Take 100 to 150 milligrams two to three times daily.

Cautions

Standardized Extracts: Pine bark extracts may be synergistic with "blood-thinning" medications such as warfarin, heparin, clopidogrel, pentoxi-fylline, and aspirin and should, therefore, be used with caution or under the supervision of a health-care practitioner if you are using these drugs. Side effects are rare: mild allergic reactions and digestive upset have been reported.

Herbal Extracts: Some people are sensitive to pine products—seeds, pollen, bark, resin, and so on. Negative reactions can run from mild aller-gies to anaphylactic shock. **If you have a history of allergies to pollen or severe reactions to bee stings, you should proceed with caution to make sure that your reactions do not extend to pine products.**

DHEA AND ANDROGEN ENHANCEMENT

DHEA, DHEA-sulfate, and other androgens are low in people with asthma. Adult-onset asthma begins around age forty, the same age that androgens and DHEA levels begin declining in the body. Forty percent of adults with asthma have levels of DHEA as low as those suffering adrenal atrophy. Testosterone levels have also been discovered to be low in people with COPD.

Studies have shown that DHEA lowers the allergen sensitivity of the lungs, reduces inflammation in airways, and suppresses the release of chemistries in the lungs that leads to airway constriction and mucus buildup. DHEA dramatically reduces the proliferation of smooth-muscle cells in rat trachea (a factor leading to obstruction of the fixed airways and causing hyperresponsiveness of smooth-muscle tissue in severe chronic asthma). In rats, DHEA has been found to completely reverse airway hyper-reactivity.[12]

Dosage

Take 25 to 50 milligrams of DHEA daily at minimum; a natural androgen replacement protocol should be considered for those with severe chronic asthma.

Cautions

Some clinicians think DHEA can exacerbate the mania stage of manic depression, others believe it is contraindicated for men whose PSA (prostate-specific antigen—an indicator for prostate disease level) is high. The only literature-noted side effect is masculinization (facial hair, etc.) in some women and the case of one woman who developed jaundice and liver problems after one week of use. It is not known if the latter side effect was related to the use of DHEA. Women seem most at risk of side effects.

MAGNESIUM

There is increasing evidence that magnesium deficiency is a major contributing factor in asthma, bronchitis, and sinusitis. Magnesium has significant regulatory impacts on the stimulatory effects of intracellular calcium; *it is one of the primary regulators of calcium activity in the body.* Magnesium inhibits the formation of calcium-based kidney and bladder stones and inhibits the buildup of calcium in blood vessel walls, in heart ventricles, and within cellular membranes. This is important in asthma and other COPDs because high intracellular calcium is directly related to bronchospasm and constriction in the muscles that make up the bronchial passageways. Sufficient dietary magnesium is absolutely necessary for healthy cellular functioning and lung homeostasis. Even disregarding other factors, increased calcium intake in the United States from calcium-enriched foods such as milk (generally because of fears about poor bone growth) has thrown cellular functioning toward the calcium side of the equation.

Studies have shown that low intake of dietary magnesium directly increases bronchial reactivity. Supplementation reduces reactivity, alleviates bronchial constriction, lowers pressure in pulmonary hypertension, and increases the force of respiratory muscles. In *in vivo* experiments, magnesium supplementation prevents the lung changes found in adult respiratory distress syndrome. Because some asthma medications (e.g., theophylline) increase magnesium loss from the body, magnesium supplementation is even more important for asthmatics who use synthetic medications.

A study in *The Lancet* reported that an examination of 2,633 English adults (ages eighteen to seventy) found that magnesium levels are inversely proportional to asthma incidence, lung function, wheezing, and airway hyperreactivity. The more magnesium, the lower the incidence of pulmonary problems. Other studies have shown that people with asthma consistently have lower levels of intracellular magnesium, even though their blood serum levels might be normal. People with low levels of magnesium have a much higher concentration of intracellular calcium, higher histamine concentrations, and higher tissue prostanoid concentrations. All are factors that contribute to bronchial hyperreactivity and bronchial spasming. Among other things, low magnesium has also been shown to cause muscle cramps, irregularities of the autonomic nervous system, and excitability of the central nervous system.

Very few studies have been conducted with magnesium supplementation in the treatment of asthma, though intravenous magnesium will reliably halt most acute asthma attacks. Given magnesium's essential role in regulating intracellular calcium and potassium levels in the body, that it is a calcium antagonist in cellular tissues, and that low magnesium is consistently found in chronic obstructive pulmonary diseases, including asthma, there is probably no more essential supplement to take on a daily basis if you suffer chronic respiratory problems.[13]

Dosage
Take 200 to 400 milligrams three times daily.

Cautions
Magnesium is normally well tolerated; however, people with certain kinds of severe heart disease, such as high-grade atrioventricular block, should only use magnesium under the supervision of a health-care provider.

N-ACETYL CYSTEINE (NAC)

Researchers have consistently noted that antioxidant levels are significantly depressed in the lung fluids of people with asthma. Levels of superoxide dismutase and glutathione are especially low and drop even lower during acute attacks. Levels remain significantly lower than baseline for up to forty-eight hours after an acute episode. This makes the lungs even more susceptible to injury from pollutants. The lungs' natural system of antioxidant production and defense, once overwhelmed by oxidants, allows tissue injury to occur unimpeded by these natural defense mechanisms. This contributes significantly to the thickening of the respiratory epithelium and its hyperreactivity. Glutathione is especially important in lung function because it has strong mucus-thinning actions and it breaks down inflammatory leukotrienes.

Supplementation with N-acetyl cysteine (from which glutathione is made) has been found to significantly help both bronchitis and chronic bronchopulmonary diseases in a number of double-blind trials. Because low antioxidant levels are a primary indicator of injury to the respiratory system, supplementation with glutathione precursors is important.[14]

See "Selenium" below for more information.

Dosage
Take 1,200 milligrams daily.

VITAMIN C

Because antioxidants are so important to lung health, it is not surprising that low vitamin C levels have been found in many people with asthma and other bronchopulmonary diseases. Vitamin C is, in general, inversely correlated to the incidence of asthma. Asthma is higher in those whose vitamin C intake is low. Vitamin C is a primary antioxidant, commonly present in the lining of the bronchial passages. Vitamin C prevents the secretion of histamines by mast cells and increases the detoxification of histamines once they are released. In one study, people with chronic asthma were given either 2 grams of vitamin C or a placebo over a five-week span. During the periods of vitamin C supplementation, blood histamine levels decreased by 38 percent.[15] While vitamin C can be useful in some kidney conditions, you should not use vitamin C if you are on hemodialysis, or suffer from recurrent kidney stones, severe kidney disease, or gout.

Dosage
Take 1 to 2 grams daily.

SELENIUM

Selenium is essential for the formation of glutathione; without it, NAC supplementation will be only minimally effective. Selenium levels, not surprisingly, have been found to be chronically low in people with asthma. Some studies have shown improvements in asthma following supplementation with selenium.[16]

Dosage
Take 200 micrograms daily.

Cautions
Selenium can be highly toxic. Although dosages can range as high as 400 micrograms per day, this may become toxic over the long run. The dosage range for safety should be between 50 and 200 micrograms daily. Signs of toxicity are nausea and vomiting and emotional instability. The metabolism of N-acetyl cysteine can deplete the body's zinc and copper, so take it with a zinc supplement that also includes copper.

VITAMIN B$_6$

Asthmatics have problems with tryptophan metabolism and reduced platelet transport of the serotonin—a bronchoconstrictor—produced by the lungs' Kulchitsky cells. Vitamin B_6 is necessary (as is magnesium) for both the metabolism of tryptophan and the transport of serotonin. To make matters worse, the asthma medication theophylline reduces the body's levels of vitamin B_6. Double-blind studies have consistently shown that B_6 supplementation in asthma helps correct blocked tryptophan metabolism. Another study with B_6 supplementation (50 milligrams twice daily) resulted in a dramatic decrease in the frequency and severity of wheezing and asthmatic attack.[17]

Note: Vitamin B_{12} may also be of benefit. It has been found to help prevent the onset of allergic reactions in a number of studies, especially allergic reactions to sulfites. The usual dosage is 1,000 micrograms daily.[18]

Dosage
Take 50 to 100 milligrams twice daily.

SINUPRET

Sinupret has been shown to be reliably effective in treating sinusitis, both acute and chronic. Sinupret is a combination herbal formula that is in fact Germany's top-selling phytomedicinal and tenth most prescribed medication, pharmaceutical or herbal. Sinupret, normally sold as a tablet, contains 6 milligrams gentian root and 18 milligrams each of cowslip flowers, sorrel, elder flowers, and European vervain. There is also a proprietary alcohol/water tincture that contains the same proportion of herbs.

Sinupret has been tested in at least twelve clinical trials, four against placebo and eight against pharmaceuticals. In all trials it was found statistically superior to both placebo and pharmaceuticals in the treatment of sinusitis. It is equally effective for children and adults.[19]

Dosage
Normal dosage in trials was 156 milligrams of the tablet, 76 milligrams of the liquid tincture. Sinupret, while it has been licensed to Warner-Lambert for production in the United States, has not yet been released here. It can be very hard to find. Some American herbal companies are making identical-ratio tincture combinations of these same herbs, which may work just as well.

BROMELAIN

Bromelain has been found to be effective in treating both chronic bronchitis and sinusitis. Bromelain is highly anti-inflammatory, reducing edema in respiratory tissues. It stimulates the production of anti-inflammatory prostaglandin E1 and inhibits the synthesis of pro-inflammatory prostaglandin E2.

Bromelain is one of the chemical compounds found in pineapple and acts to decrease bronchial secretions and make them more liquid. Trials in the treatment of chronic bronchitis have shown that bromelain decreases coughing incidence and reduces the thickness of mucus in the lungs. Testing with a spirometer (which measures air volume from the lungs) after bromelain supplementation showed increased lung capacity and function. In sinusitis trials, bromelain has been found to provide excellent results for 87 percent of those with acute sinusitis.[20]

Dosage
Take 250 to 750 milligrams three times daily.

DIETARY ADDITIONS AND CONSIDERATIONS

There are a number of additives, foods, or common analgesics that can trigger asthma attacks: aspirin (or other NSAIDs such as indomethacin and ibuprofen), yellow dye #5 (tartrazine), eggs, fish, shellfish, nuts, peanuts, milk, chocolate, wheat, citrus, apples, chlorinated water, and other food colorings.

People with asthma also commonly have a defect in their tryptophan metabolism. While vitamin B_6 supplementation can help alleviate this problem, tryptophan-containing foods should be eliminated. These include pumpkin seeds, turnip greens, collard greens, potatoes, and milk.

Studies with people who have altered their diet to strictly avoid all these substances have shown either a significant alleviation of symptoms or even complete remission of asthma. Generally, the diets need to be followed for twelve months to produce significant results.

The diet outlined in Chapter 12 can be modified for asthma and other bronchial problems by simply eliminating any of the items listed above. Foods that have been found especially supportive of asthma remission are garlic, anise, fennel, tomato, coriander, bell pepper, green tea, cayenne, cabbage, carrot, cranberry, currant, eggplant, oregano, sage, cardamom, purslane, wasabi, spinach, steamed nettles, onions, and omega-3 fatty acids (flaxseed oil). Once the symptoms have alleviated or the asthma is in remission, foods that have been removed from the diet can be added back one at a time. Those that do not provoke a negative response can become a regular part of the diet.

Perhaps the most important food to include liberally in the diet is onions. Onions have been found to have significant impacts on asthma and other bronchopulmonary problems, such as chronic sinusitis and bronchitis. A number of *in vitro, in vivo*, and human trials have been conducted with impressive results.

Onions naturally reduce the release of histamines and leukotrienes in bronchial tissues. They inhibit mast cell degranulation, allergen-induced bronchial constriction, and PAF release in lung tissue.

A number of clinical studies have shown that onions are highly effective in the treatment of asthma. Alcohol extracts of the dried bulb produce a potent and specific bronchodilator activity in human lung tissue. In human trials, one study of one hundred people with asthma found significant relief from symptoms with daily consumption of the fresh, cooked bulb. Another trial with three hundred asthmatics revealed that the administration of 500 milligrams daily of an alcohol extract of the dried bulb provided significant relief of symptoms.[21]

YOGA AND MASSAGE

Yoga has been effectively used for bronchopulmonary disorders for millennia. It lowers stress levels, increases body levels of DHEA, and reduces bronchial asthmatic attacks.[22] These same kinds of effects have been found with massage, deep tissue bodywork, and meditation. Massage and yoga have both shown direct positive effects on the health of the bronchopulmonary system. There is less tendency for the bronchi to spasm, deeper respiration in general, and much lower stress. (For more see Chapter 13.)

SUGGESTED

Have a massage once a week. Practice yoga and meditate daily.

Part III

Diet, Exercise, and Other Unmentionables

We would have no objection to people who eat like sparrows if they would only stop that everlasting chirping about it. —Changing Times

A thin man may live longer than a fat one, but he usually makes a bigger fuss about it. —Anonymous

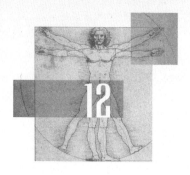

Food

Everybody, sooner or later, sits down to a banquet of consequences. —Robert Louis Stevenson

Nature does her best to teach us. The more we overeat, the harder she makes it for us to get close to the table.
—Earl Wilson

The potent chemistries in plants can be brought powerfully into the body through the foods that make up everyday meals. While less than ten vegetables are regularly included in the typical American diet, human beings have historically consumed between one hundred and one thousand plants during an average yearly cycle.[1] James Duke, in his book *The Green Pharmacy* (Rodale 1997), explores the relationship of foods to health perhaps more thoroughly than any other author. As he says, he would rather eat his medicine than take it.

One of the best approaches to reestablishing a higher level of health in the body (and to begin bringing in more potent plant chemistries) is to do a ten-week cleansing diet each year. If one of your organ systems has finally sent you notice that changes will now be occurring (one way or another), this type of diet can have even more benefit. This type of food regimen helps reduce stress on the body and assists the body's innate processes as it begins healing itself.

It is especially important to make a dietary alteration of some sort in conditions such as inflammatory bowel disease (IBD) or diabetes. Diet changes, especially so-called elimination diets, have been found to significantly alleviate both Crohn's disease and ulcerative colitis. Many people with IBD have been found to be allergic to both wheat and dairy. Eliminate both of these if you have IBD. If you have diabetes, drink only moderate amounts of fruit juices and do not fast or reduce meals unless you are working with a health-care practitioner.

If you wish, you can, by the sixth week, begin reducing your meals slowly until you only eat once per day by the eighth week. Then fast for one day and then slowly begin increasing the amount of food you eat daily. It is normal, on this diet, to lose from five to ten pounds.

This diet is especially good if you are overweight or have been eating a poor diet. Too much body fat causes increases in estrogen and decreases in testosterone levels. If your diet has been poor, this regimen allows your body to detox and prepare itself for a better, more testosterone-supportive diet.

To maintain high testosterone levels, however, it is important to note that people on vegetarian diets (NO meat) consistently show higher SHBG levels, lower testosterone levels, and lower levels of free testosterone. Lowering fat intake lowers the available cholesterol that the body needs to make testosterone. The optimum testosterone diet has been found to consist of 55 percent carbohydrate, 15 percent protein, and 30 percent fat. As politically incorrect as it is, meat consumption one to three times per week is positively correlated with higher testosterone levels. I generally prefer a mix of wild or organic meats during the week, such as one chicken, one fish, and one red meat.[2]

THE TEN-WEEK LOW-FAT CLEANSING DIET

It is best to establish a routine for meals and a list of meals *before* you start on the diet. Cook a large pot of a grain of your choice and keep it in the refrigerator. This way if you get hungry there is already something available.

Eat as much as you wish throughout the day. Fruit is good as a snack food. Have it available to eat whenever you feel hungry. It is helpful to get a good vegetarian cookbook and plan out a week's meals.

Sample Daily Menus

- BREAKFAST: (1) Herbal tea, oatmeal with raisins, and maple syrup; (2) fruit salad; (3) Green drink.

- LUNCH: (1) Vegetable soup, sprouted bread; or (2) rice and steamed vegetables with tamari.

- DINNER: (1) Steamed vegetables or vegetable casserole, grain of choice, salad with herbed vinegar; (2) steamed salmon with dill and lime, steamed asparagus, wild green salad with snow peas, and radish.

1. Drink six to eight glasses of water every day. Do not use tap water.

2. Eliminate dairy products, eggs, sweets.

3. Eat only *whole* grains (brown rice, millet, barley, oats, quinoa, and so on), organic beans, lightly steamed organic vegetables and fruit, and minimal wild or free-range meats. Tempeh and tofu are excellent. *Do not cook any grains with oil.*

4. Use only olive oil for cooking. Use no more than two tablespoons of oil per day. Do not use butter or margarine of any kind.

5. Drink all the fresh vegetable and fruit juices you like (except for grapefruit juice).

6. Do not use salt. Any other spices you wish are okay as are small amounts of tamari and soy.

7. Do not use any caffeinated drinks (except green tea); alcohol (except for tinctures); or recreational drugs during the diet. If you are a heavy caffeine drinker, instead of stopping cold turkey, go from coffee to black tea to green tea over a one- to two-week period of time.

8. Eat fruits first and alone. They digest rapidly and when eaten with other foods are held in the stomach, where they can cause gas and intestinal upset.

9. Do not eat any fried foods.

10. Consider consuming a "green drink" each morning. See below.

Food List

Buy only organic, pesticide-free foods. This is important. The chemistries in nonorganically farmed foods are all too often estrogen mimics. They can have highly negative impacts on the male reproductive system. Further, by only eating organic, you reduce synthetic chemistries that are hard for the liver to process. This takes the load off the liver and allows it to work more efficiently.

FRUITS

Use any fruits you wish except grapefruit.

VEGETABLES

acorn squash	corn	romaine
artichoke	cucumber	rutabagas
asparagus	daikon greens	snow peas
avocados	eggplant	spinach
beets	jicama	sprouts (all)
broccoli	kale	string beans
Brussels sprouts	mustard greens	summer squash
burdock	onion	sweet potatoes
butternut squash	parsley	Swiss chard
cabbage	parsnips	tomatoes
carrots	potatoes, red or white	turnip greens
cauliflower	pumpkin	turnips
celery	red leaf lettuce	watercress
collards	red radish	zucchini

Minimize legumes because of their actions in the gastrointestinal tract.

OIL

Use olive oil for cooking. Flaxseed oil, because of its high levels of omega-3 oils, is a very good oil to use (uncooked) for such things as salad dressings.

SALAD DRESSING

Use herbed vinegar, champagne, wine, or fruit vinegars only. Combine with flaxseed oil if desired.

SEASONINGS

Use any seasoning except salt.

BEVERAGES

- Water: filtered or artesian spring water. Do not use distilled water. Avoid all frozen concentrated juices.
- Herbal teas: especially ginger, peppermint, and chamomile.

MEAT

Fish from the sea, especially cold-water fish, is excellent. If you feel you want fowl, use only range-fed, pharmaceutical-free, organic chickens (or other birds). Wild meats such as venison or elk are excellent; if they are farmed they should be organic. Meat should be eaten only once or twice a week during the diet. *Note:* Salmon is almost always raised in pens in the sea. These fish are highly dosed with growth stimulants and antibiotics. They should be avoided. Eat only wild sea salmon. (Catfish is also farm-raised.)

BREAD

Use only sprouted grain breads.

COOKING

Use only stainless steel, enameled, or earthenware cooking utensils. Never use aluminum.

SWEETENER

Use pure maple syrup. Maple syrup contains enough essential ingredients that it is possible to live on it for extended periods of time. It supplies nearly all the essential vitamins and minerals necessary for health.

Green Drinks

"Green drinks" have become more popular of late and a number are readily available in health-food stores and on the Internet. You can buy them pre-mixed (follow directions on container) or make them yourself. The one I make contains spirulina, chlorella, bladderwrack (a seaweed), turmeric, milk thistle seed, dandelion root, burdock, Siberian ginseng, ashwaghanda, nettle leaf, and astragalus. I add ⅓ cup of the powdered mixture to 12 ounces of apple juice and 1 tablespoon of flaxseed oil and blend, then drink. It is more effective if you begin blending the apple juice first, then add the oil and powdered herbs. Otherwise it clumps. This drink is just about as healthy a thing as you can take and it is very filling, especially if taken at breakfast.

Things to Remember

1. It is normal to feel a sensation that is usually described as hunger no matter how much you eat in the early days (up to two weeks) of this kind of diet. It is not actually hunger but the shift away from the foods you are used to eating. During this time your body fat will decrease and you will move from a catabolic, cortisol-based metabolism to an anabolic DHEA-based metabolism. By the end of the diet most people generally feel increased energy, more mental alertness, little hunger, eat smaller portions, are highly relaxed, and have low stress levels.

2. You may feel lightheaded. This is also normal.

3. Since eating is such a social event it is normal to feel left out when others go out to eat. Go with them and convince them to go to a good health-food restaurant. Order food that comes from this list and that is light on oils.

4. When others order alcohol and you also wish to drink, order sparkling water with a lime in a champagne glass.

5. Emotional issues often arise during any change in eating patterns, especially when the body is using up its stores of fat. Remember that this is normal and make no major life decisions during this time. Remember, you are only doing this for ten weeks; it will pass.

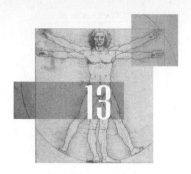

Helpful Physical Processes

*The trouble with some self-made men is that they
insist on giving everybody their recipe.*

—MAURICE SEITTER

*I often have the urge to exercise. Usually I lie down
until it passes.* —ANONYMOUS

I often walk up to ten miles looking for medicinal
plants. If my wife wants me to go for a walk I can hardly make it four blocks
without whining. I can work for weeks remodeling a house, lifting heavy
bags of concrete, or smoothing and shaping wood for hours on end. Fifteen
minutes on an exercise machine and my temper is ruined. I hate exercise
and I always have. It's a nasty, brutish way to spend valuable time. The
things I like to do aren't exercise, they're *fun*. It took me a long time to realize that most people think them exercise. And of course, the next thing that
occurred to me was that a lot more people might "exercise" if people weren't
endlessly carping at them about it all the time, if, in fact, they were encour-
aged to do something fun. (After all, no one likes to have their mother
telling them what to do all the time.)

So . . . find something fun to do that uses your body. It doesn't really
matter what it is. The natural movement of the body as it works at any physical task increases muscle mass, keeps the joints and bones strong and flexible, and improves the circulation of both the lymph system and the blood.

Here are some things that can be helpful. Some of them are even fun.

MASSAGE

The ancient Chinese, Egyptians, Hindus, Japanese, Greeks, and Romans all used massage; it's been around for at least six thousand years. Julius Caesar had massage every day to relieve neural pain, reduce stress, and help prevent epileptic attacks. (Unfortunately, things still worked out badly.)

There are a number of types of massage: Swedish, sports, Shiatsu, Trager, acupressure, and Reiki are some of the more popular. Sports massage is usually used to help enhance performance or heal sports-related injuries. Shiatsu is an oriental form of massage that uses a lot of finger pressure on trigger points, much like acupressure massage does. It can be painful (though invigorating). Trager (created by Milton Trager), among other things, uses a gentle rocking motion that is very relaxing. Some studies have indicated that it may help regenerate the nerve sheaths in the brain that degenerate during multiple sclerosis and other central nervous system disorders.

Swedish massage is a relaxation massage that, in the hands of a good practitioner, works each muscle group in the body, relieving deeply held muscle tension. This type of massage was formalized by Per Henrik Ling in the early nineteenth century and imported to the United States in 1856. Ling integrated a number of massage styles and other body therapies (e.g., yoga) to create the Swedish technique.

The best massage therapists are caring and attentive in their work, talk very little during sessions, and are generally able to gauge the exact amount of pressure needed to produce benefit. They often enter a mild trance state and the massage then becomes a remarkably sophisticated dialogue between their hands and your body. An expert massage should feel like a nonsexual orgasm of the entire body. At its conclusion you should feel slightly sleepy, completely relaxed, and joyful in an ungrandiose, early-morning, butterscotch-sunshine sort of way. The best health effects come from having at least one to two massages per month.

Swedish massage is my favorite form of massage for a variety of reasons: touch, reducing stress, and enhancing immune health.

Touch

Touch is one of the most basic needs that we have, one that, unfortunately, men rarely experience. Of all the things a man can do to increase his level of health, touch is perhaps the simplest, and hardest.

Researchers have found, not surprisingly, that children who are touched and held regularly show increased levels of health and immune function, greater alertness, more mental clarity, higher IQ, and less emotional depression and uncertainty. Touch is in fact one of the most basic ways that we are told we matter and are cared about. It is as ancient and basic to us as the caress of our mother's womb. Human beings respond to touch at a much deeper level than that of the conscious mind. The heart takes in some meaning from it that is essential to our health; its entire pattern of activity alters in response.

In many respects, we in the United States have been trained as a nation of emotional ascetics—wide ranges of strong feeling are suspect, so is any deep emotional needing of others. This is especially true of men and it expresses itself directly in a general reluctance to be touched (except in shaking hands). Touch, however, is a basic human need and is strongly connected to healthy and full-bodied emotional development. Perhaps no better exploration of its importance exists than Ashley Montagu's *Touching: The Human Significance of the Skin* (Harper & Row, 1971). Examining the clinical data on the importance of touch he remarks:

> Tactile stimulation appears to be a fundamentally necessary experience for the healthy development of the individual. Failure to receive tactile stimulation in infancy results in a critical failure to establish contact relations with others. Supplying that need, even in adults, may serve to give the individual the reassurance he needs, the conviction that he is wanted and valued, and thus involved and consolidated in a connected network of values with others. . . . Body contact is a basic mammalian need which must be satisfied if the individual is to develop those movements, gestures, and body-relatednesses which will be normally developed during the growth of one's experience in relation to one's mother's body. Deprivation of this experience has been experimentally shown to produce the most atypical movements and postures.[1]

As the industrial revolution gained momentum in our country in the late nineteenth century, touch between mothers (and other family members) and infants began to disappear. Rocking infants in any form, in a cradle *or* by holding, was highly discouraged by medical experts. Breastfeeding, once a major component of touch between babies and their mothers was also discouraged in favor of bottle feeding. New generations of children, it is now understood, began to exhibit behaviors consistent with long-term touch deprivation. Montagu notes that these new children (especially the boys) took on attitudes "which usually assumed the form of an elaborate denial of the need for closeness."[2] They had become emotional ascetics. He goes on to say that:

> The benefits of rocking are considerable. When the infant is too warm, the rocking has a cooling effect, hastening evaporation from the skin. When the infant is too cold the rocking helps to warm him. The warming has a hypnotic effect on the infant, it is soothing to his nervous system. Above all, the rocking motion produces a gentle stimulation of almost every area of his skin, with consequential beneficial physiological effects of every kind.[3]

Infants who are not rocked have been found to experience many intestinal problems in later life including irritable bowel disease. The intestine, loosely attached by folds of the peritoneum to the back wall of the abdominal cavity, moves like a pendulum while being rocked. Rocking enhances its tone. The contents of the intestine, liquid chyle and gas, move back and forth when the infant is rocked, also helping to increase the intestine's tone and aiding in digestion and absorption. Further, certain nerve sheaths in the brain form early in infancy and research has found their formation is enhanced, even stimulated, by rocking.[4]

As with our hearts, the knowledge of the importance of touch is embedded in our language. If someone we love calls on us when we are sick we are "touched by their concern"; if we are too sensitive to others, we are "touchy"; if emotionally hurt, "touched to the quick"; an emotionally moving story can be "touching"; and most of us like to "keep in touch" even if it is not physical.

Reducing Stress

A Swedish massage, like most massages, usually lasts from one to one and a half hours. During that time, a good practitioner can relieve a majority of the tension and stress that people now tend to hold in their bodies. Each person holds tension in different places—wrists, forearms, shoulders, neck, back, etc. As your massage therapist gets to know you, he or she will become more and more efficient in helping reduce body-held tension. This produces a number of benefits, including reduced anxiety, deeper respiration, less tendency to become depressed, enhanced immune function, and increased mental alertness. Adults, it has been found, show the same benefits from deep and caring touching as young children.

Although important for many reasons, relieving depression and reducing stress levels have a strong impact on testosterone health. Men with major depression tend to have 40 percent lower testosterone and higher cortisol levels than men without depression. Male medical residents, who experience extreme levels of stress on the job, have 80 percent lower testosterone and much higher cortisol levels than men who work at less stressful jobs. Feeling good does increase testosterone levels.[5]

Enhancing Immune and Physiological Function

The lymph system of the body, a parallel circulatory system to the blood, does not have a muscular pump to keep things moving. Instead, the lymph system is "worked" by the movement of the muscles. The lymph system moves white blood cells and cellular debris, especially the debris that occurs during disease, through and out of the body. One of the reasons that the lymph nodes swell during disease is that they are filled with old white blood cells and dead bacteria. The more efficiently the lymph system moves dead bacteria and old white blood cells, the more quickly people get well. Some form of movement of the muscles of the body is needed for the lymph system to remain healthy. In addition to stimulating the health of the lymph system, massage has been shown to produce direct increases in white blood cell and other immunoactive cells of the immune system. Other physiological alterations include a 10 to 15 percent increase in oxygen capacity of the blood after a massage, increased excretion of nitrogen, phosphorus, and salt in the urine, and improved skin health.

MAJOR HEALTH BENEFITS OF MASSAGE

- Intimate human contact
- Enhanced immune function
- Lowered blood pressure
- Reduced anxiety
- Deeper respiration
- Less depression
- Improved alertness

- Reduced heart rate
- Reduced tension levels
- Increased blood circulation
- Increased lymph flow
- Enhanced joint flexibility and range of motion
- Lower pain levels in chronic disease

YOGA

Yoga is the oldest form of formalized exercise in the world. It was developed in India, where it has been practiced for six to seven thousand years. Originally intended as a technique to enhance spiritual development, most people now use it as a daily form of exercise and meditation.

The different yoga postures have been developed to work every muscle system in the body. They keep every muscle toned, reduce tension, free or open up habituated muscle tension and holding patterns, keep flexibility levels high, and lower stress. Stress reduction is enhanced by the deep breathing meditation that is an integral part of the exercises. Yoga is, in a sense, self massage and provides all of the benefits (and more) of massage except that of touch. People who do yoga daily are usually as flexible as a twenty-year-old well into their nineties. Yoga is very popular and classes are easy to find throughout the United States.

Yoga has a great many healthy benefits and an associated branch of the discipline trains practitioners to treat disease. There are a number of yoga hospitals in India that treat acute and chronic diseases with great success.

Health Benefits of Yoga

The health benefits of yoga have been intensively studied and generally fall into three areas: physiological benefits, psychological benefits, and biochemical effects. The longer yoga is practiced as a daily part of life, the more pervasive these benefits become.[6]

PHYSIOLOGICAL BENEFITS

- Moves the body to anabolic rather than catabolic functioning
- Decreases pulse rate
- Decreases respiration
- Decreases blood pressure
- Increases galvanic skin response
- Increases alpha brain wave activity
- Cardiovascular efficiency increases
- Respiratory efficiency increases
- Gastrointestinal function normalizes
- Muscle and joint flexibility improves
- Improves asthma
- Increases strength
- Increases endurance
- Increases energy levels
- Weight normalization
- Improves sleep
- Enhances immunity
- Lowers pain in chronic or acute disease
- Improves grip strength
- Improves dexterity
- Improves balance
- Improves eye-hand coordination

PSYCHOLOGICAL BENEFITS

- Improves overall mood and sense of well-being
- Enhances socialization and human interaction
- Lowers anxiety and depression
- Decreases hostility
- Enhances attention, concentration, memory
- Enhances learning efficiency

BIOCHEMICAL EFFECTS

Decreases commonly occur in:

- Blood glucose
- Sodium
- Total cholesterol levels
- LDL cholesterol

Increases commonly occur in:

- HDL cholesterol
- Cholinesterase
- Catecholamines
- Hemoglobin
- Thyroxin
- Vitamin C

DEEP TISSUE BODYWORK

Rolfing, Feldenkrais, and Hellerwork

There are a number of bodywork techniques that go deeper than massage. Most of them are somewhat painful but they can be of tremendous benefit. They are especially good after major life changes, when you have let go of one way of being and have entered another.

All of us develop patterns of holding our bodies and muscles that come out of our primary, daily emotional states. For example, if we spend a lot of time afraid or highly stressed, the muscles in our bodies begin to naturally hold that kind of pattern—it is very different from a relaxed, happy holding pattern. Over time, the patterns lock in. They do not automatically change if, years later, a person suddenly begins leading a totally different kind of life. And unfortunately, all muscle and body-holding patterns generate specific emotional and mental states irrespective of what is going on in the external world. They literally can recreate those old states of mind and feeling even if the circumstances out of which they arose are gone. (Sit slumped with your mouth hanging open and you will see what I mean. Your IQ will drop twenty points.) Yoga can change these kinds of holding patterns over time; deep tissue bodywork does it faster.

The two fastest forms of deep bodywork for changing held patterns are Rolfing and Hellerwork. Feldenkrais takes a bit longer, is less invasive, less painful, and was intentionally developed to increase the intelligence of the body, to retrain its ways of moving, holding, and receiving the impacts of the world. They all have benefits; I have done all of them, more than once.

ROLFING

Rolfing was developed by the German-born Ida Rolf between 1930 and 1970. It integrates techniques from yoga, massage, chiropractic, osteopathy and Ida's own unique insights. In 1971 she founded the Rolf Institute in Boulder, Colorado, and began training practitioners in the technique. There are now several thousand practitioners throughout the world.

Rolfing is much like yoga in many of its effects except that it is done to you ("Ve haf vays of making you release tension"). Usually, Rolfing consists of a series of ten one- to two-hour sessions; they can sometimes be very painful. I feel that its greatest benefit is the freeing up of old patterns of holding tension in the body. Ida Rolf described her work as "structural integration" and, in fact, the process allows a restructuring of the body that is more integrated, whole, and balanced. Benefits include increased mobility, enhanced respiration, lowered stress, heightened energy, and improved well-being. It has been found to be especially effective for chronic back, neck, shoulder, and joint problems, repetitive stress injuries, sports injuries, headaches, digestive problems, and asthma.

HELLERWORK

After Ida Rolf died in 1979, Joseph Heller directed the institute for many years before developing his own program. The primary difference between the two systems is his incorporation of movement re-patterning in Hellerwork. Movement re-patterning retrains people in how they move their bodies through space, how they stand, and how they hold themselves. This helps to integrate the restructured muscle patterns more completely into everyday life. In my opinion, Hellerwork is a trifle less painful than Rolfing and the movement training is of tremendous benefit. The health benefits are similar to Rolfing; however, in my experience, there is a significant increase in motor, movement, and joint flexibility, physical coordination, and physical confidence that is not usually found after Rolfing.

FELDENKRAIS

The Feldenkrais Method was developed by the Israeli scientist Moshe Feldenkrais; its primary training institute is still located in Tel Aviv. He referred to his work as "awareness through movement" and, indeed, the method is an elegant mixture of increasing body intelligence, enhancing conscious relationship with the body, healer-based aid for bodily problems, and personal instruction in a series of exercises that retrain and then maintain the body's health and flexibility. Feldenkrais's book, *Awareness Through Movement*, is a classic in the field, not only because of his insights into the body but his insights into the development of a full human life. He comments:

> Many of our failings, physical and mental, need not be considered
> as diseases to be cured, but rather as an acquired result of a learned

mode of doing. Actions repeated innumerable times for years on end, such as all habitual actions, mold even the bones, let alone the muscular envelope. The physical faults that appear in our body long after we were born are mainly the result of activity we have imposed on it. Faulty modes of standing and walking produce faulty feet, and it is the mode of standing and walking that must be corrected, not the feet. . . . [Faulty behavior] will remain largely so unless the nervous paths producing the undesirable pattern of motility are undone and reshuffled into a better configuration.[7]

Feldenkrais has been found to be helpful for a very large range of problems, especially if there are central nervous system elements. These include autism, back pain, balance difficulty, cerebral palsy, chronic anxiety, chronic fatigue, chronic pain, closed and open head injuries, stroke, systonia, fibromyalgia, irritable bowel syndrome, multiple sclerosis, muscular dystrophy, neurologic disorders, orthopedic injuries, postsurgical tissue trauma, repetitive stress injuries, stress, TMJ, whiplash, hypertension, insomnia, osteoarthritis, osteoporosis, sleep disorders, and tinnitus. His exercises for lower back spasms are exceptionally effective. If you have this problem on any kind of a regular basis, learning this technique can eliminate lengthy recoveries, trips to the chiropractor, or even the episodes themselves.

WALKING

Walking is probably the simplest form of beneficial exercise that exists. Walking for thirty minutes six days a week (or one hour three days per week) at a moderate pace of three miles per hour will produce all the health benefits that can be had from jogging, aerobics, or intense workouts. The only thing you need is a comfortable pair of walking shoes. A large number of studies have shown that walking for this minimal length of time will:

- Enhance cardiovascular health (it will cut the risk of heart attack by 40 percent)

- Enhance respiration

- Improve circulation

- Enhance immune function

- Lower depression

- Lower stress levels in the body

- Keep muscles toned

- Enhance lymph system function

- Help prevent osteoporosis

- Help prevent and control Type II diabetes

- Help control weight gain

WEIGHT LIFTING

As noted in Chapter 7, seventy-year-old infirm men who engage in power lifting three times per week (*for only fifteen minutes each time*) have experienced significant improvement in mobility, balance, bone density, and flexibility. (Those who had only been able to walk with canes no longer needed them.) Studies have found that such power-lifting workouts increase testosterone levels 32 percent, which is probably why impacts are so readily apparent in mobility, balance, bone density, and flexibility.[8] These same kinds of benefits have been found with many kinds of regular, minimal resistance training. Yoga is, in a sense, a type of resistance training using the weight of the body instead of weights, which is why it is so good for osteoporosis. Feldenkrais is similar to yoga in this respect as well.

Part IV

Final Words, Suggested Readings, and Resources

If the head and body are to be well, you must begin by curing the soul.
                                                                —PLATO

. . . a broken spirit drieth up the bones.
                                                —HEBREW SAYING

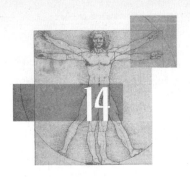

Final Words

You might have noticed as you perused the book that many of the same herbs and supplements show up no matter the nature of the physical problem. So here is a tonic regimen, not for any particular problem, but to help your vitality remain high and help prevent future problems.

Natural Care for Men in Daily Life

Pine pollen, 5 grams daily
Nettle root, 300 milligrams daily
Tribulus, 250 milligrams daily
Hawthorn, 160 milligrams daily
Ginkgo, 80 milligrams daily
Asian ginseng, 1 gram daily (or ¼ teaspoon tincture)
Pine bark or grape seed extract, 100 milligrams daily
Flaxseed oil, 1 tablespoon daily
Alpha lipoic acid, 100 milligrams daily
Androstenedione, 50 to 100 milligrams daily
DHEA, 25 to 50 milligrams daily
Magnesium, 200 milligrams daily
Selenium, 100 micrograms daily
Vitamin B complex, 1 to 2 tablets daily
Vitamin C, 0.5 to 3 grams daily
Zinc, 20 to 40 milligrams daily

Garlic, celery, oatmeal, ginger, onions, corn, blueberries, yogurt, pineapple, turmeric, tofu, cold-water fish, and green leafy vegetables in the diet regularly

In the end, it is perhaps not so important that bad things happen to us but what we do with them after. The challenge of a full life is not in having the safest length of it but in becoming one's self, in filling the life we have with richness, in deeply savoring the life and attendant experiences we are given. Sometimes, this is a very difficult proposition. For all of us, there are times that are hard, times when we find ourselves going down a dark street not knowing if it will open out again into the light. The transition through the stages of our lives often contain periods of such darkness. These final words come from people who have found their way through the dark. It is my hope that their wisdom and this book ease your journey.

Man's main task in life is to give birth to himself. —ERIC FROMM

What on earth would a man do with himself if something did not stand in his way? —H. G. WELLS

We grow neither better nor worse as we get old, but more like ourselves.
—MAY LAMBERTON BECKER

As you know, my friend, a gem is not polished without rubbing nor a man perfected without trials. —EARL DERR BIGGERS

You must do the thing that you cannot do. —ELEANOR ROOSEVELT

What lies behind us and what lies before us are tiny things to what lies within us. —UNKNOWN

Must the soul be properly aged before it leaves? —JAMES HILLMAN

Those we respect as our great teachers from a certain distance, were faithful. They did not break faith with their beliefs, they remained dedicated to something outside the self. As far as we know, they never became the enemies of their souls or their memories. —BARRY LOPEZ

Although men are accused of not knowing their own weaknesses, yet perhaps as few know their own strength. It is in men as in soils, where sometimes there is a vein of gold which the owner knows not of.

—JONATHAN SWIFT

Life is like an onion; you peel it off one layer at a time, and sometimes you weep. —CARL SANDBURG

Illigitimi non carborundum. —JOHN DUNNING

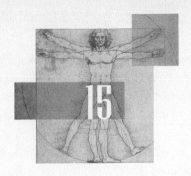

Suggested Readings and Resources

*Because I'm afraid of worms, Roxanne, worms! Oh,
wait! I mean words!*

—COMMENT IN THE MOVIE *ROXANNE*

I reviewed a little over 150 books and several thousand review articles during my research for this book. These are the books I think you will find most useful. Of special note are those marked with an asterisk.

SUGGESTED READINGS

James Balch and Phyllis Balch, *Prescription for Nutritional Healing* (New York: Avery, 1997).

Stephen Harrod Buhner, *Herbal Antibiotics: Natural Alternatives for Drug-Resistant Bacteria* (Pownal, VT: Storey Publishing, 1998).

———, *Herbs for Hepatitis C and the Liver* (Pownal, VT: Storey Publishing, 1999).

Malcolm Carruthers, *The Testosterone Revolution* (London: Thorsons, 2001).

Doc Childre and Howard Martin, *The Heartmath Solution* (San Francisco: HarperSanFrancisco, 1999).

Jared Diamond, *Male Menopause* (Naperville, IL: Sourcebooks, 1998).

* James Duke, *The Green Pharmacy* (New York: Rodale Press, 1997).

* James Hillman, *The Force of Character and the Lasting Life* (New York: Random House, 1999).

David Hoffmann, *An Elder's Herbal* (Rochester, VT: Healing Arts Press, 1993).

———, *The Holistic Herbal* (Rockport, MA: Element, 1990).

Mark McClure, *Smart Medicine for a Healthy Prostate* (New York: Avery, 2000).

John Morganthaler and Mia Simms, *The Smart Guide to Better Sex: From Andro to Zinc* (Petaluma, CA: Smart Publications, 1999).

* Michael Murray and Joseph Pizzorno, *Encyclopedia of Natural Medicine* (Roseville, CA: Prima, 1998).

Andrew Weil, *8 Weeks to Optimum Health* (New York: Knopf, 1998).

———, *Spontaneous Healing* (New York: Fawcett Columbine, 1995).

* Jonathan V. Wright and Lane Lenard, *Maximize Your Vitality and Potency (for Men Over 40)* (Petaluma, CA: Smart Publications, 1999).

Donald Yance, *Herbal Healing, Medicine, and Cancer* (Chicago: Keats, 1999).

SOURCES FOR SUPPLEMENTS AND HERBS MENTIONED IN THE BOOK

Some of the herbal supplements mentioned in this book may be difficult to find. If you can't find them at your local pharmacy or health-food store, you can try contacting the manufacturer directly. Following are some manufacturers of some of the harder-to-find supplements that I recommend.

The Internet is a good source for everything. If you can't find something discussed in this book, try the search engine www.google.com.

Herbs, retail

Dandelion Botanicals
708 North 34th Street
Seattle, WA 98103
1-206-545-8892

Woodland Essence
P.O. Box 206
Cold Brook, NY 13524
1-315-845-1515

Dry Creek Herb Farm
14245 Edgehill Lane
Auburn, CA 95603
1-530-888-0889
info@drycreekherbfarm.com

Herbs, wholesale

Trinity Herb
P.O. Box 1001
Graton, CA 95444
1-888-874-4372
www.trinityherb.com

Chinese Pine Pollen
  Bee Fit Herbs
  4710 Yelm Highway
  Lacey, WA 98503
  1-888-842-2049
  www.1stchineseherbs.com

  Herbal Remedies
  1-866-467-6444 (USA)
  1-307-577-6444 (outside USA)
  www.herbalremedies.com

  Pharm East
  326 North Stone Street Avenue
  Suite 205
  Rockville, MD 20850
  1-301-610-5620

Pine Pollen (Pinus sylvestris) and
David's Lily Flower
  Woodland Essence
  P.O. Box 206
  Cold Brook, NY 13524
  1-315-845-1515

Kidney Teas and Tinctures
  Dry Creek Herb Farm
  14245 Edgehill Lane
  Auburn, CA 95603
  1-530-888-0889

Rye Grass Pollen (Cernilton)
  Graminex
  95 Midland Road
  Saginaw, MI 48603

  1-877-472-6469
  www.cernitinamerica.com
  www.abcernelle.com/
    products.html

Japanese Dogwood (Cornus fructi)
  Bee Fit Herbs
  4710 Yelm Highway
  Lacey, WA 98503
  1-888-842-2049
  www.1stchineseherbs.com

  Herb Cupboard
  P.O. Box 552
  Elk Grove, CA 95759
  1-916-502-2911
  www.herbcupboard.com

  NL Acupuncture and Herbal
    Supplies
  1-888-991-2288
  1-604-438-2913
  www.nl-supplies.com

Speman
  Lynx Ayurvedics
  P.O. Box 14-084
  Hamilton, New Zealand
  64-7-855-4555
  www.world-lynx.com

  Natural Cure
  47/48 Hawley Square
  Margate, Kent CT9 1NY UK
  01-843-866-792
  www.natural-cure.co.uk

ENDNOTES

CHAPTER I

1. James Hillman, *The Force of Character and the Lasting Life* (New York: Random House, 1999), 54.
2. Peter Montague, "The Challenge of Our Age," *Rachel's Health and Environment Weekly* (hereinafter *Rachel's*) 447, June 22, 1995, 2.
3. J. Toppari, et al., "Male Reproductive Health and Environmental Xenoestrogens," *Environmental Health Perspectives* 104(4) (1995): 741–803; Theo Colburn, et al., *Our Stolen Future* (New York: Plume, 1997), chapters 5 and 10.
4. R. Bergstrom, et al., "Increase in testicular cancer incidence in six European countries," *Journal of the National Cancer Institute* 88(11) (1996): 727–33; J. McKiernan, et al., "Increasing risk of developing testicular cancer by birth cohort in the United States," *Dialogues in Pediatric Urology* 23(1) (2000): 7–8, cited in Colburn, et al., *Our Stolen Future*.
5. Louise Guillette, "Endocrine Disruptors and Pharmaceutically Active Compounds in Drinking Water Workshop," Center for Health Effects of Environmental Contamination, April 19–21, 2000, 4; online: www.cheec.uiosa.edu/edc_2000/guillette.html.
6. Ibid., 6.
7. Stephen Harrod Buhner, *The Lost language of Plants* (White River Junction, VT: Chelsea Green, 2002), 96.
8. Guillette, "Endocrine Disruptors and Pharmaceutically Active Compounds in Drinking Water Workshop," 5.
9. Anonymous, "Environmental Estrogens Differ from Natural Hormones," Center for Environmental Studies, Tulane and Xavier Universities, 3; online: www.tmc.tulane.edu/ecme/eehome.basics/eevshorm/default.html.
10. Montague, "The Challenge of Our Age," *Rachel's* 447, 3; W. Kelce, et al., "Persistent DDT metabolite p,p'-DDE is a Potent Androgen Receptor Antagonist," *Nature*, 375 (1995): 581–85.

11. Montague, "The Challenge of Our Age," *Rachel's* 447, 4; L. Gray, et al., "Developmental Effects of an Environmental Antiandrogen; The Fungicide Vinclosolin Alters Sex Differentiation of the Male Rat," *Toxicology and Applied Pharmacology* 129 (1994): 46–52.

12. Gerald LeBlanc, "Are Environmental Sentinels Signaling?" *Environmental Health Perspectives* 103(10) (October 1995): 888–90.

13. Theo Colburn, et al., *Our Stolen Future,* 85.

14. J. Ostby, et al., "Perinatal exposure to the phthalates DEHP, BBP, but not DEP, DMP, or DOTP permanently alters androgen-dependent tissue development in Sprague-Dawley rats," *Biology of Reproduction* 62 (2000): 184.

15. Ted Schettler, "Phthalate Esters and Endocrine Disruption," *The Science and Environmental Health Network,* 2; online: www.sehn.org/pubhealthessays.html.

16. Greenpeace, "Taking back our stolen future," April 1996; online: www.greenpeace.org/~uk/science/stolen.txt.

17. Theo Colburn, et al., *Our Stolen Future,* 178.

18. Peter Montague, "Warning on Male Reproductive Health." *Rachel's* 438, April 20, 1995, 1.

19. Ibid, 2.

CHAPTER 2

1. Most of these comparisons are from Jonathan Wright and Lane Lenard, *Maximize Your Vitality and Potency (for Men Over 40)* (Petaluma, CA: Smart Publications, 1999), 24.

2. Wright and Lenard, *Maximize Your Vitality and Potency;* Eugene Shippen and William Fryer, *The Testosterone Syndrome* (New York: Evans, 1998).

3. M. Saden-Krehula, et al., "17-Ketosteroids in *Pinus nigra* Ar. Steroid Hormones in the Pollen of Pine Species IV," *Naturwissenschaften* 70(10) (1983): 520–522; M. Saden-Krehula, M. Tajic, D. Kolbah, "Sex Hormones and Corticosteroids in Pollen of *Pinus nigra,*" *Phytochemistry* 17 (1978): 345–6; Saden-Krehula, et al., "Testosterone, Epitestosterone, and Androstenedione in the Pollen of Scotch Pine, *Pinus sylvestris* L.," *Experientia* 27 (1971): 108; *Phytochemical Dictionary: A Handbook of Bioactive Compounds from Plants,* Jeffery Harborne, et al. (eds.) (London: Taylor and France, 1999), 2944, 2976; Maurice Hanssen, *The Healing Power of Pollen* (Wellingborough, Northhamptonshire, UK: Thorsons, 1979), Appendix: A Comparative Analysis of Three Pollens: *Zea mays, Alnus spp.,* and *Pinus montana;* online at www.graminex.com; James Duke, Dr. Duke's Phytochemical and Ethnobotanical Databases, USDA-ARS-NGRL, Beltsville Agricultural Research Center, Beltsville, MD; online at www.ars-grin.gov/cgi-bin/duke/.

4. Z. H. Yanhg, Y. Tang, and Z. X. Cao, "The Changes of Steroidal Sex Hormone-Testosterone Contents in Reproductive Organs of *Lilium davidii* Duch.," *Chih Wu Hsueh Pao* 36(3) (1994): 215–20; Shilan Feng, et al., "Studies on the chemical constituents of the flower of David lily," *Zhongguo Zhongyao Zazhi* 19(10) (1994): 611–12, 639; K. Stransky, et al., "Unusual alkanes pattern of some plant cuticular waxes," *Collection of Czechoslovak Chemical Communications* 56(5) (1991): 1123–29; Duke, Dr. Duke's Phytochemical and Ethnobotanical Databases; Dan Bensky and Andrew Gamble, *Chinese Herbal Medicine: Materia Medica, Revised Edition* (Seattle, WA: Eastland Press, 1986), 363–64.

5. Steven Foster, *Herbal Emissaries* (Rochester, VT: Healing Arts Press, 1992), 102–12; G. Salvati, et al., "Effects of *Panax ginseng* C. A. Meyer Saponins on Male Fertility," *Panminerva Med* 38(4) (1996): 249–54; Paul Bergner, *The Healing Power of Ginseng* (Rocklin, CA: Prima, 1996), 102; M. S. Fahim, et al., "Effect of *Panax ginseng* on testosterone level and prostate in male rats," *Arch Androl* 8 (1982): 261–63.

6. Q. H. Chen, et al., "Pharmacology of total saponins of the fibrous roots of *Panax notoginseng*," *Chung Yao T'ung Pao* 12(3) (1987): 173–75.

7. Duke, Phytochemical Database; I. Y. Kuntsman, "A Study of the gonadotropic activity of the leaves of *Eleutherococcus senticosus*," *Lek Sredstva Dal'Nego Vostoka* 7 (1966): 129–32; I. V. Dardymov, "Gonadotropic action of *Eleutherococcus* glycosides," *Lek Sredstva Dal'Nego Vostoka* 11 (1972): 60.

8. E. Bombardelli and P. Morazzoni, "Urtica dioica L.," *Fitoterapia* 68(5) (1997): 387–402; D. J. Hryb, et al., "The effect of extracts of the root of the stinging nettle (*Urtica dioica*) on the interaction of SHBG with its receptor on human prostatic membranes," *Planta Med* 61(1) (1995): 31–32; F. C. Lowe and E. Fagelman, "Phytotherapy in the treatment of benign prostatic hyperplasia: an update," *Urology* 53(4) (1999): 671-78; K. Schmidt, "The effect of an extract of Radix Urticae and various secondary extracts on the SHBG of blood plasma in benign prostatic hyperplasia," *Fortschr Med* 101(21) (1983): 713–16; Matthias Schottner, Gerhard Spireller, and Dietmar Gansser, "Lignans Interfering with 5a-Dihydrotestosterone Binding to Human Sex Hormone-Binding Globulin," *J Nat Prod* 61 (1998): 119–21; R. W. Hartmann, et al, "Inhibition of 5 alpha-reductase and aromatase by PHL-00801 (Prostatonin), a combination of PY 102 (*Pygeum africanum*) and UR 102 (*Urtica dioica*) extracts," *Phytomedicine* 3(2) (1996): 121–8; "(10E,12Z)-9-Hydroxy-10,12-Octadecadienoic Acid, an aromatase inhibitor from roots of Urtica dioica," *Liebigs Ann Chem* 1991(4) (1991): 335–39.

9. W. Pangkahila, "*Tribulus terrestris* (protodioscin) increases men's sex drive," Proceedings of the Xth National Congress on New Perspectives of Andrology on Human Production (1993); Stefan Popov, "Trilovin—a preliminary evaluation after 2 years of clinical experience." Both online at: www.pharmabul.com/ research.htm; A. Adimoelja and P. Ganeshan Adaikan, "Protodioscin from herbal plant *Tribulus terrestris* L improves male sexual function probably via DHEA," *International Journal of Impotence Research* 9 (Supplement 1) (1997); I. Viktorof, et al., "Pharmacological, pharmacokinetic, toxicological and clinical studies on protodioscin," *IIMS Therapeutic Focus*, Vol. 2 (1994), cited at www.nutrica.com/Libilov/LMR1.htm.

10. Ray Sahelian, *Pregnenolone* (New York: Avery, 1997), 23–31. Beverly Greenberg, *The DHEA Discovery* (Los Angeles: Majesty Press, 1996), 74–77.

11. D. Armanini, et al., "Reduction of serum testosterone in men by licorice," *N Engl J Med* 341(15) (1999): 1158; A. Mostbeck and M. Studlar, "Experimental studies of a plant extract from *Echinacea purpurea* Moench as an unspecific antibody stimulant with special consideration of the influence on the kidney cortex," *Wien Med Wochenschr* 112 (1962): 255; Lane Lenard, *The Smart Guide to Andro* (Petaluma, CA: Smart Publications, 1999), 19; Karlis Ullis, et al., *Super T* (New York: Simon & Schuster), 48–49.

12. Lenard, *The Smart Guide to Andro;* Ullis, et al. *Super T,* 50; J. Blaquier, et al., (no title) *Acta Endrocrinologica* 55 (1996): 697–704; F. Unger, et al., (no title) *J. Biol. Chem* 224 (nd): 191–200; U.S. patent application 5578588.

13. Wright and Lenard, *Maximize Your Vitality and Potency,* 157–66; Nakhla, et al., 1994, online at: http://herkules.oulu.fi/isbn9514253868/html/x1060.html; The Endocrine Society, "Dihydrotestosterone Gel Increases Muscle, Decreases Fat in Older Men," September 14, 2001, press release, reporting on the results of a study conducted at the University of Sydney and published in the September 2001 issue of the *Journal of Clinical Endocrinology and Metabolism;* see also Wright and Lenard, *Maximize,* 157–66; William Llewellyn, "DHT and the Athlete: Is It the Enemy?," www.hononline.com/dht.html; Patrick Arnold, "DHT—Is It All Bad?," www.mesomorphosis.com/articles/arnold. dht.htm (reprinted from *Muscle Monthly Magazine;* Patrick Arnold, "DHT—Is It All Bad?," 2; P. Negri-Cesi, et al., "Metabolism of Steroids in the Brain: A new Insight into the Role of 5 alpha Reductase and Aromatase in Brain Differentiation and Functions," *J. Steroid Biochem. Mol. Biol* 58 (1996): 455–66; Negri-Cesi, et al., "Metabolism of Steroids in the Brain: A New Insight into the Role of 5 alpha Reductase and Aromatase in Brain Differentiation and Functions," *J Steroid Biochem Mol Biol* 58 (1996): 455–66; A. Poletti, et al., "The 5 alpha reductase isozymes in the Central Nervous System," *Steroids* 63 (1998): 246–51; A. Poletti and L. Martini, "Androgen-activating enzymes in the Central Nervous System," *J Steroid Biochem Mol Biol* 65 (1998): 295–99; D. M. Avila, et al., "Identification of genes expressed in the rat prostate that are modulated differently by castration and finasteride treatment," *Journal of Endocrinology* 159 (Part 3), abstract online, www.journals.endocrinology.org.

14. *DHEA: A Comprehensive Review.* J. H. H. Thijssen and H. Nieuwehnhuyse, eds. (New York: Parthenon, 1999) 14, 138, chs. 2, 3; Beverly Greenberg, *The DHEA Discovery* (Los Angeles: Majesty Press, 1996); Stephen Cherniske, *The DHEA Breakthrough* (New York: Ballantine, 1998); Hasnain Walji, *DHEA:The Ultimate Rejuvenating Hormone* (Prescott, AZ: Hohm Press, 1996); Ray Sahelian, *DHEA: A Practical Guide* (New York: Avery, 1996).

15. A. Netter, et al., "Effect of Zinc Administration on Plasma Testosterone, Dihydrotestosterone, and Sperm Count," *Arch Androl* 7 (1981): 69–73.

16. J. B. Härborne, *Introduction to Ecological Biochemistry* (London: Academic Press, 1982), 191.

17. J. T. Bradbury, "The rabbit ovulating factor of plant juice," *Am J Physiol* 142 (1944): 487–93; M. O. Curruba, et al., "Stimulatory effect of a maize diet on sexual behavior of male rats," *Life Sci* 20 (1977): 159–64.

18. Ullis, et al., *Super T,* 39; Bradbury, "The rabbit ovulating factor of plant juice."

19. O. Sodimu, et al., "Certain biochemical effects of garlic oil on rats maintained on fat-high cholesterol diet," *Experientia* 40(1) (1984): 78–79; S. Kasuga, et al., "Recent advances on the nutritional effects associated with the use of garlic as a supplement. Pharmacologic activities of aged garlic extract in comparison with other garlic preparations," *J Nutr* 131(3S) (2001): 1180S–84S; Paul Bergner, *The Healing Power of Garlic* (Rocklin, CA: Prima, 1996), 173; Melvyn Werbach and Michael Murray, *Botanical Influences on Illness* (Tarzana, CA: Third Line Press, 1994), 61–65, 115, 145–46, 185–86, 192–93.

20. www.birdways.com; www.medicalmeals.com; www.nat.uiuc.edu; www.vegsoc.org.

21. M. R. Gutierrez-Fernandez, et al., "Methods for the study of estrone, estradiol and testosterone in the seeds of *Pinus pinea* L.," *An R Acad Farm* 47(1) (1981): 97–112.

22. Daniel Reid, *Chinese Herbal Medicine* (Boston, MA: Shambhala, 1986), 61.

23. M. Schambelan, "Licorice ingestion and blood pressure regulating hormones," *Steroids* 59(2) (1994): 127–30; P. M. Stewart, et al., "Mineralocorticoid activity of carbenoxolone: Contrasting effects of carbenoxolone and liquorice on 11-beta-hydroxysteroid dehydrogenase activity," *Clin Sci* 78(1) (1990): 49–54; C. R. W. Edwards, "Lessons from licorice," *N Engl J Med* 325(17) (1991): 1242–43; Doc Childre, *The Heartmath Solution* (San Francisco: HarperSanFrancisco, 1999), 55; Ullis, *Super T*, 98; Wright and Lenard, *Maximize Your Vitality and Potency*, 143; Suzanne, Shepherd, "Plant Poisoning, Licorice," *eMedicine Journal* 2(4) (2001 April 17): 2; D. Armanini, et al., "Reduction of serum testosterone in men by licorice," *N Engl J Med* 341(15) (1999): 1158; Duke, Phytochemical Database.

24. M. M. Seidl and D. E. Stewart, "Alternative treatments for menopausal symptoms: A systematic review of scientific and lay literature," *Can Fam Phys* 44 (1998): 1299–1308.

25. Rudolf Weiss, *Herbal Medicine* (Gothenberg, Sweden: AB Arcanum, 1988), 286; Duke, Phytochemical Database; W. H. Moger, "Direct effects of estrogens on the endocrine function of the mammalian testis," *Can J Physiol Pharmacol* 58(9) (1980): 1011–22; M. Namiki, et al., "Direct inhibitory effect of estrogen on the human testis *in vitro*," *Arch Androl* 20(2) (1988): 131–35; J. E. Damber, et al., "The acute effect of estrogens on testosterone production appears not to be mediated by testicular estrogen receptors," *Mol Cell Endocr* 31(1) (1983): 105–16; W. Stammel, et al., "Tetrahydroisoquinoline alkaloids mimic direct but not receptor-mediated inhibitory effects of estrogens and phytoestrogens on testicular endocrine function. Possible significance for Leydig cell insufficiency in alcohol addiction," *Life Sci* 49(18) (1991): 1319–29.

26. Stephen Harrod Buhner, *Sacred and Herbal Healing Beers: The Secrets of Ancient Fermentation* (Boulder, CO: Siris Press, 1998), 169–74.

27. S. Tazuke, et al., "Exogenous estrogen and endogenous sex hormones," *Medicine* 71 (1992): 44–50; *DHEA: a Comprehensive Review*. Thijssen and Nieuwenhuyse (eds.) 46; *DHEA: a Comprehensive Review*. Thijssen and Nieuwenhuyse (eds.) 45; Stammel, et al., "Tetrahydroisoquinoline alkaloids mimic direct . . ."

CHAPTER 3

1. H. Jeng, et al., "A substance isolated from *Cornus officinalis* enhances the motility of human sperm," *American Journal of Chinese Medicine* 25(3–4) (1997): 301–06; Q. L. Peng, et al., "Fructus corni enhances endothelial cell antioxidant defenses," *Gen Pharmacol* 31 (1998): 221–25.

2. I. Viktorof, et al., "Pharmacological, pharmacokinetic, toxicological, and clinical studies on protodioscin," *IIMS Therapeutic Focus* Vol. 2 (1994), cited at www.nutrica.com/Libilov/LMR1.htm; K. M. Arsyad, "Effect of protodioscin on the quantity and quality of sperms from males with moderate oligozoospermia," *Medika* 22(8) (1996): 614–18; L. Se-

tiawan, "*Tribulus terrestris* L. extract improves spermatozoa motility and increases the efficiency of acrosome reaction in subjects diagnosed with oligoasthenoteratozoospermia," Aialangga University (1996); A. Adimoelja, et al., "*Tribulus terrestris* (protodioscin) in the treatment of male infertility with idiopathic oligoasthenoteratozoospermia," Proceedings of the First International Conference of Medical Plants for Reproductive Medicine held in Taipei, Taiwan, 1995; N. Moeloek, et al., "Trials of *Tribulus terrestris* (Protodioscin) on oligozoospermia," Proceedings of the VIth National Congress and IIIrd International Symposium on New Perspectives of Andrology on Human Reproduction, 1994; A. Adimoelja and P. Ganeshan Adaikan, "Protodioscin from herbal plant *Tribulus terrestris* improves the male sexual functions, probably via DHEA," *Int J Impotence Research* 9(1) (1997); Adimoilja and Adaikan, "Protodioscin from herbal plant *Tribulus terrestris* improves the male sexual functions, probably via DHEA"; S. Milanov, et al., "Tribestan effect on the concentration of some hormones in the serum of healthy subjects," online: www.tribestan.com; D. Obreshkova, et al., "Comparative analytical investigation of *Tribulus terrestris* preparations," *Pharmacia* 15(11), vol. 2, 1998.

3. D. S. Pardanani, et al., "Study of the Effects of Speman on Semen Quality in Oligospermic Men," *Indian J Surg* 38 (1976): 34–39; P. G. Jayatilak, et al., "Effect of an indigenous drug (Speman) on human accessory reproductive function," *Indian J Surg* 38 (1976): 12–15; H. R. Limaye and C. S. Madkar, "Management of oligozoospermia, asthenospermia, and necrozoospermia by treatment with 'Speman,'" *Antiseptic* (November 1984): 612; Sabuj Sengupta, "A clinico-pathological study of the effect of Speman on spermatogenesis in cases of oligozoospermia," *Probe* 21(4) (1982): 275–76; K. N. Gour and Sudhir Gupta, "Speman in Male Sexual Disorders," *Current Medical Practice* 3 (1959): 135; S. Madaan and T. R. Madaan, "Speman in Oligospermia," *Probe* 24(2) (1985): 115–17; S. E. Mukher, et al., "Effect of Speman on prostatism—a clinical study," *Probe* 25 (1986): 237–40; K. P. Gaur, "Evaluation of Speman in prostatitis," *Capsule* 1 (1982): 2; P. Bannerjee, "Speman and Cystone in Benign Prostatic Enlargement," *Probe* 13(2) (1974): 88–90; V. K. Agarway and R. K. Gupta, "Clinical Studies with Speman in Cases of Benign Enlargement of the Prostate," *The Indian Practitioner* 6 (1971): 281; Mir Nazir Ahmed, et al., "Speman in Patients of Benign Prostatomegaly," *Current Medical Practice* 9 (1983): 257; H. S. Rathore and V. Saraswat, "Protection of Mouse Testes, Epididymis, and Adrenals with Speman against Cadmium Intoxication," *Probe* 25 (1986): 257–68; P. G. Jayatilak, et al., "Effect of an indigenous drug (Speman) on accessory reproduction functions in mice," *Indian J Exp Biol* 14 (1976): 170.

4. G. Salvati, et al., "Effects of *Panax ginseng* C. A. Meyer, saponins on male fertility," *Panminerva Med* 38(4) (1996): 249–54; I. M. Popov and C. F. Hering III, "The use of ginseng extract as an adjunct in different types of treatment for male impotency," *Abstr Third Int Ginseng Symp Korea*, Res Inst, Seoul, Korea, Sept 8–10, 1980, 10; J. C. Chen, et al., "Effect of *Panax notoginseng* saponins on sperm motility and progression in vitro," *Phytomedicine* 5(4) (1998): 289–92; J. C. Chen, et al., "Effects of *Panax notoginseng* polysaccharide and aqueous fraction on human sperm motility *in vitro*," *China Med Coll J* 7(4) (1998): 39–46; J. C. Chen, et al., "Effect of *Panax notoginseng* extracts on inferior sperm motility *in vitro*," *Amer J Chinese Med* 27(1) (1999): 123–28.

5. A. Schacter, J. A. Goldman, Z. Zuckerman, "Treatment of Oligospermia with the Amino Acid Arginine," *J Urol* 110 (1973): 311–13; D. W. Keller and K. L. Polakoski, "L-arginine stimulation of human sperm motility *in vitro*," *Biol Reprod* 13 (1975): 154–57.

6. G. Vitali, R. Parente, C. Melotti, "Carnitine supplementation in Human Idiopathic Asthenospermia: Clinical results," *Drugs Exp Clin Res* 21 (1995): 157–59.

7. B. Sandler and B. Faragher, "Treatment of Oligospermia with Vitamin B$_{12}$," *Infertility* 7 (1984): 133–38; Y. Kumamato, et al., "Clinical Efficacy of Mecobalamin in Treatment of Oligospermia: Results of a Double-Blind Comparative Clinical Study," *Acta Urol Japan* 34 (1988): 1109–32; John Morgenthaler and Mia Simms. *Better Sex: From Andro to Zinc* (Petaluma, CA: Smart Publications, 1999), 49–58.

8. Michael Murray and Joseph Pizzorno, *Encyclopedia of Natural Medicine* (Roseville, CA: Prima, 1998), 581–83, 891; Shippen and Fryer, *The Testosterone Syndrome*, 132.

9. M. Tikkiwal, "Effect of zinc administration on seminal zinc and fertility of oligospermic males," *Ind Journal Physiol Pharmacol* 31 (1987): 30–34; Murray and Pizzorno, *Encyclopedia of Natural Medicine*, 583, 891.

10. S. Kasuga, et al., "Recent advances on the nutritional effects associated with the use of garlic as a supplement: Pharmacologic activities of aged garlic extract in comparison with other garlic preparations," *J Nutr* 131(3S) (2001): 1180S–84S.

11. Murray and Pizzorno, *Encyclopedia of Natural Medicine*, 583, 891.

12. R. Sikora and R. Sikora, "Ginkgo biloba extract in the therapy of erectile dysfunction," *J Urol* 141 (1989): 188A.

13. C. Pepe, et al., "Video capillaroscopy evaluation of efficacy Ginkgo biloba extract with L-arginine and magnesium in the treatment of trophic lesions in patients with Stage 4 peripheral arterial occlusive disease," *Minerva Cardioangiol* 47(6) (1999): 223–30.

14. Melvyn Werbach and Michael Murray, *Botanical Influences on Illness* (Tarzana, CA: Third Line Press, 1994), 200.

15. A. W. Nasution, "Effect of *Tribulus terrestris* treatment on impotence and libido disorders," Andalas University, School of Medicine, (1993); W. Pangkahila, "*Tribulus terrestris* (protodioscin) increases men's sex drive," Proceedings of the Xth National congress on New Perspectives of Andrology on Human Reproduction (1993); A. Adimoelja and P. Ganeshan Adaikan, "Protodioscin from herbal plant *Tribulus terrestris* improves the male sexual functions, probably via DHEA," *Int J Impotence Research* 9(1) (1997); A. Adimoelja, "Treatment of Sexual dysfunction in diabetes mellitus subjects using orally administered protodioscin and injection of vasoactive compounds," Proceedings from the Seminar of Erectile Dysfunction of Diabetes in Bandung, Indonesia (1997); K. M. Arsyad, "Effect of protodioscin (*Tribulus terrestris*) on the well-being and sexual response of men with diabetes mellitus." All are available online at www.nutrica.com/Libolov/ClinicalStudies/LLibilovTrialsSummary.htm; J. R. Sankaran, "Problem of male virility— an oriental therapy," *J Natl Integ Med Ass* 26(11) (1984): 315–17; A. Adimoelja, "Phytochemicals and the breakthrough of traditional herbs in the management of sexual dysfunction," *Int J Androl* 23(2) (2000): 82–84; A. Gauthaman, et al., "Pro-erectile pharmacological effect of *Tribulis terrestris* on the rabbit corpus cavernosum," *Ann Acad Med Singapore* 29(1) (Jan. 2000): 22–26; Adimoelja and Adaikan, "Protodioscin from herbal

plant *Tribulus terrestris* improves the male sexual functions, probably via DHEA"; Adimoelja, "Treatment of Sexual dysfunction in diabetes mellitus subjects using orally administered protodioscin and injection of vasoactive compounds."

16. V. Yoram and G. Illan, "Oral pharmacotherapy in erectile dysfunction," *Curr Opin Urol* 7(6) (1997): 349–53; A. W. Zorgniotti and E. F. Lia, "Effect of large doses of nitric oxide precursor, L-arginine, on erectile dysfunction," *Int J Impot Rev* 1 (1994): 33–35; Morgenthaler and Simms, *Better Sex from Andro to Zinc,* 13–21, 117–18.

17. Durk Pearson and Sandy Shaw, "Sexual effects of nutrients: arginine and choline," *Lifenet News* 2 (1999): 6, cited in Morgenthaler and Simms, *Better Sex from Andro to Zinc,* 20.

18. Yoram and Illan, "Oral pharmacotherapy in erectile dysfunction," Morgenthaler and Simms, *Better Sex from Andro to Zinc,* 20–23, 117–18.

19. Yoram and Illan, "Oral pharmacotherapy in erectile dysfunction," A. W. Zorgniotti and E. F. Lia, "Effect of large doses of nitric oxide precursor, L-arginine, on erectile dysfunction," *Int J Impot Rev* 1 (1994): 33–35; Morgenthaler and Simms, *Better Sex from Andro to Zinc,* 52–57, 119–20.

20. Duke, *The Green Pharmacy,* 187–88.

21. Quoted in Wright and Lenard, *Maximize Your Vitality and Potency,* 157.

22. R. J. Cote, et al., "The effect of finasteride on the prostate gland in men with elevated serum prostate-specific antigen levels," *Br J Cancer* 78 (1998): 413–18, cited in Wright and Lenard, *Maximize Your Vitality and Potency,* 160.

23. P. C. Walsh, et al., "Tissue content of dihydrotestosterone in human prostatic hyperplasia is not supranormal," *J Clin Invest* 72 (1983): 1772–77, cited in Wright and Lenard, *Maximize,* 161.

24. S. J. Janter, et al., "Comparative rates of androgen production and metabolism in Caucasian subjects," *J Clin Endocrinol Metab* 83(6) (1998): 2104–09.

25. H. Yamanaka and S. Honma, "Endocrine environment of benign prostatic hyperplasia: prostate size and volume are correlated with serum estrogen concentration," *Scand J Urol Nephrol* 29(1) (1995): 65–68; P. H. Gann, et al., "A prospective study of plasma hormone levels, nonhormonal factors, and development of benign prostatic hyperplasia," *Prostate* 26(1) (1995): 40–49; N. N. Stone, "Estrogen formation in human prostatic tissue from patients with and without benign prostatic hyperplasia," *Prostate* 9(4) (1986): 311–18.

26. B. R. Konety, et al., "The role of vitamin D in normal prostate growth and differentiation," *Cell Growth Differ* 7 (1996): 1563–70.

27. H. Ehara, et al., "Expression of estrogen receptor in diseased human prostate assessed by non-radioactive in-situ hybridization and immunohistochemistry," *Prostate* 27(6) (1995): 304–13; K. D. Voigt and W. Bartsch, "The role of tissue steroids in benign hyperplasia and prostate cancer," *Urologe* [A] 26(6) (1987): 349–57; Mark MCClure, *Smart Medicine for a Healthy Prostate* (New York: Avery, 2001), 22–23.

28. W. E. Farnsworth, "Roles of estrogen and SHBG in prostate physiology," *Prostate* 28(1) (1996): 17–23; A. M. Nakkla, et al., "Estradiol causes the rapid accumulation of cAMP in human prostate," *Proc Natl Acad Sci USA* 91(12) (1994): 5402–05.

29. J. J. Lichiu and C. Muth, "The inhibiting effects of *Urtica dioica* root extracts on experimentally induced prostatic hyperplasia in the mouse," *Planta Med* 63(4) (1997): 307–10;

A. Friesen, *Statistical analysis of a multicenter long-term study with ERU1*, 1988, 121–30 (Napralert citation); M. Oberholzer, et al., "Results obtained by electron microscopy in medicamentously treated benign prostatic hyperplasia (BPH)," in *Benigne Prostatahyperplasie*, H. W. Bauer (ed), 1986, 13–17 (Napralert citation); J. Djulepa, "A two year study of prostatic syndrome. The results of a conservative treatment with Bazoton," *Arztl Praxis* 63(7) (1982): 2199–05; G. Dathe and H. Schmid, "Phytotherapy of the benign prostatic hyperplasia (BPH): A double-blind study with an extract of radicis urticae (ERU)," *Urologe* 27 (1987): 223–26; H. P. Vontobel, et al., "The results of a double-blind study on the efficacy of ERU capsules in the conservative treatment of benign prostatic hyperplasia," *Urologe* 24 (1985): 49–51; K. Maar, "Retrogression of the symptomatology of prostate adenoma. Results of a six-month conservative treatment with ERU capsules," *Fortschr Med* 105 (1987): 1–5; U. Tosch and H. Mussiggang, "The Medicamentous treatment of the benign prostatic hyperplasia," *Euromed* 6 (1983): 1–8; H. Fieber, "Sonographical observations of the course concerning the influence of the medicamentous therapy of the benign prostatic hyperplasia (BPH)," in H. W. Bauer (ed.), *Klinische und Experimentelle Urologie 19. Benigne Prostatahyperplasie II* (np, nd Napralert database citation), 1988: 75–82; P. Goetz, "Treatment of Benign Prostatic Hyperplasia with Urticae Radix," *Z Phytother* 10 (1989): 175–78; H. P. Stahl, "Therapy of prostatic nocturia with a standardized extract of urtica root," *Z Allg Med* 60 (1984): 128–32; I. Romics, "Observations with Bazoton in the management of prostatic hyperplasia," *Int Urol Nephrol* 19(3) (1987): 293–97; E. Montanari, et al., "Benign prostatic hyperplasia randomized study with 63 patients," *Informierte Arzt* 6A (1991): 593–98; F. C. Lowe, et al., "Review of recent placebo-controlled trials utilizing phytotherapeutic agents for the treatment of BPH," *Prostate* 37(3) (1998): 187–93; W. Vahlensieck, "Konservative Behandlung der benignen Prostatahyperplasie (BPH)," *Therapiewoche* 35 (1985): 4031–40; T. Krzeski, et al., "Combined extracts of *Urtica dioica* and *Pygeum africanum* in the treatment of benign prostatic hyperplasia: double-blind comparison of two doses," *Clin Ther* 15(6) (1993): 1011–20; D. J. Hryb, et al., "The effect of extracts of the roots of the stinging nettle (*Urtica dioica*) on the interaction of SHBG with its receptor on human prostatic membranes," *Planta Med* 61(1) (1995): 31–32; H. Wagner, et al., "Search for the antiprostatic principle of stinging nettle (*Urtica dioica*) roots," *Phytomedicine* 1(3) (1994): 213–24; N. Suh, et al., "Discovery of natural product chemopreventative agents utilizing HL-60 cell differentiation as a model," *Anticancer Res* 15(2) (1995): 233–39; P. Goetz, "Treatment of benign prostatic hyperplasia with nettle root," *Z Phytother* 10 (1989): 175–78; R. W. Hartmann, et al., "Inhibition of 5 alpha-reductase and aromatase by PHL-00801 (Prostatonin), a combination of PY 102 (*Pygeum africanum*) and UR 102 (*Urtica dioica*) extracts," *Phytomedicine* 3(2) (1996): 121–28; F. C. Lowe and E. Fagelman, "Phytotherapy in the treatment of benign prostatic hyperplasia: An update," *Urology* 53(4) (1999): 671–78; P. Belaiche and O. Lievoux, "Clinical studies on the palliative treatment of prostatic adenoma with extract of urtica root," *Phytother Res* 5(6) (1991): 267–69; J. J. Lichius, et al., "The inhibiting effects of components of stinging nettle roots on experimentally induced prostatic hyperplasia in mice," *Planta Med* 65(7) (1999): 666–68; E. Bombardelli and P. Morazzoni, "*Urtica dioica* L.," *Fitoterapia* 68(5) (1997): 387–402; H. Zieglar, "Investigations of prostate cells under effect of extract Radix Urticae (ERU) by fluorescent microscopy," *Fortschr Med* 45 (1983): 2112–14; M. Oberholzer, et al., "Results obtained by electron microscopy in medicamentously treated benign prostatic hyperplasia (BPH)," in *Benigne Prostatahyperplasie*, H. W. Bauer (ed.), (Np, nd) 1986, 13–17 (Napralert citation); V. H. Ziegler, "Zytomorphologische verlaufskontrolle einer therapie der residivierenden prostatis durch eine landzeit-kombinations behandlung," *Fortschr Med* 39(21) (1982): 1832–34; H. Wagner, et al., "Biologically active compounds from the aqueous extract of *Urtica dioica*," *Planta Med* 55(5) (1989): 452–54; H. Wagner, et al., "Search for the antiprostatic principle of stinging nettle (*Urtica dioica*) roots," *Phytomedicine* 1(3) (1994): 213–24.

30. L. S. Marks, et al., "Effects of a saw palmetto herbal blend in men with symptomatic benign prostatic hyperplasia," *J Urol* 163(5) (2000): 1451–56; J. Sokeland, "Combined Sabal and Urtica extract compared with finasteride in men with benign prostatic hyperplasia: an analysis of prostate volume and therapeutic outcome," *Brit J Urol Int* 86(4) (2000): 439–42; E. Koch, "Pharmacology and modes of action of extracts of palmetto fruit (*Sabal fructus*), stinging nettle roots (*Urticae radix*), and pumpkin seed (*Curcurbitae peponis semen*) in the treatment of benign prostatic hyperplasia," *Phytopharmaka forsch Klin Anwend* 1995 (1995): 57–79; E. Koch and A. Biber, "Pharmacological effects of saw palmetto and urtica extracts for benign prostatic hyperplasia," *Quart Rev Nat Med* 1995 (1995): 281–89; H. J. Schneider, et al., "Treatment of benign prostatic hyperplasia. Results of a surveillance study in the practices of urological specialists using a combined plant-based preparation (Sabal extract WS 1473 and urtica extract WS 1031)," *Fortschr Med* 113(3) (1995): 37–40; D. V. C. Awang, "Saw palmetto, African prune, and stinging nettle for benign prostatic hyperplasia (BPH)," *Can Pharm J* 130(9) (1997): 37–44–62 [sic]; J. Stokeland and J. Albrecht, "Combined Sabal and urtica extract vs finasteride in BPH (Alken Stage I-II)," *Urology* 36 (1997): 327–33.

31. L. S. Marks, et al., "Tissue effects of saw palmetto and finasteride: use of biopsy cores for *in situ* quantification of prostatic androgens," *Urology* 57(5) (2001): 999–1005; F. Di Silverio, et al., "Effects of long-term treatment with *Serenoa repens* (Permixon) on the concentrations and regional distribution of androgens and epidermal growth factor in benign prostatic hyperplasia," *Prostate* 37(2): 77–83; F. Di Silverio, et al., "Evidence that *Serenoa repens* extract displays an antiestrogenic activity in prostatic tissue of benign prostatic hypertrophy patients," *Eur Urol* 21(4) (1992): 309–14; M. Caponera, et al., "Antiestrogenic activity of *Serenoa repens* in patients with BPH," *Acta Urol Ital* 1992(4) (1992): 271–72; Lowe and Fagelman, "Phytotherapy in the treatment of benign prostatic hyperplasia: An update"; Winston, *Saw Palmetto for Men and Women* (Pownal, VT: Storey, 1999), 57–58; G. Strauch, et al., "Comparison of finasteride (Proscar) and *Serenoa repens* in the inhibition of 5 alpha reductase in healthy male volunteers," *Eur Urol* 26(3) (1994): 247–52; D. E. McKinney, "Saw Palmetto for Benign Prostatic Hyperplasia," *J Amer Med Ass* 281(18) (1999): 1699; S. Broccafoschi and S. Amnoscia, "Comparison of *Serenoa repens* Extract with Placebo in Controlled Clinical Trial in Patients with Prostatic Adenomatosis," *Urologia* 50 (1983): 1257–68; G. Champault, et al., "Medical Treatment of Prostatic Adenoma: Controlled Trial: PA 109 vs Placebo in 110 patients," *Ann Urol* 18 (1984): 4–7, 10; Murray

and Pizzorno, *Encyclopedia of Natural Medicine*, 758–59, 911–12; J. Braeckman, et al., "Efficacy and safety of the extract of *Serenoa repens* in the treatment of benign prostatic hyperplasia," *Phytotherapy Research* 11 (1997): 558–63; J. Braeckman, "The Extract of *Serenoa repens* in the Treatment of Benign Prostatic Hyperplasia: A Multicenter Open Study," *Curr Ther Res* 55 (1994): 776–85; Vahlensieck, et al., "Benign Prostatic Hyperplasia: Treatment with Sabal Fruit Extract," *Fortschritte Med* 111 (1993): 323–26.

32. F. K. Habib, et al., "*In vitro* evaluation of the pollen extract, Cernitin T-60, in the regulation of prostate cell growth," *Br J Urol* 66 (1990): 393–437, cited in Volker Schulz, et al., *Rational Phytotherapy* (Berlin: Springer, 1998), 230; R. Yasumoto, et al., "Clinical evaluation of long-term treatment using Cernilton pollen extract in patients with benign prostatic hyperplasia," *Clinical Therapeutics* 17 (1995): 82–86; A. C. Buck, et al., "Treatment of outflow tract obstruction due to benign prostatic hyperplasia with the pollen extract, Cernilton: A double-blind, Placebo-controlled Study," *Br J Urol* 66(4) (1990): 398–404; Mark McClure, *Smart Medicine for a Healthy Prostate*, 54–55, 85–86; Volker Schulz, et al., *Rational Phytotherapy* (Berlin: Springer, 1998), 230–31; E. W. Rugendorff, et al., "Results of treatment with pollen extract (Cernilton N) in chronic prostatitis and prostatodynia," *Br J Urol* 71 (1993): 433–38; A. Jodai, et al., "A long-term therapeutic experience with Cernilton in chronic prostatitis," *Hinyokika Kiyo* 34 (1988): 561–68; J. Wojcicki, et al., "Effect of flower pollen in patients with rheumatoid arthritis and concomitant diseases of the gastroduodenal and hepatobiliary systems," *Likarska Sprava* 4 (1998): 151–54.

33. A. P. Lanier, et al., "Cancer in Alaskan Indians, Eskimos, and Aleuts, 1969–1983: Implications for etiology and control," *Public Health Rep* 27 (1989): 798–803; J. Hart and W. Cooper, *Vitamin F in the treatment of prostatic hypertrophy*, Milwaukee, WI: Lee Foundation for Nutritional Research, 1941.

34. Murray and Pizzorno, *Encyclopedia of Natural Medicine*, 755–56; Wright and Lenard, *Maximize*, 196.

35. G. Derosa, et al., "Prolactin secretion after beer," *Lancet* 2(1981): 934.

36. J. J. Lichius, et al., "Antiproliferative effect of a polysaccharide fraction of a 20% methanolic extract of stinging nettle roots upon epithelial cells of the human prostate (LNCAP)," *Pharmazie* 54(10) (1999): 768–71; L. Konrad, et al., "Antiproliferative effect on human prostate cancer cells by a stinging nettle root (*Urtica dioica*) extract," *Planta Med* 66(1) (2000): 44–47; F. C. Lowe and E. Fagelman, "Phytotherapy in the treatment of benign prostatic hyperplasia: an update," *Urology* 53(4) (1999): 671–78; McClure, *Smart Medicine for a Healthy Prostate*, 138; Winston, *Saw Palmetto*, 74; K. P. Roberts, et al., "Cyclic hydroxamic acid inhibitors of prostate cancer cell growth: selectivity and structure activity relationships," *Prostate* 34 (1996): 92–99; X. Zhang, et al., "Isolation and characterization of a cyclic hydroxamic acid from a pollen extract, which inhibits cancerous cell growth *in vitro*," *J Med Chem* 38 (1995): 735–38; Zi Xiaolin, et al., "A flavonoid antioxidant, Silymarin, inhibits activation of erbB1 signaling and induces cyclin-dependent kinase Inhibitors, GI arrest, and anticarcinogenic effects in human prostate carcinoma DU145 cells," *Cancer Research* 58(9) (1998): 1920–29; cited in McClure, *Smart Medicine for a Healthy Prostate*, 138; Donald Yance, *Herbal Medicine Healing and Cancer* (Chicago, IL: Keats, 1999), 350; Wright and Lenard, *Maximize*, 198–206, also chapter 8; especially also

see James Brooks, et al., "Plasma selenium level before diagnosis and the risk of prostate cancer development," *Journal of Urology* 166 (2001): 2034–38.

37. B. de Ligniereres, "Transdermal dihydrotestosterone treatment of 'andropause,'" *Ann Med* 25 (1993): 235–41; Wright and Lenard, *Maximize,* Chapter 8.

CHAPTER 4

1. Doc Childre, *The Heartmath Solution* (San Francisco: HarperSanFrancisco, 1999).
2. Jonathan Wright and Lane Lenard, *Maximize Your Vitality and Potency (for Men Over 40)* (Petaluma, CA: Smart Publications, 1999), Chapter 7.
3. Eugene Shippen and William Fryer, *The Testosterone Syndrome* (New York: Evans, 1998), 82.
4. Wright and Lenard, *Maximize,* Chapter 7; Shippen and Fryer, *The Testosterone Syndrome,* Chapter 7.
5. Ibid.
6. Wright and Lenard, *Maximize,* 129–33.
7. Stephanie Nano, "Heart May Be Able to Repair Itself," Associated Press, America Online, January 2, 2002, citing *New England Journal of Medicine.*
8. Dan Bensky and Andrew Gamble, *Chinese Herbal Medicine: Materia Medica,* Revised Edition (Seattle: Eastland Press, 1993), 224; Volker Schulz, et al., *Rational Phytotherapy* (Berlin: Springer, 1998), 90–99; W. L. Weng, et al., "Therapeutic effect of crataegus on 46 cases of angina pectoris—a double-blind study," *J Trad Chin Med* 4(4) (1984): 293–94; U. Schmidt, et al., "Efficacy of the hawthorn (Crataegus) preparation LI 132 in 78 patients with chronic congestive heart failure defined as NYHA Functional Class II," *Phytomedicine* 1(1) (1994): 17–24; G. Nemecz, "Hawthorn—This herb dilates coronary vessels, lowers blood pressure, and reduces lipid levels," *US Pharmacist* 1999 (1999): 52–60; M. Tauchert, et al., "High dose crataegus (Hawthorn) extract WS 1442 for the treatment of NYHA Class II heart failure patients," *Herz* 24(6) (1999): 465–74.
9. Wright and Lenard, *Maximize,* Chapter 7; Shippen and Fryer, *The Testosterone Syndrome,* Chapter 7.
10. Jens Moller and H. Einfeldt, *Testosterone Treatment of Cardiovascular Disease* (Berlin: Springer-Verlag, 1984); M. Lesser, "Testosterone propionate therapy in one hundred cases of angina pectoris," *J Clin Endocrinol* 6 (1946): 549–57; Wright and Lenard, *Maximize,* Chapter 7, 127–28; Shippen and Fryer, *The Testosterone Syndrome,* Chapter 7.
11. *DHEA: A Comprehensive Review,* J. H. H. Thijssen and H. Nieuwenhuyse (eds.) (New York: Parthenon, 1999), 113–15.
12. Michael Murray and Joseph Pizzorno, *The Encyclopedia of Natural Medicine* (Roseville, CA: Prima, 1998), 502–04.
13. Ibid., 504–05.
14. Ibid, 505–06.
15. Schulz, et al., *Rational Phytotherapy,* 90–99.
16. Heinrich Koch and Larry Dawson, *Garlic: The Science and Therapeutic Application of Allium Sativum and Related Species* (Baltimore, MD: Williams and Wilkins, 1996), 135–62;

Melvyn Werbach and Michael Murray, *Biological Influences on Illness* (Tarzana, CA: Third Line Press, 1994).

17. F. A. Arustamova, "Hypotensive effect of *Leonarus cardiaca* on animals in experimental chronic hypertension," *Izvestiya Akademii Nauk Armyanski SSR, Biologicheski Nauki,* 16(7) (1963): 47–52; Y. X. Xia, "The inhibitory effect of motherwort extract on pulsating myocardial cells *in vitro*," *J Trad Chin Med,* 3(3), 185–88; Daniel Mowrey, *The Scientific Validation of Herbal Medicine* (New Canaan, CT: Keats, 1986), 138, 142.

18. Rudolf Weiss, *Herbal Medicine* (Gothenburg, Sweden: AB Arcanum, 1988), 180–81.

19. Murray and Pizzorno, *Encyclopedia of Natural Medicine,* 527–31.

20. Ibid., 533.

21. Ibid., 533–34.

22. Ibid., 526–27.

23. Wright and Lenard, *Maximize,* 44, 139–40.

24. Werbach and Murray, *Botanical Influences on Illness,* 66–67; Murray and Pizzorno, *Encyclopedia of Natural Medicine,* 356–57; Robyn Landis and K. P. Khalsa, *Herbal Defense* (New York: Warner, 1997), 413.

25. Murray and Pizzorno, *Encyclopedia of Natural Medicine,* 351–54; Andrew Weil, *8 Weeks to Optimum Health* (New York: Knopf, 1997), 241–44.

26. Schulz, et al., *Rational Phytotherapy,* 128.

27. Murray and Pizzorno, *Encyclopedia of Natural Medicine,* 249; Werbach and Murray, *Biological Influences on Illness,* 69–70.

28. Murray and Pizzorno, *Encyclopedia of Natural Medicine,* 248.

29. Ibid., 246–47.

30. Schulz, *Rational Phytotherapy,* 128–36.

31. M. R. Cesarone, et al., "Microcirculatory activity of Centella asiatica in venous insufficiency: A double-blind study," *Minerva Cardioangiol* 42(6) (1994): 299–304; Murray and Pizzorno, *Encyclopedia of Natural Medicine,* 828, 920.

32. James Duke, *The Green Pharmacy* (Emmaus, PA: Rodale, 1997), 251.

33. Wright and Lenard, *Maximize,* Chapter 7.

CHAPTER 5

1. Anonymous, "UI researchers use intestinal worms to treat inflammatory bowel disease," University of Iowa Healthcare, *UI Health Care News,* Weeks of August 9 and 16, 1999; Anonymous, "We need the worms," *Discover* 20 (December 1999): 12.

2. Michael Murray and Joseph Pizzorno, *The Encyclopedia of Natural Medicine* (Roseville, CA: Prima, 1998), 591.

3. K. Mitsuyama, et al., "Treatment of ulcerative colitis with germinated barley foodstuff feeding: A pilot study," *Aliment Pharmacol Ther* 12(12) (1998): 1225–30.

4. Melvyn Werbach and Michael Murray, *Biological Influences on Illness* (Tarzana, CA: Third Line Press, 1994), 266–67; Bing Yang and Paul Schwarz, "Factors Involved in the Formation of Two precursors of Dimethylsulfide During Malting," *Am Soc Brew Chem* 56(3) (1998): 85–92.

5. Thomas Newmark and Paul Schulick, *Beyond Aspirin* (Prescott, AZ: Hohm Press, 2000), Chapter 14.

6. W. Shive, et al., "Glutamine in the treatment of peptic ulcer" *Texas State Journal of Medicine,* 53 (1957): 840–43.

7. B. A. Lashner, et al., "Effect of folate supplementation on the incidence of dysplasia and cancer in chronic ulcerative colitis," *Gastroenterol* 97 (1989): 255–59; B. A. Lashner, et al., "The effect of folic acid supplementation on the risk for cancer or dysplasia in ulcerative colitis," 112 (1997): 29–32; Murray and Pizzorno, *Encyclopedia of Natural Medicine,* 597.

8. A. Belluzzi, "Effect of an enteric-coated fish oil preparation on relapses in Crohn's disease," *New England Journal of Medicine* 334 (1996): 1557–60; A. Asian, et al., "Fish oil fatty acid supplementation in active ulcerative colitis: a double-blind, placebo-controlled, crossover study," *Am J Gastroenterol* 87 (1992): 432–37; P. Salomon, et al., "Treatment of ulcerative colitis with fish oil N-3-omega-fatty acid: an open trial," *J Clin Gastroenterol* 12 (1990): 157–61.

9. Murray and Pizzorno, *Encyclopedia of Natural Medicine,* 597.

10. Ibid., 597–98.

11. I. Gupta, et al., "Effects of *Boswellia serrata* gum resin in patients with ulcerative colitis," *Eur J Med Res* 2 (1997): 37–43.

12. G. Cheney, "Vitamin U therapy of peptic ulcer," *Calif Med* 77(4) (1952): 248–52; V. V. Trusov and IaM [sic] Vakhrushev, "Therapeutic use of vitamin U in gastroenterological practice," *Vrach Delo* 10 (1978): 101–04.

13. S. Meyers and H. D. Janowitz, "Natural History of Crohn's Disease: An Analytical Review of the Placebo Lesson," *Gastroenterol* 87 (1984): 1189–92; H. Malchow, et al., "European Cooperative Crohn's Disease Study (ECCDS): Results of Drug Treatment," *Gastroenterol* 86 (1984): 249–66.

14. Buhner, *Herbal Antibiotics,* 53–55; Murray and Pizzorno, *Encyclopedia of Natural Medicine,* 815; Werbach and Murray, *Biological Influences on Illness,* 261–66.

15. H. S. Shin, et al., "Clinical trials of Madecassol (*Centella asiatica*) on gastrointestinal ulcer patient," *Korean J Gastroenterol* 14(1) (1982): 49–56; J. C. Rhee and K. W. Chow, "Clinical effect of titrated extract of *Centella asiatica* (Madecassol) on peptic ulcer," *Korean J Gastroenterol* 13(1) (1981): 35–40; K. H. Cho, et al., "Clinical experiences of Madecassol (*Centella asiatica*) in the treatment of peptic ulcer," *Korean J Gastroenterol* 13(1) (1981): 49–56; Werbach and Murray, *Biological Influences on Illness,* 316–18.

16. Ibid., 266–67; Duke, *Green Pharmacy,* 435–41.

17. W. J. Jiang, et al., "Effects of raw and processed Da Huang on experimental gastric ulcer in rats," *Bull Chinese Mater Med* 10 (1985): 65–67; D. A. Sun, et al., "Comparison of the clinical effects of *R. palmatum* and cimetidine in upper gastrointestinal bleeding," *Chin J Integrat Trad West Med* 6 (1986): 458–59; H. Zhou and D. Jiao, "312 cases of gastric and duodenal ulcer bleeding treated with three kinds of alcoholic extract of rhubarb tablets," *Chung Hsi Chieh Ho Tsa* 10(3) (1990): 150–51.

18. Mark Blumenthal, et al., *The Complete German Commission E Monographs* (Austin, TX: American Botanical Council, 1998), 190–92.

CHAPTER 6

1. I. Goutal, et al., "Expression of the genes of arginine-synthesizing enzymes in rat kidney during development," *Biol Neonate* 76(4) (1999): 253–60.

2. Lindsey Tanner, "Birth Control Pill, Urine Protein, Linked to Kidney and Heart Disease," Associated Press, September 9, 2001, www.mindfully.org.

3. J. T. Bradbury, "The rabbit ovulating factor of plant juice," *Am J Physiol* 142 (1944): 487–93.

4. Stephen Harrod Buhner, *Sacred and Herbal Healing Beers; The Secrets of Ancient Fermentation* (Boulder, CO: Siris Press, 1998), 108–09.

5. Michael Murray and Joseph Pizzorno, *Encyclopedia of Natural Medicine* (Roseville, CA: Prima, 1998), 186–87.

6. Mark Blumenthal, et al., *The Complete German Commission E Monographs* (Austin, TX: American Botanical Council, 1998), 216.

7. Murray and Pizzorno, *Encyclopedia of Natural Medicine*, 186.

8. Blumenthal, et al., *German Commission E Monographs*, 224–25.

9. Ibid., 155–56.

10. James Duke, *The Green Pharmacy* (Emmaus, PA: Rodale, 1997), 81.

11. Blumenthal, et al., *German Commission E Monographs*, 118–20.

12. Ibid., 118.

13. H. Hirayama, et al., "Effect of *Desmodium styracifolium-triterpenoid* on calcium oxalate renal stones," *British J Urol* 71(2) (1993): 143–47; H. Z. Li, et al., "Inhibition of the crystallization of calcium oxalate monohydrate by constituents of *Desmodium styracifolium* and *Lysimachia christinae*," *Journal of Shenyang College of Pharmacy* 5(3) (1988): 208–12; C. S. Ho, et al., "The Hypotensive action of *Desmodium styracifolium* and *Clematis chinensis*," *American Journal of Chinese Medicine* 17(3–4) (1989): 189–202.

14. Blumenthal, et al., *German Commission E Monographs*, 154–55; Rudolf Weiss, *Herbal Medicine* (Gothenburg, Sweden: AB Arcanum, 1988), 240; Zhari Ismail and Norhayati Ismail, Report presented at the 29th Malaysia-Singapore Congress of Medicine, August 1995; M. Nirdnoy and V. Muangman, "Effects of Folia orthosiphonis on urinary stone promoters and inhibitors," *Journal of the Medical Association of Thailand* 74(6) (1991): 318–21; I. M. Lyckander and K. E. Malterud, "Lipophilic flavonoids from *Orthosiphon spicatus* prevent oxidative inactivation of 15-lipoxygenase," *Prostaglandins, Leukotrienes, and Essential Fatty Acids* 54(4) (1996): 239–46; Duke, *The Green Pharmacy*, 208.

15. Weiss, *Herbal Medicine*, 241–43; Blumenthal, et al., *German Commission E Monographs*, 139–40.

16. Murray and Pizzorno, *Encyclopedia of Natural Medicine*, 616; M. K. Li, et al., "Effects of magnesium on calcium oxalate crystallization," *J Urol* 133 (1985): 123–25; F. Parivar, et al., "The influence of diet on urinary stone disease," *J Urol* 155 (1996): 432–40; G. Johansson, et al., "Biochemical and clinical effects of the prophylactic treatment of renal calcium stones with magnesium hydroxide," *J Urol* 124 (1980): 770–74.

17. P. Barcelo, et al., "Randomized double-blind study of potassium citrate in idiopathic hypocitrauric calcium nephrolithiasis," *J Urol* 150 (1993): 1761–64; B. Ettinnger, et al., "Potas-

sium-magnesium citrate is an effective prophylaxis against recurrent calcium oxalate nephrolithiasis," *J Urol* 158 (1997): 2069–73; C. Y. Pak, "Citrate and renal calculi: an update," *Miner Electrolyte Metab* 20 (1994): 371–77; M. A. Seltzer, et al., "Dietary manipulation with lemonade to treat hypocitrauric calcium nephrolithiasis," *J Urol* 156 (1996): 907–09.

18. R. Nath, et al., "Role of pyridoxine in oxalate metabolism," *Ann NY Acad Sci* 585 (1990): 274–84; R. W. E Watts, et al., "The effect of pyridoxine on oxalate dynamics in three cases of primary hyperoxaluria (with glycolic aciduria)," *Clin Sci* 69 (1985): 87–90; S. N. Gershoff and E. L. Prien, "Effect of daily MgO and Vitamin B_6 administration to patients with recurring calcium oxalate kidney stones," *Am J Clin Nutr* 20(5) (1967): 393–99; G. C. Curhan, et al., "Intake of vitamins B_6 and C and the risk of kidney stones in women," *J Am Soc Nephrol* 10 (1999): 840–45; E. L. Prien and S. F. Gershoff, "Magnesium oxide-pyridoxine therapy for recurrent calcium oxalate calculi," *J Urol* 112 (1974): 509–12; Murray and Pizzorno, *Encyclopedia of Natural Medicine,* 616.

19. Murray and Pizzorno, *Encyclopedia of Natural Medicine,* 617.

20. Zhari Ismail and Norhayati Ismail, Report presented at the 29th Malaysia-Singapore Congress of Medicine, August 1995.

21. G. C. Curhan, et al., "Beverage use and risk for kidney stones in women," *Ann Intern Med* 128 (1998): 534–40.

22. F. Moattar, et al., "Antiurolithiasis activities from selected medicinal plants. I. Extraction, clinical and pharmacological studies," *Internat Res Cong Nat Prod,* College of Pharmacy, University of North Carolina, Chapel Hill, July 7–12, 1985. Abstract 197.

23. M. P. Lan, "Treatment of 32 cases of urolithiasis with Yiqi paishi Tang," *Shandong Journal of Traditional Chinese Medicine* 6 (1986): 29, 24; W. B. Wang and J. H. Dai, "Treatment of 38 cases of urolithiasis by integrated Chinese and Western medicine," *Zhejiang Journal of Traditional Chinese Medicine* 22(5) (1987): 203; M. Y. Li and B. Li, "Treatment of urolithiasis with Yishi Huatong Tang," *Journal of Traditional Chinese Medicine* 29(8) (1988): 605–07; X. J. Wang, "Treatment of 215 cases of urolithiasis with Paishi Tang: *Hunan Journal of Traditional Chinese Medicine* 2 (1987): 8–9; X. M. Jiang, "Treatment of 32 cases of urolithiasis with Rongshi Tang," *Hunan Journal of Chinese Medicine* 2 (1987): 10; G. L. Pan, "Report on 1,001 cases of urolithiasis treated by Chinese medicine," *New Journal of Traditional Chinese Medicine* 21(4) (1989): 37–39; all cited in Subhuti Dharmananda "Traditional Chinese Specific Condition Review: Shrinking and Eliminating Urinary Tract Calculi," *Protocol Journal of Botanical Medicine* 1(3) (Winter 1996): 175–78.

24. V. S. Suphakarn, et al., "The effect of pumpkin seeds on oxalcrystalluria and urinary compositions of children in hyperendemic urea," *Am J Clin Nutr* 45 (1987): 115–21; V. Suphiphar, et al., "The effect of pumpkin seeds snack on inhibitors and promoters of urolithiasis in Thai adolescents," *J Med Assoc Thai* 76 (1993): 487–93.

25. H. Z. Li, et al., "Inhibition of the crystallization of calcium oxalate monohydrate by constituents of *Desmodium styracifolium* and *Lysimachia christinae,*" *Journal of Shenyang College of Pharmacy* 5(3) (1988): 208–12; X. Y. Mao, et al., "Report on the plant Kunming Jinqiancao," *Journal of the American College of Traditional Chinese Medicine* (Beijing: Higher Education Press, 1990).

26. Weiss, *Herbal Medicine,* 247.

CHAPTER 7

1. Jonathan Wright and Lane Lenard, *Maximize Your Vitality and Potency (for Men Over 40)* (Petaluma, CA: Smart Publications, 1999), Chapter 10; *DHEA: A Comprehensive Review,* J. H. H. Thijssen and H. Nieuwenhuyse (eds.) (New York: Parthenon, 1999), 135–36.

2. Michael Murray and Joseph Pizzorno, *Encyclopedia of Natural Medicine* (Roseville, CA: Prima, 1998), 708.

3. Wright and Lenard, *Maximize;* Eugene Shippen and William Fryer, *The Testosterone Syndrome* (New York: Evans, 1998).

4. *DHEA: A Comprehensive Review,* Thijssen and Nieuwenhuyse (eds.), 91, 136; Hasnain Waljii, *DHEA: The Ultimate Rejuvenating Hormone* (Prescott, AZ: Hohm Press, 1996), 46–49; Ray Sahelian, *DHEA: A Practical Guide* (New York: Avery, 1996), 68–69.

5. Michael Murray, *Total Body Tune Up* (New York: Bantam, 2001), 282.

6. L. Kotkowiak, "Behavior of selected bio-elements in women with osteoporosis," *Ann Acad Med Stetin* 43(1997): 225–38; R. K. Rude and M. Olerich, "Magnesium deficiency: possible role in osteoporosis associated with gluten-sensitive enteropathy," *Osteoporosis Int* 6(6) (1996): 451–63; Murray and Pizzorno, *Encyclopedia of Natural Medicine,* 719, 906.

7. Ira Dreyfuss, "Power Lifts Urged for Older Men," The Associated Press, November 19, 2001, America Online.

8. Murray and Pizzorno, *Encyclopedia of Natural Medicine,* 714.

9. Thomas Newmark and Paul Schulick, *Beyond Aspirin* (Prescott, AZ: Hohm Press, 2000), 40–41.

10. Ibid., 41.

11. James Duke, *The Green Pharmacy* (Emmaus, PA: Rodale, 1997), 57; Murray and Pizzorno, *Encyclopedia of Natural Medicine,* 784; Newmark and Schulick, *Beyond Aspirin,* Chapter 14.

12. Melvyn Werbach and Michael Murray, *Botanical Influences on Illness* (Tarzana, CA: Third Line Press), 214–18, 252, 255, 294–95.

13. Ibid., 218, 253–54, 295–96.

14. E. Bombardelli and P. Morazzoni, "*Urtica dioica* L.," *Fitoterapia* 68(5) (1997): 387–402.

15. Duke, *The Green Pharmacy,* 58; Werbach and Murray, *Botanical Influences on Illness,* 252–53, 294–95.

16. Ray Sahelian, *Pregnenolone* (New York: Avery, 1997), 57–64.

17. Sahelian, *DHEA: A Practical Guide,* 59–64.

18. Murray and Pizzorno, *Encyclopedia of Natural Medicine,* 698–99.

19. Paul Bergner, *The Healing Power of Echinacea and Goldenseal* (Rocklin, CA: Prima, 1997), 111.

20. C. di Padova, "S-adenosylmethionine in the treatment of osteoarthritis: Review of the clinical studies," *Am J Med* 83(5A) (1987): 60–65; Murray and Pizzorno, *Encyclopedia of Natural Medicine,* 701–02; G. Stramentinoli, "Pharmacologic effects of S-adenosylmethionine. Pharmacokinetics and pharmacodynamics," *Am J Med* 83(5A) (1987): 35–42; M. F. Harmand, et al., "Effects of S-adenosylmethionine on human articular

chondrocyte differentiation. An *in vitro* study," *Am J Med* 83(5A) (1987): 48–54; H. A. Barcelo, et al., "Experimental osteoarthritis and its course when treated with S-adenosyl-L-methionine" *Rev Clin Exp* 187(2) (1990): 74–78; Murray and Pizzorno, *Encyclopedia of Natural Medicine*, 701–02.

21. Ibid., 781; Allan Sosin and Beth Ley Jacobs, *Alpha Lipoic Acid* (New York: Kensington, 1998), Chapter 11; Stephen Harrod Buhner, *Herbs for Hepatitis C and the Liver* (Pownal, VT: Storey, 2000), 76–78.

22. Ibid., Murray and Pizzorno, 781; ibid., Buhner, 79–80.

23. Ibid., Murray and Pizzorno, 703.

24. Newmark and Schulick, *Beyond Aspirin*, Chapter 14.

25. Michael Moore, *Herbal Repertory in Clinical Practice* (Albuquerque, NM: Southwest School of Botanical Medicine, 1994), citation 12.9; Bergner, *The Healing Power of Echinacea and Goldenseal*, Chapters 2, 3, and 6; Murray and Pizzorno, *Encyclopedia of Natural Medicine*, 160.

26. Werbach and Murray, *Botanical Influences on Illness*, 216–17; Murray and Pizzorno, *Encyclopedia of Natural Medicine*, 807.

27. Werbach and Murray, *Botanical Influences on Illness*, 214–16; Murray and Pizzorno, *Encyclopedia of Natural Medicine*, 807.

28. Ibid., 807.

CHAPTER 8

1. Anita Manning, "Depression may double diabetes risk," *USA Today*, May 24, 2001.

2. T. W. Balon and J. L. Nadler, "Evidence that nitric oxide increases glucose transport in skeletal muscle," *J Appl Phyisiol* 82(1) (1997): 359–63; M. E. Young and B. Leighton, "Evidence for altered sensitivity of the nitric oxide/cGMP signaling cascade in insulin-resistant skeletal muscle," *Biochem J* 329(Part 1) (1998): 73–79; G. R. Etgen, et al., "Nitric oxide stimulates skeletal muscle glucose transport through a calcium/contraction-and phospharidylinositol-3-kinase-independent pathway." *Diabetes* 46(11) (1997): 1915–19.

3. B. K. Chakravarthy, et al., "Pancreatic Beta-Cell Regeneration in Rats by (-)-Epicatechin," *Lancet* 2 (1981): 759–60; B. K. Chakravarthy, et al., "Functional Beta-Cell regeneration in the Islets of Pancreas in Alloxan Induced Diabetic Rate by (-)-epicatechin," *Life Sci* 31 (1982): 2693–97; S. S. Subramanian "(-)-Epicatechin as an Anti-Diabetic Drug," *Ind Drugs* 18 (1981): 259: all cited in Michael Murray and Joseph Pizzorno, *Encyclopedia of Natural Medicine* (Roseville, CA: Prima, 1998), 427; S. Rajasekharan, et al., (title not available), *Ind Jour Med Res* (55)2 (1976): 166–68; Sheehan, et al., (title not avail.), *J Nut Prod* 46(2) (1983): 232–34: both cited at www.pancreastonic.com.

4. Murray and Pizzorno, *Encyclopedia of Natural Medicine*, 425–26, 875; Mitra, et al., (title not avail.), *Bull Calcutta Trop Med* 23(1–4) (1975): 6–7, cited at www.pancreastonic.com; Melvyn Werbach and Michael Murray, *Biological Influences on Illness* (Tarzana, CA: Third Line Press, 1994), 147; E. R. B. Shanmugasundaram, et al., "Possible regeneration of the islets of Langerhans in Streptozotocin-diabetic rats given *Gymnema sylvestre* leaf ex-

tracts," *Journal of Ethnopharmacology* 30 (1990): 265–79; "Gymnema Research Statistics," online at www.pharmaterra.com.

5. Murray and Pizzorno, *Encyclopedia of Natural Medicine*, 426; James Duke, *The Green Pharmacy* (Emmaus, PA: Rodale, 1997), 163; Werbach and Murray, *Biological Influences on Illness*, 144; R. D. Sharma, "Effect of extracted fenugreek on postprandial glucose levels in human diabetic subjects, *Nutr Res* 9(6) (1989): 693; see also: R. D. Sharma, *Nutrition Research* (December 6, 1986): 1353–64.

6. Murray and Pizzorno, *Encyclopedia of Natural Medicine*, 425; Werbach and Murray, *Biological Influences on Illness*, 139–41; A. Raman and C. Lau, "Anti-diabetic properties and phytochemistry of *Momordica charantia* L. (Cucurbitaceae)," *Phytomedicine* 2(4) (1996): 349–62.

7. *DHEA: A Comprehensive Review,* J. H. H. Thijssen and H. Nieuwenhuyse (eds.) (New York: Parthenon, 1999), 111–13, 116–18, 133–35; Jonathan Wright and Lane Lenard, *Maximize Your Vitality and Potency (for Men Over 40)* (Petaluma, CA: Smart Publications, 1999), 120–38; Eugene Shippen and William Fryer, *The Testosterone Syndrome* (New York: Evans, 1998), 87–89.

8. Burt Berkson, *Alpha Lipoic Acid* (Rocklin, CA: Prima, 1998), Chapter 7.

9. Murray and Pizzorno, *Encyclopedia of Natural Medicine*, 416–17.

10. Ibid., 419.

11. Ibid., 421.

12. Ibid., 420.

13. Ibid., 421–22.

14. Ibid, 419–20; Berkson, *Alpha Lipoic Acid*, 117.

15. *Garlic: The Science and Therapeutic Application of* Allium sativum *and Related Species* (2nd edition), Heinrich Koch and Larry Lawson (eds.) (Baltimore: Williams and Wilkins, 1996), Chapter 5; Werbach and Murray, *Biological Influences on Illness*, 145; Murray and Pizzorno, *Encyclopedia of Natural Medicine*, 424–25.

16. Ibid., Murray and Pizzorno, 414–15; Duke, *The Green Pharmacy*, 163–64.

17. Werbach and Murray, *Botanical Influences on Illness*, 147.

18. A. C. Frati-Munari, et al., "The effect of different doses of prickly-pear cactus (*Opuntia streptacantha lemaire*) on the glucose tolerance test in healthy individuals," *Arch Invest Med (Mex)* 19(2) (1988): 143–48; Frati-Munari, et al., "Influence of Nopal intake upon fasting glycemia in Type II diabetics and healthy subjects," *Arch Invest Med (Mex)* 1983(14) (1983): 269–74; Frati-Munari, et al., "Effects of Nopal (*Opuntia spp.*) on serum lipids, glycemia, and body weight," *Arch Invest Med (Mex)* 1984(14): 117–25; Werbach and Murray, *Biological Influences on Illness*, 148.

19. J. Hallfrisch, et al., "Diets containing soluble oat extracts improve glucose and insulin responses of moderately hypercholesterolemic men and women," *Amer J Clin Nutr* 61(2) (1995): 379–84; J. T. Braaten, et al., "Oat gum lowers glucose and insulin after an oral glucose load 1-4," *Amer J Clin Nutr* 53(6) (1991): 1425–30; A. C. Frati-Munari, et al., "Effect of *Plantago psyllium* mucilage on the glucose tolerance test," *Arch Invest Med (Mex)* 1985(16) (1985): 191–97; J. G. Pastors, et al., "Psyllium fiber reduces rise in postprandial glucose and insulin concentrations in patients with non-insulin dependent diabetes,"

Amer J Clin Nutr 53(6) (1991): 1431–35; R. Hopewell, et al., "Soluble fiber: effect on carbohydrate and lipid metabolism," *Progress Food Nutr Sci* 17(2) (1993): 159–82.

20. Murray and Pizzorno, *Encyclopedia of Natural Medicine*, 423.

CHAPTER 9

1. Michael Murray and Joseph Pizzorno, *Encyclopedia of Natural Medicine* (Roseville, CA: Prima, 1998), 626.

2. Michael Murray, *Total Body Tune Up* (New York: Bantam, 2001), 245.

3. Werbach and Murray, *Botanical Influences on Illness* (Tarzana, CA: Third Line Press, 1994), 292.

4. Murray and Pizzorno, *Encyclopedia of Natural Medicine*, 95; C. Corbe, J. P. Boissin, A. Siou, "Light vision and chorioretinal circulation: Study of the effect of procyanidolic oligomers," *J Fr Ophthalmol* 11 (1988): 453–60; J. P. Boissin, C. Corbe, A. Siou, "Chorioretinal circulation and dazzling: Use of procyanidol oligomers," *Bull Soc Ophthamol Fr,* 88 (1988): 173–79.

5. Rudolf Weiss, *Herbal Medicine* (Gothenburg, Sweden: AB Arcanum, 1988), 180–81.

6. Murray and Pizzorno, *Encyclopedia of Natural Medicine*, 322, 624–25; James Duke, *The Green Pharmacy* (Emmaus, PA: Rodale, 1997), 129.

7. Murray and Pizzorno, *Encyclopedia of Natural Medicine*, 625.

8. Ibid., 626.

9. Ibid., 427.

10. Werbach and Murray, *Botanical Influences on Illness*, 170.

11. Murray and Pizzorno, *Encyclopedia of Natural Medicine*, 95; C. Corbe, J. P. Boissin, A. Siou, "Light vision and chorioretinal circulation: Study of the effect of procyanidolic oligomers," *J Fr Ophthalmol* 11 (1988): 453–60; J. P. Boissin, C. Corbe, A. Siou, "Chorioretinal circulation and dazzling: Use of procyanidol oligomers," *Bull Soc Ophthamol Fr* 88 (1988): 173–79.

12. Rudolf Weiss, *Herbal Medicine*, 180–81.

13. Richard Barrett, "Naturopathic specific condition review: Glaucoma," *Protocol Journal of Botanical Medicine,* 2(2) (1997): 68.

14. Werbach and Murray, *Botanical Influences on Illness*, 170.

15. Murray and Pizzorno, *Encyclopedia of Natural Medicine*, 486.

16. Ibid., 487.

17. Ibid., 323; Subhuti Dharmananda, "Traditional Chinese specific condition review: Cataracts," *Protocol Journal of Botanical Medicine* 2(2) (1997): 40–44.

18. Murray and Pizzorno, *Encyclopedia of Natural Medicine*, 323.

19. Ibid., 321.

20. Burt Berkson, *Alpha Lipoic Acid* (Rocklin, CA: Prima, 1998), 119.

21. Murray and Pizzorno, *Encyclopedia of Natural Medicine*, 320.

22. Duke, *The Green Pharmacy,* 127.

23. Werbach and Murray, *Botanical Influences on Illness*, 170, 225.

24. Rudolf Weiss, *Herbal Medicine*, 180–81.

25. Melvyn Werbach, *Nutritional Influences on Illness,* cited in Duke, *The Green Pharmacy,* 423.

26. Murray, *Total Body Tune Up,* 265.

27. J. Attias, et al., "Oral magnesium intake reduces permanent hearing loss induced by noise exposure," *Am J Otolaryngol* 15(1) (1994): 26–32; T. Gunthes, et al., *Am J Otol* 10(1) (1989): 36–41.

28. Werbach and Murray, *Botanical Influences on Illness,* 224–25.

29. Weiss, *Herbal Medicine,* 180–81.

30. Werbach and Murray, *Botanical Influences on Illness,* 223–24.

CHAPTER 10

1. Quoted in James Hillman, *The Force of Character* (New York: Random House, 1999), 84–85.

2. Hasnain Walji, *DHEA:The Ultimate Rejuvenating Hormone* (Prescott, AZ: Hohm Press, 1996), 8.

3. *DHEA: A Comprehensive Review,* J. H. H. Thijssen and H. Nieuwenhuyse (eds.) (New York: Parthenon, 1999), 170.

4. Eugene Shippen and William Fryer, *The Testosterone Syndrome* (New York: Evans, 1998), 147.

5. Subhuti Dharmananda, "Traditional Chinese Specific Condition Review: Alzheimer's Disease," *Protocol Journal of Botanical Medicine* 2(1) (1996): 114–18; D. H. Cheng, et al., "Huperzine A, a novel, promising acetylcholinesterase inhibitor," *Neuroreport* 8 (1996): 97–101; D. L. Bai, et al., "Huperzine A, a potential therapeutic agent for treatment of Alzheimer's disease," *Curr Med Chem* 7(3) (2000): 355–74; S. S. Xu, et al., "Efficacy of tablet huperzine A on memory, cognition, and behavior in Alzheimer's disease," *Zhongguo Yao Li Xue Bao* 16(5) (1995): 391–95; R. W. Zhang, et al., "Drug evaluation of huperzine A in the treatment of senile memory disorders," *Chung Kuo Yao Li Hsueh Pao* 12(3) (1991): 2502; Q. Q. Sun, et al., "Huperzine A capsules enhance memory and learning performance in 34 pairs of matched adolescent students," *Zhongguo Yao Li Xue Bao* 20(7) (1999): 601–03.

6. B. Hofferberth, "Ginkgo biloba special extract in patients with cerebro-organic syndrome," *Muench Med Wochenschr* 133 (1991): S30–S33; E. Ernst, "Herbal medications for common ailments in the elderly," *Drugs Aging* 15(6) (1999): 423–28; G. Burkard and S. Lehrl, "Ratio of multi-infarct dementia and Alzheimer's dementia in practices of established physicians," *Muench Med Wochenschr* 133 (1991): S38–S43; L. E. Bars, et al., "A 26-week analysis of a double-blind, placebo-controlled trial of the Ginkgo biloba extract EGB 761 in dementia," *Dement Geriatr Cogn Disord* 11(4) (2000): 230–37; A. Wettstein, "Cholinesterase inhibitors and Ginkgo extracts—are they comparable in the treatment of dementia?," *Phytomedicine* 6(6) (2000): 393–401; Murray and Pizzorno, *Encyclopedia of Natural Medicine,* 231–32.

7. Ibid., 230, 854.

8. Hasnain Walji, *DHEA: The Ultimate Rejuvenating Hormone* (Prescott, AZ: Hohm Press, 1996), 26; S. S. Yen, et al., "Replacement of DHEA in Aging Men and Women: Potential Remedial Effects," *Ann NY Acad Sci* 774 (1995): 128–42; A. J. Morales, et al., "Effects of

Replacement Dose of Dehydroepiandrosterone in Men and Women of Advancing age," *J Endocrinol Metab* 78(6) (1994): 1360–67; L. Bologa, et al., "DHEA and its sulfate derivative reduce neuronal death and enhance astrocytic differentiation in brain cell cultures," *J Neurosci Res* 17 (1987): 225–34.

9. Shippen and Fryer, *The Testosterone Syndrome*, 147.

10. Murray and Pizzorno, *Encyclopedia of Natural Medicine*, 228–29, 854.

11. Michael Murray, *Heart Disease and High Blood Pressure* (Rocklin, CA: Prima, 1997), 102–04.

12. Weiss, *Herbal Medicine*, 180–81; P. K. Fischhof, et al., "Therapeutic efficacy of vincamine in dementia," *Neuropsychobiology* 34(1) (1996): 29–35.

13. Mark Blumenthal, et al., *The Complete German Commission E Monographs* (Austin, TX: American Botanical Council, 1998), 364–65.

Chapter ii

1. William Agosta, *Bombardier Beetles and Fever Trees* (New York: Addison-Wesley, 1996), 166, 168.

2. E. M. Schwiebert, et al., "CFTR is a conductance regulator as well as a chloride channel," *Physiol Rev* 79(1) (1999): 145–66; V. Urbach, and B. J. Harvey, "Regulation of intracellular Ca(2+) by CFTR in Chinese hamster ovary cells," *J Membr Biol* 171(3) (1999): 255–65; Neil Sweezey, et al., "Sex hormones regulate cystic fibrosis transmembrane conductance regulator in developing fetal rat lung epithelial cells," *Am J Physiol* 272 (1997): 844–51; Neil Sweezey, et al., "Female gender hormones regulate the expression of the lung epithelial Na channel and CFTR," *American Journal of Physiology* 274 (1996): 379–86; Neil Sweezey, et al., "Progesterone and estradiol inhibit CFTR-mediated ion transport by pancreatic epithelial cells," *American Journal of Physiology* 271 (1996): G747–54.

3. The U.S. Centers for Disease Control (CDC) estimates that in the under-forty-five age groups, the ratio of women to men with asthma is 3:2; from forty-five to sixty-four, the ratio is about 5:2, and in the over-sixty-four group, the ratio is about 2:1. Boys under ten years of age have asthma at about three times the rate of girls. However as both groups move into puberty this begins to change rapidly until women outnumber men with asthma in young adulthood at about 3:2.

4. T. Quinlan, et al., "Regulation of Antioxidant Enzymes in Lung after Oxidant Injury," *Environmental Health Perspectives* 102 (Supplement 2) (1994): 79–87.

5. H. P. T. Ammon, et al., "Forskolin: From Ayurvedic remedy to a modern agent," *Planta Medica* 51 (1985): 473–77; K. B. Seamon and J. W. Daly, "Forskolin: A unique diterpene activator of cAMP-generating systems," *Journal of Cyclic Nucleotide Research* 7 (1981): 201–24; G. Marone, et al., "Forskolin inhibits the release of histamine from human basophils and mast cells," *Agents Actions* 18 (1986): 96–99; M. H. Yousif and O. Thulesius, "Forskolin reverses tachyphylaxis to the bronchodilator effects of salbutamol: an *in vitro* study on isolated guinea pig trachea," *J Pharm Pharmacol* 51 (1999): 181–86; S. Wong, et al., "Forskolin inhibits platelet-activating factor binding to platelet receptors independently of adenylyl cyclase activation," *Eur J Pharmacol* 245 (1993): 55–61; R. W. Kreutner,

et al., "Bronchodilator and antiallergy activity of forskolin," *European Journal of Pharmacology* 111 (1985): 1–8; J. F. Burka, "Effects of selected bronchodilators on antigen- and AZ3187-induced contraction of guinea pig trachea," *Journal of Pharmacology and Experimental Therapeutics* 225 (1983): 427–35; E. M. Schwiebert, et al., "CFTR is a conductance regulator as well as a chloride channel," *Physiol Rev* 79 (Supplement 1) (1999): 145–66; V. Urbach and B. J. Harvey, "Regulation of intracellular Ca(2+) by CFTR in Chinese Hamster ovary cells"; Barbara Renaudon and Valerie Urbach, "Forskolin stimulation of CFTR and outwardly rectifying chloride channels," *Journal of Physiology* 527 (2000): 124; S. Kimura, et al., "Cyclic AMP-dependent long-term potentiation of nitric oxide release from cerebellar parallel fibers in rats," *J Neurosci* 18 (1998): 8551–58; J. H. Poulson, et al., "Bicarbonate conductance and pH regulatory capability of cystic fibrosis transmembrane regulator," *Proc Natl Acad Sci* (91) (1994): 5340–44; Michael Welsh and Jeffrey Smith, "cAMP stimulation of HCO3—Secretion Across Airway Epithelia," *J. Pancreas (Online)* 2 (Supplement 4) (2001): 291–93; J. Smith and M. Welsh, "cAMP stimulates bicarbonate secretion across normal, but not cystic fibrosis airway epithelia," *J Clin Invest* 89 (1992): 1148–53; I. M. Bird, et al., "Regulation of 3B-hydroxysteroid dehydrogenase expression in human adrenocortical H295R cells," *Journal of Endocrinology* 150 (1996): 165–73; Y. C. Chiao, et al., "Regulation of thyroid hormones on the production of testosterone in rats," *J Cell Biochem* 73(4) (1999): 5554–62; "Inhibin and activin differentially regulate androgen production and 17alpha-hydroxylase expression in human ovarian thecal-like tumor cells," *Journal of Endocrinology* 148(2) (1996); Christopher De Ponge, "The cAMP-dependent kinase pathway and human sperm acrosomal exocytosis," *Frontiers in Bioscience* 1 (1996): 234–40; J. P. Mulhall, et al., "Intracavernosal forskolin: Role in management of vasculogenic impotence resistant to standard 3-agent pharmacotherapy," *J Urol* 158(5) (1997): 1752–59; www.forslean.com/clinical.html.; anonymous, "Harvard study links obesity to asthma," *Health Story Page Online,* April 26, 1998, www.cnn.com; anonymous, "Asthma and obesity link," *BBC News online,* October 18, 2001; Barbara Berg, "PHS/UW study links asthma, obesity," FHCR Center News 7(15) (2001); J. A. Menninger and B. Tabakoff, "Forskolin-stimulated platelet adenylyl cyclase activity is lower in persons with major depression," *Biol Psychiatry* 42(1) (1997): 30–38; Y. Bersudsky, et al., "A preliminary study of possible psychoactive effects of intravenous forskolin in depressed and schizophrenic patients," *J Neural Transm* 103(12) (1996): 1463–67; K. Bauer, et al., "Pharmacodynamic effects of inhaled dry powder formulations of fenoterol and colforsin [forskolin] in asthma," *Clin Pharmacol Ther* 53(1) (1993): 76–83; G. Kaik and P. U. Witte, "Protective effect of forskolin in acetylcholine provocation in healthy probands. Comparison of 2 doses with fenoterol and placebo," *Wien Med Wochenschr* 136(23–24) (1986): 637–41; N. J. DeSouza, "Industrial development of traditional drugs: the forskolin example, a mini review," *Journal of Ethnopharmacology* 38 (1993): 177–80; Joanne Snow, "Coleus forskohlii," *Protocol Journal of Botanic Medicine* 1(2) (1995): 39–42.

6. P. S. Haranth and S. Shyamalakumari, "Experimental study on mode of action of Tylospora asthmatica in bronchial asthma," *Ind J Med Res* 63 (1975): 661–70; C. Gopalakrishnan, et al., "Effect of tylophorine, a major alkaloid of Tylospora indica, on immunopathological and inflammatory reactions," *Indian J Med Res* 71 (1980): 940–48;

H. Wagner, "Search for new plant constituents with potential antiphlogistic and antial-lergenic activity," *Planta Med* 55 (1989): 235–41; A. L. Udupa, et al., "The possible site of anti-asthmatic action of *Tylospora asthmatica* on pituitary-adrenal axis in albino rats," *Planta Med* 57 (1991): 409–13; C. Gopalakrishnan, et al., "Pharmacological investigations of tylophorine, the major alkaloid of *Tylospora indica*," *Ind J Med Res* 69 (1979): 513–20; D. N. Shivpuri, et al., "Treatment of asthma with an alcoholic extract of *Tylospora indica*: A cross-over, double-blind study," *Ann Allergy* 30 (1972): 407–12; S. Gupta, et al., "*Tylospora indica* in bronchial asthma—a double-blind study," *Ind J Med Res* 69 (1979): 981–89; K. V. Thiruvengadam, et al., "*Tylospora indica* in bronchial asthma (a controlled comparison with a standard anti-asthmatic drug)," *J Ind Med Assoc* 71(7) (1978): 172–76; K. V. Gore, et al., "Physiological studies with *Tylospora asthmatica* in bronchial asthma," *Ind J Med Res* 71 (1980): 144–48; D. N. Shivpuri, et al., "A crossover, double-blind study on *Tylospora indica* in the treatment of asthma and allergic rhinitis," *J Allergy* 43(3) (1969): 145–50.

7. O. B. McManus, et al., "An activator of calcium-dependent potassium channels isolated from a medicinal herb," *Biochemistry* 32(24) (1993): 6128–33; M. E. Addy and J. F. Burka, "Effect of *Desmodium adscendens* fractions on antigen- and arachidonic acid–induced contractions of guinea pig airways," *Can J Pharmacol* 66(6) (1988): 820–25; M. E. Addy and J. F. Burka, "Effect of *Desmodium adscendens* fraction 3 on contractions of respiratory smooth muscle," *J Ethnopharmacol* 29(3) (1990): 325–35; M. E. Addy and E. M. Awmey, "Effect of the extracts of Desmodium adscendens on anaphylaxis," *J Ethnopharmacol* 11(3) (1984): 283–92; M. E. Addy and W. K. Dzandu, "Dose-response effects of *Desmodium adscendens* aqueous extract on histamine response, content and anaphylactic reactions in the guinea pig," *J Ethnopharmacol* 18(1) (1986): 13–20; M. E. Addy, "Some secondary plant metabolites in *Desmodium adscendens* and their effects on arachidonic acid metabolism," *Prostaglandins, Leukotrienes, and Essential Fatty Acids* 47(1) (1992): 85–91; O. Ampofo, "Plants That Heal," *World Health* 1977 (1977): 26–30.

8. Rudolf Weiss, *Herbal Medicine* (Gothenburg, Sweden: AB Arcanum, 1988), 221–22; M. C. S. Kennedy and J. P. P. Stock, "The bronchodilator action of khellin," *Thorax* 7 (1952): 43–65.

9. M. Makarewicz-Plonska, et al., "BN 52021, PAF-receptor antagonist, improves diminished antioxidant defense system of lungs in experimentally induced hemorrhagic shock," *Pol J Pharmacol* 50 (1998): 265–69; M. H. Li, et al., "Effects of Ginkgo leaf concentrated oral liquor in treating asthma," *Chung-kuo Chung Hsi I Chieh Ho Tsa Chih* 17(4) (1997): 216–18.

10. Christopher Hobbs, *Medicinal Mushrooms* (Loveland, CO: Interweave Press, 1996), 96–108; Terry Willard, *Reishi* (Seattle, WA: Sylvan Press, 1990), Chapter 5.

11. Michael Murray and Joseph Pizzorno, *Encyclopedia of Natural Medicine* (Rocklin, CA: Prima, 1998), 268; H. Kakegawa, et al., (no title given), *Chem Pharm Bull* 33 (1985): 5079.

12. P. J. Dunn, et al., "Dehydroepiandrosterone sulphate concentrations in asthmatic patients: pilot study," *New Zealand Med J* 97 (1984): 805–08; J. M. Nogueira, et al., "Soluble CD30, dehydroepiandrosterone sulfate and dehydroandrosterone in atopic and non atopic children," *Allerg Immunol* 30 (1998): 3–8; R. E. Weinstein, et al., "Decreases adrenal sex steroid levels in the absence of glucocorticoid suppression in postmenopausal

asthmatic women," *J Allergy Clin Immunol* 97(1 pt1) (1996): 1–8; C. K. Yu, et al., "Attenuation of house dust mite dermatophagoides farinae-induced airway allergic responses in mice by dehydroandrosterone is correlated with down-regulation of TH2 response," *Clin Exp Allergy* 29 (1999): 414–22; no author given, "DHEA inhibits smooth muscle proliferation," *Journal of Pharmacology and Experimental Therapeutics* 285(2) (1998): 876–83, cited in *Life Extension* magazine, May 1999.

13. R. A. Landon, "Role of magnesium in regulation of lung function," *J Am Diet Assoc* 93(6) (1993): 674; T. Bohmer, "Magnesium in lung diseases," *Tidsskr Nor Laegeforen* 115(7) (1995): 827–28; J. Britton, et al., "Dietary magnesium, lung function, wheezing, and airway hyperreactivity in a random adult population sample," *Lancet* 344(8919) (1994): 357–62; P. Fantidis, et al., "Intracellular (polymorphonuclear) magnesium content in patients with bronchial asthma between attacks," *J R Soc Med* 88(4) (1995): 441–45; Murray and Pizzorno, *Encyclopedia of Natural Medicine,* 269.

14. Serpil Erzurum, et al., (no title listed), *The Lancet* 355(9204) (2000): 624, cited in Lerner Research Institute News, March 2000, "LRI Researchers Link Decline of Lung Antioxidant Levels to Asthma"; N. L. A. Miso, et al., "Reduced platelet glutathione peroxidase activity and serum selenium concentration in atopic asthmatic patients," *Clinical Exp Allergy* 26 (1996): 838–47; Murray and Pizzorno, *Encyclopedia of Natural Medicine,* 268; G. Boman, et al., "Oral acetylcysteine reduces exacerbation rate in chronic bronchitis: a report of a trial organized by the Swedish Society for Pulmonary Diseases," *Eur J Respir Dis* 64 (1983): 405–15; Multicenter Study Group, "Long-term oral acetylcysteine in chronic bronchitis. A double-blind controlled study," *Eur J Respir Dis* 61 (1980): 93–108; E. M. Grandjean, et al., "Efficacy of long-term N Acetylcysteine in chronic bronchopulmonary disease: A meta-analysis of published double-blind, placebo-controlled clinical trials," *Clin Ther* 22 (2000): 209–21.

15. Murray and Pizzorno, *Encyclopedia of Natural Medicine,* 267–68; see also bibliography of vitamin C studies listed at www.usyoga.org/yogasthma/ nutrition_bibliography.htm.

16. J. Stone, "Reduced selenium status of patients with asthma," *Clinical Science* 77 (1989): 495–500; Murray and Pizzorno, *Encyclopedia of Natural Medicine,* 268; L. Hasselmark, et al., "Selenium supplementation in intrinsic asthma," *Allerg* 48 (1993): 30–36.

17. Canadian Asthma Prevention Institute, online at: www.asthmaworld.org.

18. Murray and Pizzorno, *Encyclopedia of Natural Medicine,* 268–69

19. Volker Schulz, et al., *Rational Phytotherapy* (Berlin: Springer-Verlag, 1998), 163–66; G. D. Tarasova, "Sinupret in therapy of acute sinusitis in children," and T. S. Polyakova and V. V. Vladimirova, "Sinupret against nasal and paranasal diseases," both in *Bulletin of Otorhinolaringology* 2 (2001).

20. Melvyn Werbach and Michael Murray, *Botanical Influences on Illness* (Tarzana, CA: Third Line Press, 1994), 214–16; Murray and Pizzorno, *Encyclopedia of Natural Medicine,* 297–98.

21. Ibid., 261, 264, 265; L. Ho, et al., "A double-blind controlled trial of elemental diet in severe, perennial asthma," *Allergy* 36 (1981): 257–62; James Duke, *The Green Pharmacy* (Emmaus, PA: Rodale Press, 1997), 65–67; K. S. Broughton, et al., "Reduced asthma symptoms with n-3 fatty acid ingestion are related to 5-series leukotriene production," *Am J Clin Nutr* 65 (1997): 1011–17; Melvyn Werbach and Michael Murray, *Biological In-*

fluences on Illness, 85; Murray and Pizzorno, *Encyclopedia of Natural Medicine*, 270; G. Handa, et al., "Antiasthmatic principle of *Allium cepa* Linn. (Onions)," *Indian Drugs* 20(6) (1983): 239; K. C. Sharma and S. S. K. Shanmugasundram, "*Allium cepa* as an anti-asthmatic," *RRL Jammu Newsletter* 6(2) (1979): 8; V. Alma, et al., "Clinical study of *Allium cepa* Linn. in patients of bronchial asthma," *Indian J Pharmacol* 13 (1981): 63–64.

22. M. V. Bhole, "Treatment of Bronchial Asthma by Yogic Methods," *Yoga-Mimansa* 1967 (no other citation data available); Adriane Fugh-Berman *Alternative Medicine: What Works* (Tucson, AZ: Odonian Press, 1996); Alan Miller, "The etiologies, pathophysiology and alternative/complementary treatment of asthma," *Altern Med Rev* 6(1) (2001): 20–47.

Chapter 12

1. Stephen Harrod Buhner, *The Lost Language of Plants* (White River Junction, VT: Chelsea Green, 2002).
2. E. Hamalainen, et al., "Diet and serum sex hormones in healthy men," *J Steroid Biochem* 20(1) (1984): 459–64.

Chapter 13

1. Ashley Montagu, *Touching: The Human Significance of the Skin* (New York: Harper & Row, 1971), 248–49.
2. Ibid., 218.
3. Ibid., 151.
4. Stephanie Simonton, 1980, personal communication.
5. John Berardi, "The Big T—Part 2: How Your Lifestyle Influences Your Testosterone Levels," www.t-mag.com, citing W. Schweiger, et al., (no title), *Psychosomatic Med* 61 (3): 292–96, 1999; F. Singer, et al., (no title), *Steroids* 57(2) (1992): 86–89.
6. This list of the benefits of yoga is mostly from Trish Lamb Feuerstein, "Health Benefits of Yoga," online at www.iayt.org/benefits.html. Her article includes an excellent bibliography of clinical studies on the health benefits of yoga.
7. Quoted at www.movementstudies.com.
8. John Berardi, www.t-mag.com, citing W. Kraemer, et al., (no title), *Int J Sports Med* 12(2) (1991): 228–35.

INDEX